FRONTIERS OF PRIMARY CARE

Series Editor: Mack Lipkin, Jr.

Frontiers of Primary Care

Series Editor: Mack Lipkin, Jr.

Published Volumes

Barnes, Aronson, and Delbanco (eds.)
    Alcoholism: A Guide for the Primary Care Physician
Schmidt, Lipkin, Jr., de Vries, and Greep (eds.)
    New Directions for Medical Education: Problem-Based Learning and
    Community-Oriented Medical Education
Goldbloom and Lawrence (eds.)
    Preventing Disease: Beyond the Rhetoric
WONCA Classification Committee
    Functional Status Measurement in Primary Care
White
    Healing the Schism: Epidemiology, Medicine, and the Public's Health

Forthcoming Volumes

Lipkin, Jr., Putnam, and Lazare (eds.)
    The Medical Interview

Kerr L. White

Healing the Schism

Epidemiology, Medicine, and the Public's Health

With Foreword by Halfdan Mahler

Springer-Verlag

New York Berlin Heidelberg London Paris
Tokyo Hong Kong Barcelona Budapest

Kerr L. White, M.D.
Former Deputy Director for Health Sciences
The Rockefeller Foundation
New York, NY 10036, USA

Series Editor
Mack Lipkin, Jr., M.D.
Director, Primary Care
Associate Professor of Medicine
New York Univeristy Medical Center
School of Medicine,
New York, NY 10016, USA

Library of Congress Cataloging-in-Publication Data
White, Kerr L.
    Healing the schism : epidemiology, medicine, and the public's
health / Kerr L. White.
        p. cm. — (Frontiers in primary care)
    Includes bibliographical references and index.
    ISBN 0-387-97574-8
    1. Public health. 2. Epidemiology. 3. Medicine—Philosophy.
I. Title. II. Series.
    [DNLM: 1. Epidemiology. 2. Public Health. WA 105 W585h]
RA427.W48   1991
614—dc20
DNLM/DLC   91-5053
Printed on acid-free paper.

Text prepared on Ventura Publisher using author-supplied WordPerfect disk.
Printed and bound by Edwards Brothers, Inc., Ann Arbor, MI.
Printed in the United States of America.

9 8 7 6 5 4 3 2 1

ISBN 0-387-97574-8 Springer-Verlag New York Berlin Heidelberg
ISBN 3-540-97574-8 Springer-Verlag Berlin Heidelberg New York

In Memory of
John H. Knowles, M.D.
1926-1979

Foreword

My conviction is that the matters addressed in this volume are of transcendental importance if we are to face up to the challenges of the 1990s and beyond. How, for instance, are we to cope with a truly ecological approach to public health and all its concomitant changes of risk groups worldwide unless there is a full appreciation of the population perspective throughout the health establishment? The global village has achieved a measure of interdependence requiring recognition by all concerned with the health of both individuals and communities that there is an urgent need to share our knowledge and deploy our resources in the best interests of people everywhere.

The history of public health initiatives, the origins of epidemiology, and the tragic separation—virtually a divorce—of public health from medicine recounted in the chapters that follow argue strongly for an early rapprochement. Health professionals who complement each other's knowledge and skills can be reunited through their common reliance on epidemiology as a major fundamental science for the entire health enterprise. Henceforth, epidemiology should be ranked in importance with cellular and molecular biology, immunology, and the social and systems sciences; all are essential if we are to cope with the vast array of diseases and disorders that face us in both the developed and developing worlds. We need more first-rate laboratory scientists, clinicians, nurses, aides, village health workers, and managers committed to serving the public. But we also need many more epidemiologists and much more epidemiological thinking throughout our health systems to measure the burden of illness, determine priorities, elucidate causal pathways, assess risks, appraise the relative benefits of interventions, and evaluate services. A health system that consisted only of biomedical scientists, only of tertiary care clinicians, only of village health workers, or even solely of epidemiologists would be sadly distorted. The public's health is best served by balanced arrays of academic, administrative, and practicing health personnel of all types, deployed and managed with the help of epidemiologically based information systems. Only then will it become possible to build facilitating and catalytic bridges between health needs as professionals *perceive* them and needs as populations *perceive* them. The way to achieve this is to imbue undergraduate and postgraduate medical education with the population or epidemiological perspective. This perspective and its methods were born and nurtured in the heart of clinical medicine and brought to maturity and preeminence in schools of public health.

The Rockefeller Foundation has played a major role in all of this during the present century, but times and problems change and institutions must also change. The Foundation's recent initiative in establishing the International Clinical Epidemiological Network (INCLEN) is an innovative approach to *Healing the Schism*. This schism has increasingly disturbed many thoughtful medical and public health leaders faced with the avalanche of health problems—especially in the developing world—which have grown in severity since schools of public health were separated from schools of medicine by the Rockefeller Foundation 75 years ago.

INCLEN's success to date in 27 medical schools in China, Southeast Asia, India, Latin America, and East and West Africa augurs well for the future, but it too will have to change with the times, and final answers are a decade or two away. In the meantime our global health problems are so urgent, and our common destinies so intertwined, that we truly are in need of radical reflections on the many issues related to the process of bringing medicine and public health together again. The central idea in Kerr White's volume is that, in contrast to recent trends, we need to attract a much larger share of the best brains in medicine and other health-related professions to careers directed at improving the health of populations, especially the health of the disadvantaged and high risk groups everywhere. I believe the problem requires prompt attention from leaders in both the developed and developing worlds.

I commend this volume to leaders in academic medicine and public health and their junior colleagues, to officials in ministries of health and education, to my colleagues in international agencies—especially bilateral and multilateral funding agencies, to professionals in the media advocating greater social responsibility in health matters, and to students everywhere who aspire to careers in medicine and all health professions that strive to improve the health of individuals and populations wherever they be. I hope above all that the ideas presented here will stimulate a vigorous debate about new institutional arrangements for achieving our common goals.

Halfdan Mahler, M.D.
Director General, Emeritus
World Health Organization
and Secretary General
International Planned Parenthood Federation
London

Series Preface

The twentieth century in medicine has seen the development of biomolecular approaches to disease and such triumphs of public health as the elimination of small pox. Yet medicine is deeply troubled by an ongoing identity crisis related to its dual missions of healing and preventing disease and illness. The mid-century phenomenon of specialization has been answered by "modern" generalists who combine elements from both sides of the schism to dispense medicine to the sick and prevention to the healthy.

This small volume represents a much needed call to heal the schism between mainstream clinical medicine and public health. It points to primary care as the meeting ground of these two disparate and warring disciplines. It is included in this series on the Frontiers of Primary Care for its contribution to our intellectual perspective of general medicine. We require not only practical works such as the volumes in this series on preventing disease and on functional assessment but also theoretical and historical guides to the nature, past, and future of our field. This concise, eloquent treatise is a welcome addition to discussion concerning the roles and functions of primary care.

It is particularly appropriate and gratifying to have Kerr L. White contribute to the Frontiers of Primary Care series. Dr. White reintroduced the very term "primary care" in his classic 1961 article, "The ecology of medicine" and has been a major contributor to its literature and its institutional development, as recognized by the Society of General Internal Medicine which awarded the Robert Glaser Award for contributions to general internal medicine research and education to Dr. White in 1990. Once again, Kerr White is perceiving and articulating the implications of current medical practice and lending us a vision for the future.

Mack Lipkin, Jr.
Series Editor
New York, 1991

Preface

Today, the two cultures "medicine" and "public health" seem to live in different, often unfriendly, worlds. This was not always the case. Experiences with universities, health departments, and governments during four decades have convinced me that continued separation of the two enterprises greatly diminishes their combined scientific, organizational, and institutional potentials. In the face of the contemporary domination of medical education, research, and services by the enormously productive biomedical sciences, epidemiology, among the population-based disciplines, may have the greatest leverage for effecting badly needed changes in all three sectors. Broader understanding and acceptance of epidemiology (and epidemiological thinking) is but one of several promising keys to the reintegration of the medical and public health perspectives, but it may also be the most feasible and most useful at this time.

In 1978 the Rockefeller Foundation afforded me an opportunity to test aspects of this long-held hypothesis under the auspices of its proposed Health of Populations program. The strategy adopted was to train young established clinical faculty members in epidemiology, and later to train other colleagues in health economics, health statistics, and the social sciences. The historical origins of the ideas and the rationale for this decision and the origins of what became the International Clinical Epidemiology Network (INCLEN) are described in this volume.

Most of the seminal ideas in the evolution of medicine's responses to the public's health problems were generated by clinicians. If they were not formally called epidemiologists, they seem to have reasoned epidemiologically. One of my purposes, therefore, is to describe briefly the central contributions during recent centuries of physicians, especially clinical faculty members, who designed, advocated, and implemented measures to improve the health of populations using epidemiological and statistical concepts and methods. These activities were perceived as a part of the profession's overall mission until the first quarter of the twentieth century. In 1916 when the Rockefeller Foundation decided to support the creation of schools of public health separate from schools of medicine, this mission was substantially curtailed. Other major factors contributed, and there were signs of cleavage between individual- and population-based approaches to health and disease toward the end of the nineteenth century. The Foundation's decision, nevertheless, marked the formal institutionalization of what has been called the *schism.*

I am neither the first to comment on this unfortunate separation nor the first to use the term schism in this connection. In 1956 the late John B. Grant, M.D., of the Rockefeller Foundation, discussing schools of medicine and public health, observed two trends: one in which the dividing line between the two institutions appeared to be breaking down and the other where public health in the previous 10 years or more seemed to have grown further apart from the medical school. He went on to argue that a unified curriculum of the type discussed in the final chapter of this volume is the most sensible goal for the future.[1]

In 1975 John G. Freyman, M.D., at the time President of the National Fund for Medical Education, in a paper entitled "Medicine's Great Schism: Prevention vs Cure, An Historical Interpretation," traced the history of the medical profession's participation in efforts to improve the health of the public. He observed that "as recently as 1965, only 332 of the 1142 graduates of schools of public health were physicians, and a mere 157 of these came from the United States." Later Freymann commented that "the reasons for maintaining two separate disciplines today may appear to be primarily due to tradition and obsolete administration, but two separate educational systems make bridging the gap more difficult. Education has had fifty years to formalize the artificial and illogical barrier between those who seek to prevent disease and those who seek to cure it if prevention fails."[2]

For many decades the late Professor Su Delong, M.D. of Shanghai Medical University, was China's leading epidemiologist. A graduate of Oxford University and the Johns Hopkins School of Hygiene and Public Health, he was a world figure in the control of schistosomiasis, a renowned pathologist, statistician, investigator, and innovator of effective public health programs. Su Delong had this to say at the Eighth Regional Meeting of Directors or Representatives of Schools of Public Health in Bangkok in 1979:

> We ought to devote limited resources in the most judicious way possible to the training of the most appropriate type and number of health personnel to best serve the needs of the population....It is necessary to overcome the dichotomy or *schism* which exists between agencies for medical care and those for health care....The time of the classical type of schools of public health and of schools of medicine as well seems to be over and new alternatives are coming up concerning the internal structure of public health programmes and medical training programmes as well ....It is a pity that development of medical education and that of public health education should diverge.[3] (emphasis added by KLW)

Such is the power of Grant's, Freymann's, and Su Delong's observations that *schism* seemed the right term to use in the title of this volume. Saint Augustine instructed us that "heresy" is not to be confused with schism. Nowhere have I found any taint of the former in the relationships between medicine and public health. In a schism, St. Augustine said, groups "break off in brotherly charity, although they may may believe first what we believe." Distinctions between we and they are not helpful in reviewing the past 75 years of separation; my intention is rather to place this brief experience in historical context as a guide to resolving many of the health care establishment's current problems.

I argue that, to *heal the schism*, the population perspective and concerns for the public's health should be reintegrated into the clinical departments of medical schools where they once flourished. In addition to the individual patient and molecular perspectives, medicine needs the population perspective, now more than ever. The present educational arrangements are not meeting the requirements of today's local or global villages. What follows, then, is in every sense a celebration of public health's outstanding triumphs. It is a call for the health establishment, especially the medical schools, to restore the broader vision of the missions guiding them a century ago.

The ideas discussed here should be of interest not only to deans, department heads, faculty members, and those students in schools of medicine—especially those in clinical departments—and in schools of public health, hospital and health services administration programs, and to epidemiologists of all persuasions. Clinicians, house staff, and others committed to careers as generalists in primary care may gain new insights into the historic links among prevention, cure, and care as they relate to communities and populations. All whose interests encompass practice or research with groups of patients or with populations should find the accounts of those who went before them at least instructive if not inspiring. Administrators and managers of health care institutions and systems, as well as others involved with health policies and health politics, may find that the perspectives discussed help to dispel some of their bewilderment.

Chapter 1 describes the principal problems and root causes that toward the end of the twentieth century have resulted in serious neglect of public health. Before devising strategies for *healing the schism* it is important to understand something of the major ideas and events that have shaped the population perspective over the centuries. Wider recognition of their enduring importance might have prevented the impasse that now finds much of medicine and public health apparently at odds. Chapter 2, therefore, briefly describes the evolution of the central concepts and institutions that underpinned concerns for improving the public's health; those less interested in these historical summaries may wish to skip ahead. Chapter 3 describes the impact of the major paradigm shift introduced by the bacteriological era and its impact on medical education, research, and health policies. Chapter 4 discusses the proximate factors and events leading to the Rockefeller Foundation's decision to establish separate schools to train public health workers. In so doing, the Foundation also unwittingly constricted the mission of medical schools and institutionalized the *schism*. Chapter 5 reviews recent, largely unsuccessful, approaches to broadening medicine's narrowed perspective and to making the collective health enterprise more accountable to the people served. Chapter 6 discusses what may be at once the most powerful and the most neglected forces available to improve and protect the health of both individuals and populations—the Placebo and Hawthorne effects. These ubiquitous therapeutic modalities deserve much more attention than they have been accorded by epidemiologists, clinicians, public health workers, and administrators. Failure to recognize their influence also reflects a second schism between a reductionist, Cartesian view of health and disease and a broader holistic approach to the human condition as revealed, for example, through the humanities and social sciences.

These background chapters describe the rationale for the Rockefeller Foundation's Health of Populations program and the creation of INCLEN, an account of whose origins and evolution is provided in Chapters 7 and 8. The extensive preparation, false starts, and nurturance that characterized this large-scale health sciences experiment are documented. I also recount, as I experienced them, the struggles within the Foundation to change its policies and priorities.

In the course of a decade there have been two independent external reviews of INCLEN, each by three consultants. Final evaluation, already planned and under way, of the contributions made by this experiment must wait for another decade or more. Potential implications for the future of the experiences described in this volume are discussed in the final chapter. Proposals also are advanced for restructuring aspects of undergraduate and postgraduate education to encompass the population, in addition to the molecular and clinical, perspectives.

Today's institutions were preceded by others. There are few positions, priorities, or paradigms that cannot be changed.[4] The luxury of perpetuating dysfunctional scholastic duplication and rivalries is no longer constructive; there is too much to be accomplished for the people who do the suffering and pay the bills. Now may be a time for *healing the schism* between medicine and public health. I hope this volume will further that process.

Kerr L. White
Charlottesville, Virginia

References

1. Seipp C, ed. *Health Care for the Community: Selected Papers of Dr. John B.Grant.* Baltimore: Johns Hopkins, 1963:129.
2. Freyman JG. Medicine's great schism: prevention vs. cure. An historical interpretation. Med Care, 1975;13:525-536.
3. Delong Su. *To Mend the Schism Between Public Health and Clinical Medicine.* (Mimeographed). New Delhi: World Health Organization, Regional Office for South-East Asia, Eighth Meeting of Directors or Representatives of Schools of Public Health, Bangkok, March 8, 1979.
4. Kuhn T. *The Structure of Scientific Revolutions.* Chicago: University of Chicago Press, 1970.

Acknowledgments

My longtime friend, the late John Knowles, former President of the Rockefeller Foundation, provided the institutional leadership and intellectual vision that redirected the Foundation's health programs in the 1970s. Kenneth S. Warren's initial Health of Populations proposal for the Foundation provided the framework for the creation of the International Clinical Epidemiology Network (INCLEN). Without his constructive urging and vigorous advocacy, nothing would have developed. The suggestion that I describe the rationale, background, and history of our program to expand the population perspective in medical education by providing postgraduate training of young clinicians in epidemiology and related disciplines came from Scott B. Halstead. Apart from a Foundation grant, he provided invaluable encouragement and assistance. I am grateful to both these latter colleagues for supplying documents, reading drafts of the manuscript, noting omissions, and correcting mistakes.

Many other colleagues have read parts or all of several versions of this volume. They not only saved me from grievous error but helped to improve the logic and, I hope, the accuracy and clarity of the exposition; the remaining blemishes are mine. My deep thanks go to Katherine Bennett, Annette Dobson, Suzanne Fletcher, Jane Hall, Richard Heller, Michael Hensley, Nichlos Higginbotham, Stephen Leeder, Victor Neufeld, Paul Stolley, Brian Strom, and Peter Tugwell. Roy Acheson, Carol Buck, John Evans, Robert Fletcher, and John Last were especially helpful with their extended criticisms and suggestions. Sir Donald Acheson, Gordon Defriese, James H. Eagen, John Freymann, Michael B. Gregg, John Hastings, Maureen Law, the late Abraham Lilienfeld, Gordon McLachlan, John Pemberton, Orneata Prawl, Denman Scott, and Cecil Sheps each helped in special ways. Halfdan Mahler graciously agreed to write the Foreword. Daniel Fox provided strong encouragement as well as perceptive and constructive criticisms in the course of reading two complete versions of the manuscript; I am forever indebted to him for his scholarship, patience, and friendship.

Greer Williams and John Z. Bowers gave me draft copies of unpublished manuscripts that provided detailed accounts of the Rockefeller Foundation's work in the health sciences over extended periods; these and other documents bearing on the present volume are now part of the Health Services Collection in the Claude

Moore Health Sciences Library of the University of Virginia, Charlottesville. For research, data, or documents, I thank the staffs of the Australian Commonwealth Department of Health and Welfare; the Canadian Department of National Health and Welfare; in England, the Department of Health, the King's Fund Institute, and the Public Health Alliance; and in the United States, the Department of Health and Human Services, the American Public Health Association, the Association of Schools of Public Health, and the Association of State and Territorial Health Officers.

The many excellent historians, biographers, and other scholars whose writings I have consulted and identified helped enormously. I trust they will forgive the brevity of my summaries and hope that readers of this volume will be stimulated to consult their works. Interested physicians, especially clinicians and epidemiologists, as well as others unfamiliar with the evolution of population-based medicine, may wish to consult the original accounts.

Isabel, my wife, has not only listened to the arguments and lived the experiences with me for almost half a century but has spent countless hours in research, editing, and proofreading of this and many other effusions. I can never satisfactorily acknowledge her devotion and support.

The Rockefeller Foundations's Bellagio Study and Conference Center was the venue for the most important meetings that shaped the origins of INCLEN. Their success was greatly assisted by the warm hospitality provided by Ginna and the late Roberto Celli, whose gentle stewardship of the Villa Serbelloni must have few equals. The delight Isabel and I experienced during our residency there in 1989 made the task of substantially revising an early draft of this volume highly pleasurable.

KLW

Contents

1
The Unexpected Legacy

The last quarter of the twentieth century finds most of the world's personal and public health services in disarray. The costs of medical care are widely thought to be exceeding the benefits; inequitable distribution abounds. Throughout the developed and developing worlds, many earlier triumphs of public health are forgotten. In comparison with "high-tech" clinical interventions, politicians, the practicing profession, and the public now accord public health a low priority.

What exactly is meant by the term public health? Over the decades authorities have offered many definitions. One of the shortest, and I believe the most useful, is that of Professor Fraser Brockington: "The application of scientific and medical knowledge to the protection and improvement of the health of the group."[1] Most definitions also include the notion of organized collective action for removing or altering factors affecting all citizens within some geopolitical jurisdiction. These factors usually are outside the capacity of the individual citizen to control or eliminate; they affect all those exposed without regard to individual differences and preferences. To address the problems effectively requires collective action for the "public good" or to further the "community's interest," in contrast to individual action required to achieve a "private good" or pursue a "personal interest," for example, in altering dietary habits or seeking personal medical care. When referring to public health matters the terms community, society, state, and government are used frequently. The notions of sanctions, penalties, and restrictions on individual freedom in the interests of societal benefits permeate discussions, standards, regulations, and legislation.

At a more abstract level, the prevailing reference body is usually a general population. Specifically designated subsets or groups, however, such as children, the homeless, migrants, or rural peasants, frequently are the focus of attention in contrast to an individual patient or citizen. The central idea is of organized, collective, and public action to remove or control those precursors of disease or impediments to well-being affecting all citizens or substantial subgroups.

Why does the term public health evoke such an indifferent, often negative, response from so many clinicians? Why does most of the medical profession's interest in prevention of illness lag far behind that for treatment? Why do most medical schools appear to care so little about the health services available to their neighbors in surrounding bailiwicks? Why do medical school faculties show such limited concern for the plight of the poor and disenfranchised? Why do occupational, environmental, nutritional, sociocultural, and psychological influences on health and disease receive such short shrift from most academic clinicians?

Why are ministries of health placed close to the bottom of most cabinet hierarchies? Are there institutional and structural impediments to change? Are the problems related to outmoded professional hierarchies and unproductive institutional rivalries? Are they related to the availability of faculty role models and educational practices? What can be done to influence the career choices of students so more of the best and the brightest will address major health problems afflicting the community? What can be done to stimulate research that responds to the public's needs and promotes effective application of usable knowledge? If change is required, what can be done to bring it about?

Until the latter part of the nineteenth century, most leaders of academic medicine and many members of the medical establishment had a broad view of their missions. These missions included both the care of individual patients and concern for unacceptable environmental and social conditions that endangered the public's health. During the previous three centuries, methods for investigating health problems in populations, when not originating with the work of mathematicians and statisticians, were developed by physicians, almost always clinicians. They evolved concepts and skills now subsumed under the rubric of *epidemiology*—"the study of that which is upon the people."

With the advent of the "germ theory" of disease, medical academicians increasingly pursued the task of describing microorganisms while largely neglecting studies of the host and environment. Investigation in the bacteriology laboratory gradually dominated epidemiological studies in populations. When undertaken, population-based investigations focused, quite reasonably, on the diseases of greatest prevalence and virulence at the time, infectious diseases. Epidemiology became virtually synonymous with bacteriology and bacteriology synonymous with biomedical science. Such was the specificity of the diseases associated with the growing number of microorganisms described that every "disease" was considered to have a single "cause," and that cause was thought to be a microorganism. Although there is no gainsaying the success of the strategies employed for control of major scourges of the day, the long-term consequences that resulted from limiting medicine's vision to such a narrow paradigm have offset many of these benefits. Has not this nineteenth-century paradigm now outlived its usefulness?

In 1916 the Rockefeller Foundation determined that insufficient attention was being paid to environmental and social factors in disease. The population perspective was neglected domestically and abroad; appropriately trained health officers and other public health personnel were needed urgently everywhere. The Foundation's officers decided that the solution was to establish schools of public health apart from schools of medicine. Henceforth, the latter's mission was the care of individual patients and investigation of disease processes. The former were now to be responsible for studying the determinants of health and disease in populations; they were to formulate strategies requiring collective action to improve the public's health. Medical schools lost interest in epidemiology, the social sciences, and quantitative methods; fortunately, the new schools of public health embraced them energetically. Concepts and methods created by earlier clinicians, often academic clinicians, were expanded and applied with great success by faculty working in these new institutions. The world's health establishment owes a deep debt of gratitude to the early twentieth-century epidemiologists who nurtured and developed contemporary epidemiology. Major Greenwood (1880-1949), first Professor of Epidemiology and Vital Statistics at the London School of Hygiene and Tropical Medicine, and Wade Hampton Frost (1880-1938), first Professor of Epidemiology at the Johns Hopkins School of Hygiene and Public Health, were two of the most prominent.

The narrowed mission of the medical school resulted in gradual abrogation of the social contract between the medical establishment—especially its academic component—and the public from which it derives its status. Medicine lost touch with the full array of the population's health problems and needs, and many in the public health arena lost touch with developments in the mainstream of biomedical and clinical advances. Public health could have profited through closer association and, of greater importance, influenced medicine's priorities and values; the converse would undoubtedly have occurred also. Both medicine and public health were losers, to say nothing of the populations served.

The creation of two parallel educational functions, responsibilities, and sets of schools constitutes *the schism*—a schism formally institutionalized by the Rockefeller Foundation's 1916 decision. Estrangement between the two worlds of "medicine" and "public health" was one consequence. The decision legitimized a process that had started imperceptibly and proceeded gradually for about a quarter of a century. There was no conspiracy, there was no malice—decisions were taken with the best of intentions and much good has resulted. There have however also been widespread and unintended negative perturbations from the institutional and professional initiatives which that decision set in train. The task now is to strengthen positive accomplishments while overcoming the negative fallout.

The schism favored medicine's emphasis on investigating the mechanisms of disease and public health's emphasis on studying environmental and social influences on health and disease; description and explanation gradually became separate concerns. Study of diseases processes and searches for causal determinants of diseases tended to evolve apart from one another in the two different types of schools. The patient—as a person living in a natural habitat—is left dangling, almost as if disembodied from the real world of living, loving, working, and suffering beyond the confines of the hospital ward. Equally important, the public and its politicians were caught between two conflicting views of the health establishment's overall mission and how to further it.

On the one hand, the public and their representatives hear clamors for more funds to advance technological capacity to diagnose, sometimes treat, and occasionally cure complex, and complicated conditions of low frequency. On the other, they hear less about the need for effective prevention and management of conditions with high frequency and enormous social and economic costs, to say nothing of human suffering. The arguments advanced by contemporary medical establishments are more often than not couched in terms of individual compassion rather than "statistical compassion." Anecdotes describing selected patients' suffering take precedence over data derived from measures of need and disability in the population. Table thumping, shroud waving, and dire forebodings—medical terrorism—prevail over the recitation of abstract health statistics—"people with the tears wiped off," as Major Greenwood used to call them.

In spite of its unquestioned accomplishments, the 75-year-old educational experiment to train adequate numbers of health officers to deal with the public's collective health problems has not achieved the goals originally envisioned by the Rockefeller Foundation's officers and advisers. There are those who say that educating physicians and others for careers dedicated to improving the public's health, inculcating the entire medical profession with the population perspective, and informing the public and its politicians about these matters are too important to leave solely in the hands of schools of public health.[2] The entire health establishment, led by academic medicine, should be responsible for coping with the schism's unexpected legacy.

Here are two complaints voiced in 1974 by observers from the developing world:

> Because medicine limited its vision to pathology, public health was unable to find a way to integrate with it and thus remained virtually divorced from what was generally understood to be medicine. Two distinct areas were therefore established: clinical medicine and public health—a fact that had dire consequences in that it established an artificial barrier that even today is difficult to overcome. A lack of understanding between clinicians and public health personnel blocked communication between them.[3]
>
> ...[T]he health professionals shut themselves up in their schools of public health, and the physicians stayed within the walls of the medical schools and hospitals. The latter felt that public health specialists 'were no longer doctors,' while the health people believed themselves to be crusaders in a cause they had to win, imposing it if necessary *on* the community as well as on other physicians who did not understand them, either because of cultural lag or lack of social mystique.[4]

In 1976, The Milbank Memorial Fund Commission on Higher Education for Public Health had this to say:

> As with other health professions, there is currently much dissatisfaction with the training and abilities of personnel in public health, particularly in leadership positions. In addition, there are substantial manpower shortages in certain fields. Serious criticisms of the various types of graduate programs come from many quarters. State health officers, directors of large health organizations (which are quasipublic), and members of the top echelon of the [U.S.] federal government complain that they have great difficulty finding professional personnel with appropriate skills and knowledge to meet the challenge of today's public health problems.[5]

In 1986 the Institute of Medicine (IOM) of the U.S. National Academy of Sciences constituted a Committee for the Study of the Future of Public Health. Its report declared that "public health is currently in disarray."[6] After defining "the mission of public health as fulfilling society's interest in assuring conditions in which people can be healthy," the Committee identified a number of barriers to effective progress. These included:

- Lack of consensus on the content of the public health mission;
- Inadequate capacity to carry out the essential public health functions of assessment, policy development, and assurance of services;
- Disjointed decision making without necessary data and knowledge;
- Inequities in the distribution of services and the benefits of public health;
- Limits on effective leadership, including poor interaction among technical and political aspects of decisions, rapid turnover of leaders, and inadequate relationships with the medical profession;
- Organizational fragmentation or submersion;
- Problems in relationships among the several levels of government;
- Inadequate development of necessary knowledge across the full array of public health needs;
- Poor public image of public health, inhibiting necessary support; and
- Special problems that limit unduly the financial resources available to public health.[7]

The Committee attributed these "barriers" to a variety of factors that amount to ambiguity and uncertainty about the mission of public health and about leadership capacity. "...[W]hen it comes to translating broad statements into effective action, little consensus can be found. Neither among the providers nor the beneficiaries of public health programs is there a shared sense of what the citizenry should expect in the way of services..." observed the Committee.[8]

This should not come as news to anyone familiar with the historical evolution of public health, particularly in a democracy, but the Committee apparently was surprised to find "[t]ension between professional expertise and politics...throughout the nation's public health system."[9] The Committee reported that:

[P]ublic health has had great difficulty accommodating itself to...political dynamics. Technical knowledge in fact plays a much more restricted role in public health decision-making than it once did, despite the fact that we now know more. The impact of politics is clearly evident: in the rapid turnover among public health officials (the average tenure of a state health officer is now two years); in a marked shift toward political appointees as opposed to career professionals in the top ranks of health agencies; and in the gradual disappearance of state boards of health, that have dwindled by half (from nearly all states to 24) in only 25 years. Too frequently during its investigations, the Committee heard legislators and members of the general public castigate public health professionals as 'paper-shufflers, out of touch with reality, and caught up in red tape.'[10]

Later in their report the IOM Committee attributed the high turnover among state health officers to not only "political-technical conflict...[but also to] inadequate pay, the effects of reorganization, frustrations with the structure of decision-making, and low professional prestige."[11]

The Committee bemoaned the separation of responsibility for environmental health problems from the traditional concerns of public health, that is, getting rid of filth and sewage and providing clean water and air for the citizenry. In the mid-twentieth century, however, the American schools of public health were doing less and less about these essential concerns. The environmental lobby criticized the U.S. Public Health Service for its inaction about water pollution. A major school had only 1.5 engineers on its faculty while half the world's population was drinking polluted water. In 1961 the new U.S. Environmental Protection Agency was established apart from the U.S. Public Health Service, to the great dismay of the public health community.[12]

The IOM Committee also deplored the loss by public health units in the United States of responsibility for the massive flow of government funds to pay for personal health services through Medicare and Medicaid programs for the elderly and poor, respectively. Many laboring in the vineyard of public health were and continue to be among the most articulate advocates of some form of national health insurance in the United States. Another of the public health establishment's traditions, however, emphasized vertical, disease-related, categorical "programs." This strategy, understandable at the time, left many in public health leadership positions unprepared until comparatively recently to understand the concepts of horizontal levels of medical care (starting with primary medical care) integrated into balanced health care systems, as Lord Dawson and others had advocated in Britain as early as 1920.[13-15]

In 1960 the report of a Study Group on Mission and Organization of the Public Health Service presaged changes in both these major "public health" functions by observing that:

> The next great nationwide health efforts may be expected in two broad areas: the physical environment and comprehensive health care. During the present decade, 1960-70, major national efforts, comparable with the great expansion of medical research and hospitals in the 1960s, will be required in each of these areas.[16]

In the course of a long review of public health education in relation to this era, one informed commentator wrote:

> By the early 1960s there appeared to be substantial disenchantment and dissatisfaction on the part of the Administration toward the Commissioned Corps of the PHS. It was considered by many to be unwilling or unable to meet modern problems related to the administration and delivery of health services...[17]

To cope with such problems, Philip R. Lee, a clinician, was brought in as the first Assistant Secretary of Health. Following a close call with total dissolution of the U.S. Public Health Service in 1968, there were numerous reorganizations of the Service over the next few years. Under the leadership of several clinicians the U.S. Public Health Service gradually was reoriented and some of its lost self-esteem restored.[18] In spite of these initiatives, however, the IOM Committee deplored "the poor relationships [of public health workers] with the medical profession."

> A particular problem for public health leadership is the lack of supportive relationships with the medical care profession. There are numerous examples of practicing physicians being supportive of public health activities, but confrontation and suspicion too often characterize the relationship from both sides. The director of one state medical association perceived the state health department (led by a nonphysician) as failing to seek medical advice and as distrustful of private physicians. He cited the department's effort to get a mandatory data reporting system through the legislature without consulting the association. On the other hand, health department personnel—including the director—told us that it was impossible for the department to do its job without the support of private physicians. As one official put it, 'Without them, we're dead in the water.'[19]

In Britain a similar review of public health in that country, also in 1988, culminated in *The Report of the Committee of Inquiry into the Future Development of the Public Health Function.*[20] This Committee had been created as a result of two major outbreaks of communicable diseases where inquiries "pointed to a decline in available medical expertise 'in environmental health and in the investigation and control of communicable diseases' and recommended inter alia a review of the responsibilities and authority of Medical Officers of Environmental Health (MOsEH). In addition there was continuing concern about the future role of the specialty of Community Medicine and the status and responsibilities of community physicians after implementation of 'general management' in the National Health Service (NHS) in 1984..."[21] The Committee proceeded to identify the following major problems:

- A lack of coordinated information on which to base policy decisions about the health of the population at national and local levels. This has led to:
- A lack of emphasis on the promotion of health and healthy living and the prevention of disease;
- Widespread confusion about the role and responsibilities of public health doctors, both within the NHS and among the public;
- Confusion about responsibility for the control of communicable disease and poor communication between the agencies involved, in particular widespread dissatisfaction with the position of the Medical Officer of Environmental Health (MOEH);
- Weakness in the capacity of health authorities to evaluate the outcome of their activities and therefore to make informed choices between competing priorities.[22]

The English Committee as compared to the analogous U.S. Committee provided a different definition of public health, declaring it to be "the science and art of preventing disease, prolonging life and promoting health through organized efforts of society."[23] Wide variations in performance and the inadequacies of training were decried. "The out-dated approach of some community physicians, coupled with confused lines of accountability...exacerbated by the paucity of resources available in some places, impeded the proper discharge of the public health function." And later the Committee commented that "[t]he failure of some community physicians to meet...expectations...also contributed to the failure of the specialty to establish its professional standing."[24]

In 1979 Professor C.C. Chen of the West China University of Medical Sciences, Chengdu, visited a series of North American schools of medicine and schools of public health. C.C. Chen is an eminent public health leader in China, fluent in English, widely traveled, and well read. A graduate of the Peking Union Medical College (PUMC), he earned postgraduate degrees at the Harvard School of Public Health and Das Reichshaus für Hygienische Volksbelehrung in Dresden. In his capacities as Dean, first of a leading medical school and later of a prominent school of public health, as a Professor of Public Health, and as Commissioner of Health for Sichuan Province, his experience is both broad and deep.

Early in his career, C.C. Chen was responsible for the famous Dingxian model. Guided by appropriately designed epidemiological surveys, his model demonstrated that simple, inexpensive measures materially improved the health of impoverished rural peasants in China. This experiment provided the model for China's early "barefoot doctor" attempts at providing primary health care. It established the pattern for similar efforts in many other countries. As a lifelong student and teacher of public health matters, C.C. Chen's views on the field generally, and his critiques of American schools of medicine and of public health in particular, are of special interest.[25]

Throughout his observations, Professor Chen stressed the essential prerequisite of clinical training and experience for those intending to lead public health programs:

> Most [medical] academics agree on the paramount importance of [clinical] training for a public health educator. It [is] difficult for anyone with inadequate clinical training to enlist public confidence or to command respect from his colleagues.[26]

Deploring the early specialization and separation of public health students from medical students in the Soviet Union, he found that similar patterns in China seriously impede the attraction of the best students to careers in public health. Professor Chen observed that:

> Although the public health schools were on the same academic level as the schools of medicine, they ranked lower in prestige because the best students were selected for medicine, not public health. Not unexpectedly, science and clinical teachers were quite uninterested in the public health students.[27]

And later:

> Test scores on the basis of general competitive examinations determine the order in which students can select the medical, dental, pharmaceutical, or public health school of their choice. Because the public health field is not well understood, public health schools are seldom selected first.[28]

"Public health education [in China] in 1987," C.C. Chen wrote, "...continued to be based on the assumption that its work was better left to 'specialists' who are not medical doctors and whose training followed a rather narrow channel of interest, rather than to physicians trained in public health. In medical school itself, public health studies are deemed significantly less important than clinical coursework."[29]

Of American schools of public health, C.C. Chen commented:

Those I was familiar with in the United States seemed to be concerned more with theoretical knowledge and scientific research than with the practical application of knowledge for the benefit of the general population. Regrettably, decades later public health professors in the West seemed to be encouraging graduate students along the same lines.

And of a visit to his alma mater, he wrote:

At Harvard University, I visited the Schools of Public Health and Medicine. The faculty had increased enormously, and its interests seemed to revolve less around challenging the students than in generating papers on subjects of high academic interest. Many research topics, as far as I could see, had no connection with major health problems.[30]

And of medical education in the United States in 1979, he commented:

With one exception [the Medical School of the University of Missouri in Kansas City] schools I visited seemed to have changed greatly in size but to have changed their teaching methods, educational objectives, and field training activities very little. There was no evidence that the teaching of preventive medicine and public health was respected in the medical schools; possibly the separation of teaching of clinical medicine and public health contributed to this situation. Instruction seemed to be less characterized by intellectual stimulation than by reliance on audiovisual aids.[31]

The schism's unexpected legacy persists globally. The 1988 Report of the Eleventh Interregional Meeting of Directors and Representatives of Schools and Departments of Public Health stated that:

There was general agreement that the specialty of public health is not considered attractive and that it is not sufficiently appreciated by the general public or by the medical profession as a whole. Because of this, in most countries, the recruitment of candidates, especially those of high calibre, for training in the specialty is not satisfactory.[32]

There is also a poignant statement from the Association of Schools of Public Health for the European Region:

[There is] deep concern about the unfavorable image of public health in its member countries, the deplorable state of public health training, and the limited research capability in the schools.[33]

In 1977 the late John Knowles, then President of the Rockefeller Foundation, determined to develop new approaches to the problems besetting public health. Enduring solutions had not been forthcoming in the past; better ones were required. Knowles edited a widely acclaimed volume entitled *Doing Better but Feeling*

Worse: Health in the United States. This volume explored the contemporary American predicament in matters of health, disease, and the provision of health services. In his introduction Knowles observed that:

> Public health interests have been, and continue to be, isolated from American medical education and practice. Issues that influence health, such as nutrition, family size, population density, environmental mobility, poverty, racism, sexual practices, unemployment, housing, transportation, and the like, are rarely taken into account in any overall calculation of the health needs of the nation.[34]

Knowles wrote and spoke extensively about the narrow focus of medical education and its failure to address the full range of factors impinging on health. Starting in the 1970s, problems stemming from misplaced priorities and imbalances in resource allocations in the United States increased exponentially. Throughout most parts of the developing world similar distortions of their meager resources are proving catastrophic. In large measure this is because policymakers in the Third World have been mimicking colleagues and practices in the developed world, especially those in the United States.

Knowles determined that the Foundation should support fundamental changes in the way medical faculties and medical students think about the problems of health and disease. The Foundation should eschew quick fixes and ephemeral funding for institutional and professional arrangements that he believed to have failed. He wished to strengthen its long and productive association with matters subsumed under the rubrics of "health," "medicine," and "public health," including interests in the control of specific diseases (e.g., hookworm, yellow fever, and more recently, schistosomiasis), the training of public health workers, medical education, and medical research of all types. Although emphases, programs, and officers have changed over time, knowledge about the health professions and institutions was deeply enshrined in the Foundation's traditions, concerns, and archives.

Before mounting a new program the Rockefeller Foundation's officers seek to understand the root causes of problems to be addressed. The first step in response to Knowles's initiative, therefore, was to identify the principal problems that constituted the schism's unexpected legacy. A critical review of earlier experiences at home and abroad, now bolstered by subsequent findings, supported the conclusion that there are at least two; these are examined in detail next but can be summarized as follows:

- The need for the health establishment to recruit and retain adequate numbers of bright, able, and committed physicians, as well as other professionals.
- The requirement that the entire health establishment understand and apply concepts associated with the population perspective. In addition, many should understand its methods, and adequate numbers should have the skills to apply them. The concepts, methods, and skills are epidemiological.

Problem 1, then, is the apparent inability of the public health enterprise to attract and retain its essential share of the best minds in medicine. No matter how important other disciplines and professions are for protecting and improving the public's health, physicians are likely to remain essential participants. That society can cope with its collective health problems is inconceivable without professionals whom it endows with the rights, privileges, and status of "physicians." In the future, the paradigm that guides our understanding of health and disease as well as the scope and content of medical education and practice may differ radically from today's but there will still be those whom society calls "doctor." Let us grant that investigation, advocacy, and implementation of measures to improve the population's health require the talents and skills of many disciplines and professions. In the light of the past and potential contributions made by physicians, however, public health requires the commitment and active involvement of the medical profession. Can anything of real substance be accomplished without visible leadership and support from the medical profession? Can the public health enterprise operate effectively without the unequivocal understanding and enthusiastic participation of the medical profession—albeit a different kind of medical profession?

The proportions, in four countries, of senior health officials who are physicians with graduate training in public health or a closely related field illustrate the dimensions of this first problem. The existence of schools of public health for almost three-quarters of a century makes it reasonable to expect that physicians with postgraduate public health training would hold most senior appointments in national departments of health. This is not to say that nonphysicians or physicians without formal public health training should not lead health departments, and indeed many have successfully done so. It is to suggest, however, that those with such training might have found their task easier or might have done even better. As is seen in Chapter 4, the assumption underlying the creation of schools of public health was that they would train:

> Higher administrative officials, as commissioners of health and health officers in cities and districts, and divisions or bureau chiefs in the larger state and city departments of health.[35]

In Australia in 1985, about 17% of the top leadership jobs in the Commonwealth (i.e., Federal) Department of Health were filled by physicians with public health training or its equivalent. Recent Secretaries (i.e., Chief Executive Officers) of that department have not been physicians. For the whole country, including its State Departments of Health, physicians with public health (or equivalent) training filled about 20% of all the professional positions.[36]

In Canada in 1989, about 14% of the top three levels in the Department of National Health and Welfare were filled by physicians with graduate degrees or diplomas in public health or community medicine (personal communication, M. Law, Deputy Minister, Department of National Health and Welfare, Canada, June 21, 1989).

In 1989, about 16% of the physicians (who act primarily as technical advisors to the lay civil servants) among the top five levels in England's Department of Health had postgraduate qualifications in public health, community, preventive, or social medicine. In addition to the 16 individuals represented by this figure, another 5 full-time and 2 part-time staff were studying for such qualifications. In the top three echelons, 8 of 18 (about 44%) physicians have public health or equivalent degrees (personal communications, Sir Donald Acheson, Chief Medical Officer, Department of Health, May 25 and June 23, 1989).

In 1989 the United States had a much larger Public Health Service within its Department of Health and Human Services and had 24 schools of public health. Physicians with formal public health training filled about 13% of the top leadership positions (personal communication, J.H. Eagen, U.S. Department of Health and Human Services, April 11, 1989). In the past three decades only three of the Surgeons-General of the U.S. Public Health Service and, until the most recent incumbent, none of the Assistant Secretaries for Health had received postgraduate training in public health.

The status of U.S. state health departments is bleak and growing worse. The number of physicians employed in these departments across the entire country in 1986 was only 2886, a decrease since 1979 of more than 34%. Physicians with or without public health training constituted less than 4% of all state health department employees in 1986.[37]

Perhaps the situation is now improving because the current Assistant Secretary of Health in the United States is a physician with training in a school of public health. The same is true at present in England and Canada where the Chief Medical Officer and the Deputy Minister of Health, respectively, both have had postgraduate training in public health. Their Australian counterpart is not a physician. One hopes that these are not exceptions, however, to the prevailing patterns suggested by the preceding figures.

Problem 2 is the failure by most physicians, in concert with many other health professionals, to understand or appreciate the population (or public health) perspective. An international survey conducted in 1979 for the Rockefeller Foundation had this to say:

> Two consistent themes emerge from observations on the broader issues of health in countries at different stages of development. First, the resources now available are not being used effectively to achieve the maximum impact on health. In the poorer developing countries, this situation may deprive more than half the population of access to the simplest elements of basic health care. Second, although the techniques are available to manage health resources more effectively, the three groups of professionals who might have been expected to put the techniques into practice have failed to do so. Public health officers seem unable to influence the health service system, much of which lies outside their authority; health administrators have concerned themselves with administration more than health; and practicing physicians have neither the orientation nor the analytic skills to use their leadership for these broader health purposes.[38]

Four root causes underlie the two principal problems that are the schism's unexpected legacy; they are summarized as follows:

- Failure of attempts to establish "public health" as a separate profession, apart from the underlying primary professional qualifications of those committed to this essential work.

- Failure to establish epidemiology as a fundamental science for medicine, public health, and the entire health establishment; and, as a result, inability to train adequate numbers of epidemiologists.

- Failure to provide medical students, and hence all physicians, with an understanding of the population perspective and accompanying epidemiological and social science concepts in addition to molecular and clinical perspectives and concepts.

- Failure of medicine and public health to cooperate creatively in establishing new paradigms encompassing many of the complex interactions among hosts, agents, environments, health status, and health services.

Root Cause 1 has been the failure of efforts to make "public health" a distinct calling, indeed a distinct "profession," apart from other well-established health professions. Much energy has been expended on this exercise in the United States. In Britain it also has consumed reams of paper and countless hours of debate. Over the years public health workers have argued that theirs is, indeed, a distinct profession. For example, the opening sentence in a recent brochure by the American Public Health Association refers to the "public health profession."[39] In the same vein, *Accreditation Criteria for Graduate Schools of Public Health of the Council on Education for Public Health* require these schools to have "the same prerogatives and status as other professional schools..."[40]

Unfortunately, the preponderance of evidence does not support the expectation that such aspirations are likely to be realized. In 1973 an extensive and well-documented study offered these observations:

...[A]t the outset, when public health did refer to a specific occupational group, the health officer of a governmental department and his (*sic*) immediate staff, it was at least relatively easy to identify the occupation and gain its recognition by the public. However, with the major changes in public health problems, the multiplicity of specialties which have developed to deal with these problems, and the increasingly broad scope of the settings where public health practitioners work, it is apparent that the public no longer understands what public health implies. It undoubtedly does not impute to public health the qualities of *a* profession, which is still generally defined by the medical model, although that itself is misunderstood in the realities of the present changes in medicine.[41]

And later:

The common name, [public health], derives from a general orientation binding together all who are considered *in* public health. This follows the theory that a profession has an ideology, a set of shared beliefs and values held in common by its members as they work together toward a 'cause.' Public health might almost be said to *be* an ideology, as well as to have one. Its central tenet is a concern for the *health* of populations, the one-to-many focus as contrasted to the one-to-one focus of clinical practitioners and their allied partners.[42]

The author of these conclusions identifies several factors as "undoubtedly involved in accounting for the reasons why public health and its educational model are not awarded the attention they would at first glance seem to merit":

> The first has to do with...the attempt by public health to fit itself to an outmoded concept of a profession. Although this concept might have been appropriate in the past, it led public health to remain locked in a position which did not permit it to acknowledge the strengths that constant diffusion both in the location and types of its services could in fact provide...[I]ts segments were proliferating constantly, as attested by the growth from six specialized sections within the APHA [American Public Health Association] at its inception to the current twenty-three Sections, plus six Primary Interest Groups. But public health did not see how it could retain its status as a profession if it called attention to these facts...[I]t would seem that there were errors of omission resulting from a pervasive state of mind about professional status.[43]

This author lays much of the onus for the confusion surrounding the work and status of those dedicated to improving the health of populations at the feet of the schools of public health themselves:

> Too often lip service has been given to such glories as the multidisciplinary approach and interaction with the community, but these have been rendered inoperative when communication channels even within schools, much less between the schools and other parts of their universities, or between the schools and their communities, have been virtually nonexistent. The schools too often have been locked in tradition, inflexible, rigid in course requirements, blind to the needs of their students and their constituencies.[44]

Third World countries have adopted patterns and values espoused in American (and to a lesser extent in British) schools of public health. Because the majority of the former's public health schools are closely tied to their ministries of health, primarily as staff colleges, a degree from one of them has been a means of furthering career advancement. Higher university degrees, especially those obtained abroad, are accorded great respect in the developing world. This too has added to the vocational currency of public health degrees, although their acquisition has done little to allay the confusion that surrounds public health as a distinct profession.

Public health itself may not be widely recognized as a distinct profession, but there is little question that a wide range of primary disciplines and professions undertake population-based work. These include anthropologists, biologists, chemists, demographers, economists, engineers, physicists, political scientists, sociologists, and statisticians; dentists, nurses, occupational, physical, and speech therapists, physicians, psychologists, and social workers, as well as a variety of support personnel such as aides, inspectors, sanitarians, and assorted technicians. Few, if any, of the helping or caring professions are excluded from the requirement that they have some appreciation of the population perspective, in addition to the skills required by many for one-to-one care at the individual level.

Root Cause 2 is the failure, during the twentieth century, to establish epidemiology as a fundamental discipline for medicine and for public health and the failure to train adequate numbers of epidemiologists for both the personal and the environmental health services. The two reports from United States and England argue that both countries need many more epidemiologists and expanded educational resources for training in epidemiology. They might have added that there is an even greater need for much more epidemiological, or population-based, thinking throughout the medical and health care establishments of both countries. These observations are also true for Australia, Canada, the Western democracies, and the developing world.

The Institute of Medicine report, in addition to frequently emphasizing the importance of epidemiology, quotes a well-regarded professor of epidemiology as stating that "the mother science of public health is epidemiology, i.e., the systematic, objective study of the natural history of disease within populations and the factors that determine its spread.... . Epidemiology is the 'glue' that holds public health's many professions together;" and they rest "upon the scientific core of epidemiology."[45] The British document has the same message when it refers to "epidemiology [as] the science fundamental to the study and practice of community medicine."[46]

What have schools of public health been doing over the past 75 years to train epidemiologists and to provide more training in epidemiology to all those concerned with the health of populations? The answer is not nearly enough. *Public Health in England*, stressing "the key contribution of epidemiology to the achievement of improvements in public health," has this to say:

> ...First, epidemiology has sometimes been inadequately perceived as a key priority by practicing public health doctors and trainers and by trainees. If those working in the field do not perceive the need for the skill—and the reason for this stems from the type of work they are undertaking—then it is very unlikely that those aspiring to join them will do so either. The problem has thus become self-perpetuating. Secondly, the focus of interest in epidemiology in academic departments has tended to be in the application of epidemiology to the identification of causes of particular diseases or conditions rather than analysis of health needs of the population and of the provision, organization and evaluation of services which are so relevant to those working in health authorities.[47]

The Josiah H. Macy, Jr., Foundation's 1974 report, *Schools of Public Health: Present and Future,* stated that "[o]f the variety of disciplines represented [in schools of public health], the one that is basic to all activities is epidemiology, which is considered to be the core discipline." It added that "[t]here is a great need to apply the science and techniques of epidemiology to the study of the effectiveness of widely used clinical procedures in personal health care and to the monitoring of the quality and quantity of health care delivery."[48]

The 1976 report of the Milbank Memorial Fund's Commission on Higher Education for Public Health provided another judgment about the status of epidemiology in the United States during the last quarter of the twentieth century. Asserting that epidemiology is one of the central or generic disciplines underpinning the public health enterprise, the Commission observed that "[t]he basic techniques for measuring and evaluating community-wide health problems are those of epidemiology and biostatistics, the sciences of 'social (or health) arithmetic'."[49] The Commission went on to summarize succinctly the broad scope of epidemiology as follows:

> ...[E]pidemiology is more than the accumulated knowledge about the distribution of a particular disease and the factors affecting its occurrence in the population at any one time; it also delineates the chains of inference based upon these facts and other relevant facts about the disease and that population. These chains of inference or hypotheses are an integral part of the epidemiology of today. False inferences are refuted by later experience; sound inferences foretell the epidemiologic knowledge of tomorrow.
>
> Epidemiologic techniques are used to trace the causes of specific diseases and to provide a framework for comparative studies of group health behavior with regard to chronic problems such as alcoholism, smoking, and obesity. In recent decades epidemiology has moved well beyond its traditional concerns with infectious diseases to embrace the study of factors influencing the occurrence of chronic illness, accidental death and disability, and occupational and environmental diseases. Psychological and social factors have been added to biologic and physical factors as foci of investigation. In essence, epidemiology represents both a methodologic and a descriptive approach to definition of the agent-host-environment inter-relationship which determines the collective health of populations.
>
> Recently, epidemiology has been recognized to be crucial to the planning and evaluation of medical care and other health programs because of the contribution it can make to the development of methods for program surveillance in such terms as who is being reached, with what kinds of services, with what kind of quality, and with what outcomes.[50]

The 1988 Institute of Medicine Committee, in addition to reciting a long litany of problems that account for public health's perceived ineffectiveness, defines the substance of public health as: "Organized community efforts aimed at the prevention of disease and promotion of health. It links many disciplines and rests upon the scientific core of epidemiology."[51] Although acknowledging a lack of research expertise in public health, a problem "exacerbated by a shortage of epidemiologists and other trained experts," the Committee says little about the startling absence of epidemiological thinking throughout the public health and medical care establishments. Perhaps this was because there were few practicing epidemiologists on the 22-person IOM Committee.[52]

What is known about the numbers of epidemiologists currently available? Community physician posts in England, roughly synonymous with epidemiologists, numbered 534 in 1986; this represents a ratio nationally of about 11 per million population. In addition, there were 83 positions funded but vacant and 32 for which the funding had been temporarily withdrawn; of all 649 positions, 18% were unfilled. The annual output of current training programs in England is about 60 community physicians per year. The 1988 report of the Committee of Inquiry into the Future Development of the Public Health Function estimates that by 1990 there will be a shortfall of about 140 community physicians (epidemiologists). Without any expansion of responsibilities this shortage may be reduced to zero toward the end of the century.[53] A careful estimate in 1973 stated that for a population of 5 million, Scotland required 200 community medicine specialists (primarily epidemiologists), a ratio of 40 per million population, more than three times the recent estimates for England.[54] Which is the "right" ratio?

The Milbank Memorial Fund's Commission used 1970 data to estimate there were then about 1000 epidemiologists in the United States; they calculated that by 1980 there would be between 1500 and 2000 trained to the Master's level. That Commission commented that for epidemiologists:

> Requirements are expected to double. This may be an underestimate of needs, as personnel with training in epidemiology will be used in health planning and the surveillance of medical care as well as other health care services. Many large hospitals and medical centers are beginning to employ full-time epidemiologists. The growing concerns with occupational health and safety, and the effects of pollution, together with the growing appreciation of the role of epidemiologic studies in uncovering the etiology and predisposing factors of chronic disease, have already increased the demand for epidemiologists and will continue to do so.[55]

In 1975 I estimated, based on memberships in professional organizations, there were probably no more than 500 fully trained epidemiologists in the United States, of whom 300 might be physicians. My calculations suggested the need for at least 2500 epidemiologists immediately. If we were to apply the ratios proposed for Scotland, 8000 medically trained epidemiologists were required, or 1 for every 40 physicians in the country.[56] Williams and colleagues[57] have made the most recent, and probably the most accurate, calculations to date for the United States. In 1985 they estimated there were 4600 epidemiologists in the United States, of whom 2460 or 54% were physicians. The overall (physicians and others) ratio of epidemiologists was about 19 per million population or a little less than twice the projections for England but half those for Scotland. If only physician epidemiologists are considered, the U.S. ratio is about 10 per million population, very close to the figure for England. If no change in factors occurred, other than population growth, these authors project the need for an increase of 10% to 30% in the number of epidemiologists of all types by 2010. They also compare their estimates to the 25% shortfall calculated by the U.S. Graduate Medical Education National Advisory Committee (GMENAC) for physician specialists in Preventive Medicine.

On balance, in the United States there is a realistic need for about 9,500 epidemiologists in 1990 and between 10,450 and 12,400 by 2010. "Data from [the authors'] interviews with experts also suggest that the current work force of epidemiologists is quite inadequate. While there is not a complete consensus within this group, they tend to believe that there are too few epidemiologists and that the greatest deficiency is in physician epidemiologists.... Using White's second assumption that there should be one medical epidemiologist per 40 clinical physicians, we calculate an estimated need of 13,000 medical epidemiologists in 1985 and 14,100-16,900 by 2000. If projections of the requirements of physicians as proposed by GMENAC are correct, however, the need is less, i.e., 12,300 medical epidemiologists by the year 2000."[58] In short, by the end of the 1990s the United States will require at least five times the present number of physician epidemiologists.

The state of affairs in the developing world is much more difficult to assess. One approach to estimating the availability of epidemiologists in these countries is by membership in the International Epidemiological Association, undoubtedly an underestimate because membership dues are high in relation to salaries and difficulties in obtaining foreign currency are often substantial. In 1989 there were 142 members in Africa, 354 in Asia, 90 in the Eastern Mediterranean region, and 57 in the Latin and South American countries.[59] Even a tripling of these figures leaves an enormous need for trained epidemiologists in Third World countries. Because their resources are scarce, clinicians also in short supply, and the medical problems daunting, one may argue that the need for epidemiologists and epidemiological thinking is much greater in the less developed than in the developed world.

If epidemiology is a fundamental science of public health and physician epidemiologists are scarce, as they seem to be everywhere, what is available by way of role models in the faculties of schools of public health? In 1989 the U.S. Association of Schools of Public Health offered this comment:

> [There] is another distressing problem that simply must be addressed as soon as possible: the overall decline in number of physicians taking positions in academic public health. Even in 1978, only 243 (20.6 percent) of the faculty in schools of public health, were physicians. This has steadily declined, until in 1983 there were 237, or 18.8 per cent of the total faculty, and in 1988 this increased slightly to 239 but represented a decrease in percentage of overall faculty (17.3 per cent).
>
> As might be expected under these circumstances, there are relatively more senior physician faculty members. In 1978, 84 per cent of physician faculty held the senior ranks of professor or associate professor, as contrasted with all other faculty where 60 per cent held these ranks....
>
> The paucity of young physicians choosing academic public health as a career is also demonstrated when their actual numbers are tallied school by school. In 1978 there were only 39 assistant professors in the 21 schools of public health; by 1983 this had declined to 31 in the 23 schools; in 1988 there were 47 in the 23 schools, to some extent reflecting a partial replacement of some senior personnel. However, in 1988, six schools still had no physicians at this entry-level rank, nine others had one each, and three schools had only two each. Thus 18 of the 24 schools have two or fewer physician assistant professors.
>
> If the nation is actually going to experience a surfeit of physicians in 1990 and beyond, this may, and probably will serve as a stimulus to some physicians to make their career in the public sector. However, the inducement will not be as great if there are few physicians, young or old, to serve as role models in academic public health.[60]

A survey of the student body in the Master of Public Health (MPH) program at The Johns Hopkins School of Hygiene and Public Health is informative. Among a total enrollment of 175 students in 1981, there were 74 physicians of whom 39 were U.S. citizens. Of the latter group there were 12, or 6% under the age of 30.

The age of 30 years is an arbitrary break because it should include the bulk of recent medical school graduates who opted at an early stage for a career in public health or epidemiology (personal communication, the late Professor A.M. Lilienfeld, June 16, 1981). Over a 10-year record (approximately 1960-1970), only **one** graduate of The Johns Hopkins Medical School was also a graduate of the School of Hygiene and Public Health (personal communication, Professor Caroline Bedell Thomas, The Johns Hopkins Medical School, circa 1971).

Matters improved somewhat the following decade; between 1973 and 1984, 30 graduates of The Johns Hopkins Medical School also received graduate degrees from the School of Hygiene and Public Health, that is, an average of 3 per year, not an overwhelming output. The number of physicians who were U.S. citizens under the age of 30 enrolled in the MPH class in 1984 had increased by 5 to 17, or about 10% of the class, but the number of U.S. physicians in that cohort was still only 38 (personal communication, Dean D.A. Henderson to Kenneth S. Warren forwarded to KLW, April 1, 1985). There are other schools of public health with different experiences. For example, the Harvard School of Public Health has always had a high proportion of physicians in its student body. At the University of North Carolina, Chapel Hill, there has always been a close relationship between the schools of medicine and public health. As a possible by-product there has been a steady increase in the proportion of all physicians (domestic and foreign) enrolled in the latter school until it was slightly over half in 1988-1989 (personal communication, Professor Robert H. Fletcher, October 8, 1989).

Overall, however, the situation is not encouraging. In 1985 the total enrollment for the 23 schools of public health was about 9000, of whom one-third were part-time students. Fifteen percent, presumably of the full-time students, were foreign. During the same year there were 3268 graduates from these schools of whom almost 65% received the MPH degree and 10% received a doctoral degree (Doctor of Public Health, Doctor of Science, or Ph.D.) Epidemiology was the area of specialization for 14% or about 460 of the graduates with MPH, doctoral, and other degrees. There were, however, only 541 graduates from all 23 schools with prior medical degrees, that is, 17%.

The situation is equally distressing for the major health professions combined. In the early 1960s physicians, dentists, and nurses comprised more than 40% of the graduates of schools of public health but by 1985-1986 this figure had fallen to 20%.[61] A year later, a study by the Association of Schools of Public Health reported a further decline nationally; of the 1610 graduates of American schools of public health, only 228 or 14% were prior graduates of schools of medicine or osteopathy. Of equal concern, however, is the report that in 1986 less than one-fourth of all graduates of these schools (physicians and everyone else) went to work for a health department—federal, state, or local.[62]

And what have the medical schools done about these problems? In 1983 the Rockefeller Foundation commissioned a survey of the teaching of epidemiology in North American medical schools.[63] With a 96% response rate from the universe of 140 medical school deans, the authors obtained the names of 384 faculty members said to be responsible for teaching epidemiology, and from this cohort

320 (83%) returned usable questionnaires; 53 of the respondents reported that they did not teach epidemiology. (So much for the understanding of this subject by 15% of the deans!) Of the 245 respondents who provided information about their qualifications, only 76 or 31% had a degree in public health, epidemiology, or "other field relevant to epidemiology and its methods" in addition to their medical degrees. There were 83 nonphysician faculty members with graduate degrees in public health, epidemiology, or some other related field. For argument's sake, assume that the figure "76" is off by half. That means each of the 140 medical schools in the United States and Canada had, on average, about 1 qualified physician-epidemiologist on its faculty. With such staffing patterns, how is it ever going to be possible to provide medical students with an appreciation, to say nothing of a thorough understanding, of the population perspective? As for graduate programs in epidemiology based in schools of medicine, there were six in 1981-1982 with three offering a graduate degree. The mean number of faculty members was 6.2 and the mean number of students was 12.2, or about 73 students for the entire country.

In 1984 the Commission of the European Communities commissioned an extensive review of undergraduate and postgraduate education in epidemiology. Descriptions of the diverse programs suggest that although there is some reason for hope, the diffusion of this discipline throughout medical faculties and its penetration into the medical curriculum have a long way to go; unfortunately, no tables of faculty staffing patterns are included.[64] The developing countries are, of course, in far worse shape.

It may be argued that formal postgraduate training in epidemiology is not a mandatory prerequisite for teaching, research, and practice based on epidemiological concepts and methods. Nevertheless, as in the case of public health leadership, it must surely be the assumption that such training is likely to enhance skills and accelerate diffusion of the population perspective throughout the health establishment.

Root Cause 3 has been the failure of the present educational arrangements to inculcate in medical students an adequate appreciation of the population perspective. This in turn has contributed to failure in recruiting a greater proportion of bright young physicians into the field of public health where they might expect eventually to attain leadership positions. Epidemiology's separation from the mainstream of the biomedical revolution was assured when the schism relegated nurturance and development of this fundamental aspect of the scientific method to schools of public health.

A related consequence has been the slow adoption of advances in quantitative methods in medical schools; we have had successive generations of physicians in both the developed and developing world who are largely innumerate. Exposure to epidemiological concepts and methods would have broadened their perspectives and deepened their critical capacities; the loss has been enormous.

Root Cause 4 is the failure of the outmoded paradigms employed by medicine, and also by many in public health, to encompass the full panoply of influences on health and disease. This failure is perpetuated by the academic and intellectual isolation of the two faculties in different schools. Those from schools of public health argue that the primary failure has been with the medical schools, but unfortunately separation of the two institutions has left each largely bereft of the other's influence. In Chapter 6, I discuss the importance of factors other than specific maneuvers or interventions directed at improving the health of individuals or populations. The problem is not a dearth of detailed evidence on these matters as well as on the importance of social, psychological, economic, and environmental factors in health and disease;[65-67] the tragedy is that the available evidence with its revolutionary implications for the entire health enterprise seems to have influenced the thinking of only a minority in academic medicine and that few of those have been in powerful enough positions to change priorities and policies. The single-cause, single-disease, and single-treatment approaches, fostered by the dramatic contributions of bacteriology and pyramided on a seventeenth-century Cartesian view of mind and body, have prevailed.

On the other hand, preoccupation with social, economic, and environmental concerns, important as they are, too often ignores our growing biomedical knowledge about host defenses and reactions. The former interests center in schools of public health and the latter in schools of medicine. The determinants of health, health status, and health services are intimately interrelated in ways that defy the artificial barriers that academics and bureaucrats erect around people's individual and collective problems.

In the last quarter of the twentieth century, these two principal problems and their four root causes comprise the *schism's* unexpected legacy that continues to divide medicine and public health. The task we face in attempts at healing the schism is to devise strategies for effectively coping with these problems and their causes. The strategies tried during the present century have not worked as anticipated. Further failure is possible, but, as this volume argues, there is reason for optimism.

Two objectives need to be tackled. The first is to attract a larger proportion of the best brains in medicine to careers employing population-based (i.e., epidemiological and public health) concepts and methods in teaching, research, practice, and management. The second is to see that the thinking of the entire faculty and the students—as reflected in the medical curriculum, and hence throughout the health establishment—reflects an appreciation and understanding of the population-based perspective, in addition to the equally important clinical and molecular perspectives. All three are essential if individuals and the populations they comprise are to have balanced, scientific, and compassionate personal and environmental health services. Concern for the public's health should be a central part of the academic medical establishment's overall mission, priorities, and activities. It should be on a par with clinical priorities and more recent molecular priorities. Those who struggle in each sector should have an appreciation of the essential roles played by the other two. One is not more or less important; all three are required.

The origins of medicine's and public health's contemporary malaise required examination by the Foundation's officers. Of almost equal importance was the need to understand better the factors motivating change in priorities designed to improve the public's health, medical education, and research. What are the generic characteristics of experiences over the centuries that have prompted the public's recurring concerns about health and disease? What stimulates civic leaders to organize, discuss, and eventually to legislate? From whence come the information and knowledge that make collective action both essential and useful?

In 1958 Sir Geoffrey Vickers, a prominent British industrialist, secretary of the Medical Research Council and author of distinguished texts on management and conflict resolution, examined these issues in an address at the Harvard School of Public Health entitled "What Sets the Goals of Public Health?"[68] In his classic paper Vickers argued that:

> Among the forces which make history, one of the most obvious is human need. Some would say that need sets the goals of public health. New needs emerge and evoke the measures which will satisfy them. At any moment, with a more or less significant time-lag, the goals of public health reflect the dominant needs of the time and place ...[but] we cannot satisfy all the needs we recognize. Our age, with public-health services more abundant and more active than in any before it, is probably more aware than any other of unsatisfied needs. How are they resolved, the conflicts between needs fighting for satisfaction? Are they resolved by human choice? And if so by what criteria?
>
> ...To some extent at least techniques set the goals of public health. For techniques not only enlarge our responses; they mold our expectations. Most obvious is the impact of therapeutic and preventive techniques...Every new technique, by opening a possibility, awakens a need—at least in our Western culture, where in matters of health we have a highly developed sense that whatever is possible for any should be available for all. [But] techniques [also] limit us...A technological age expects to deal with its problems technologically.[69]

Vickers then provided a fanciful example of a brave new world in which commercial interests compete against personal values and adds "ideology" as a third goal-setter for public health. He continued:

> This is perhaps the moment to question whether public health has any goals. Is it not governed rather by avoiding threats? Let us confuse ourselves by saying that a threat is only a negative goal. The psychologists have wrought havoc with lay thinking by popularizing the term "goal-seeking" as if it covered all purposive behaviour. It begins now to be widely recognized that threat-avoiding differs from goal-seeking in important ways. One of the most important is this. If I successfully seek a goal, I shall ultimately find it and I shall discover whether I really like it. But if I successfully avoid a threat, I shall never experience it and so I shall never discover whether it was worth avoiding.
>
> Threat avoiding bulks large in our individual motivation; and I fancy that it plays an even larger part in the collective decisions of larger and less coherent bodies. ...The landmarks of political, economic, and social history are the moments when some condition passed from the category of the given into the category of the intolerable....I believe that **the history of public health might well be written as a record of successive redefinings of the unacceptable** (emphasis added by KLW).[70]

At some point during our evolving efforts to cope with threats to the public's health we have lost our way. In the latter 1970s, the public and its politicians lacked authoritative and credible help from clinicians in redefining the unacceptable. The academic and practicing components of the medical profession collectively lacked appreciation of the public's perspectives and understanding of the concepts and methods required to generate change. They did not even recall Abraham Flexner's views on medicine's mission when he wrote in 1910:

> The physician's function is fast becoming social and preventive, rather than individual and curative. Upon him society relies to ascertain, and through measures essentially educational to enforce, the conditions that prevent disease and make positively for physical and moral well-being."[71]

Of special interest to our analysis of the origins and consequences of the schism's unexpected legacy, then, is the role of the medical profession—especially academic clinicians—in efforts to improve the public's health. Until the schism's advent there was only one type of "medical academy" and that was the school of medicine. It assumed responsibility for clinical services, for medical education, and for the health of the population. Until the latter part of the nineteenth century, research, especially laboratory research, was embryonic. True, both lay reformers and practicing physicians pursued their concerns for the public's health with varying degrees of knowledge, influence, and energy. Overall, however, until this century the medical schools and their clinical faculties provided the professional leaders for society's efforts to improve its collective health status. The wide range of strategies and tactics they invoked in "redefining the unacceptable" is discussed in the next chapter.

References

1. Brockington F. *World Health*, 2d Ed. Boston: Little, Brown, 1968:131.
2. Spitzer WO, Mann KV. The public's health is too important to be left to public health workers. Ann Intern Med 1989;111:939-942.
3. Bowers JZ, Purcell EF, eds. *Schools of Public Health: Present and Future*. New York: Josiah H. Macy, Jr. Foundation, 1974:137.
4. Bowers JZ, ed. *Schools of Public Health in Latin America, Report of a Macy Conference*, Medellin, Colombia, November 17-19, 1974, (Mimeographed). New York: Josiah H. Macy, Jr. Foundation, 1974:3.
5. Sheps CG, chairman. *The Milbank Memorial Fund Commission on Higher Education for Public Health*. New York: Prodist, 1976:xvii.
6. Institute of Medicine. *The Future of Public Health*. Washington, DC: National Academy Press, 1988:6.
7. Ibid, pp. 107-108.
8. Ibid, p. 3.
9. Ibid, p. 4.
10. Ibid, pp. 4-5.
11. Ibid, pp. 119-120.

12. Mullan F. *Plagues and Politics: The Story of the United States Public Health Service.* New York: Basic Books, 1989:153-154.
13. Dawson of Penn. *Interim Report on the Future Provision of Medical and Allied Services.* London: His Majesty's Stationery Office, Cmd. 693, 1920.
14. Fox DM. *Health Policies, Health Politics: The British and American Experience, 1911-1965.* Princeton: Princeton University Press, 1986.
15. Mullan F. *Plagues and Politics: The Story of the United States Public Health Service.* New York: Basic Books, 1989:153.
16. Ibid, p. 145.
17. Snoke AW. The unsolved problems of the career professional in the establishment of national health policy. Am J Public Health 1969:59:1575-1588.
18. Mullan F. *Plagues and Politics: The Story of the United States Public Health Service.* New York: Basic Books, 1989:Chapters 7, 8, 9.
19. Institute of Medicine. *The Future of Public Health.* Washington, DC: National Academy Press, 1988:122.
20. Committee of Inquiry into the Future Development of the Public Health Function. *Public Health in England.* London, Her Majesty's Stationery Office, Cm 289, 1988.
21. Ibid, p. 1.
22. Ibid, p. 64.
23. Ibid, p. 1.
24. Ibid, p. 6.
25. Chen CC (in collaboration with Bunge FM). *Medicine in Rural China: A Personal Account.* Berkeley: University of California Press, 1989.
26. Ibid, p. 39.
27. Ibid, p. 127.
28. Ibid, pp. 155-156.
29. Ibid, p. 143.
30. Ibid, pp. 172-173.
31. Ibid, p. 173.
32. World Health Organization, Regional Office for the Eastern Mediterranean. *Eleventh Interregional Meeting of Directors and Representatives of Schools and Departments of Public Health, May 1988.* WHO-EM/HMD/502-E, (Mimeographed). Alexandria, WHO, Regional Office for the Eastern Mediterranean, 1988:11.
33. Evans JR. *Measurement and Management in Medicine and Health Services: Training Needs and Opportunities.* New York: Rockefeller Foundation, 1981:18.
34. Knowles JH. *Doing Better but Feeling Worse: Health in the United States.* New York: Norton, 1977:3.
35. Welch WH, Rose W. *Institute of Hygiene. Annual Report, 1916, App. V.* New York: Rockefeller Foundation, 1916:415-427.
36. White KL. Data supplied by the Commonwealth Department of Health and the State Departments of Health in connection with *Australia's Bicentennial Health Initiative: Independent Review of Research and Educational Requirements for Public Health and Tropical Health in Australia.* Canberra, Minister of Health, 1986.
37. Madden S, McClendon BJ. *State Health Agency Staff, 1979-1985.* Washington, DC: U.S. Department of Health and Human Services, Health Resources and Services Administration, Bureau of Health Professions, 1988.
38. Evans JR. *Measurement and Management in Medicine and Health Services: Training Needs and Opportunities.* New York: Rockefeller Foundation, 1981:49.
39. Association of Schools of Public Health. *Reach.* Washington, DC: Association of Schools of Public Health, 1988 (brochure).

40. Council on Education for Public Health. *Accreditation Criteria for Graduate Schools of Public Health.* Washington, DC: Council on Education for Public Health, 1988:2.
41. Matthews MR. *Accreditation as One Force in Professionalization: The Accreditation of Schools of Public Health by the American Public Health Association.* Ph.D. Dissertation. Chapel Hill, N.C: University of North Carolina, 1973:186-187.
42. Ibid, p. 187.
43. Ibid, pp. 199-200.
44. Ibid, p. 201.
45. Institute of Medicine. *The Future of Public Health.* Washington, DC: National Academy Press, 1988:40-41.
46. Committee of Inquiry into the Future Development of the Public Health Function. *Public Health in England.* London: Her Majesty's Stationery Office, Cm 289, 1988:57.
47. Ibid.
48. Bowers JZ, Purcell EF. *Schools of Public Health: Present and Future.* 1974:175.
49. Sheps CG, Chairman. *The Milbank Memorial Fund Commission on Higher Education for Public Health.* New York: Prodist, 1976:60.
50. Ibid, pp. 61-62.
51. Institute of Medicine. *The Future of Public Health.* Washington, DC: National Academy Press, 1988:41.
52. Ibid, pp. iii-iv.
53. Committee of Inquiry into the Future Development of the Public Health Function in England. *Public Health in England.* London: Her Majesty's Stationery Office, Cm 289, 1988:35-38.
54. Scottish Home and Health Department. *Community Medicine in Scotland.* Edinburgh: Her Majesty's Stationery Office, 1973.
55. Sheps CG, Chairman. *The Milbank Memorial Fund Commission on Higher Education for Public Health.* New York: Prodist, 1976:44.
56. White KL. Opportunities and needs for epidemiology and health statistics in the United States. In: White KL, Henderson MM eds. *Epidemiology as a Fundamental Science.* New York: Oxford University Press, 1976:75.
57. Williams SJ, Tyler CW, Clark L, Coleman L, Curran P. Epidemiologists in the United States: an assessment of the current supply and the anticipated need. Am J Prev Med 1988:4:231-238.
58. Ibid, p. 235.
59. International Epidemiological Association. *Membership Newsletter.* Helsinki, IEA: March 1990.
60. Bridgers WF. *Declining Faculty Strength in Academic Public Health.* Washington, DC: The Association of Schools of Public Health, February 2, 1989 (unpublished).
61. U.S. Department of Health and Human Services. *Sixth Report to the President & Congress on the Status of Health Personnel in the United States.* DHSS Publication No. HRS-P-OD-88-1. Washington, DC: U.S. 1988.
62. Magee JH. *Employment Patterns for 1986 Graduates of U.S. Schools of Public Health.* (Mimeographed). Washington, DC: Association of Schools of Public Health, 1987:19.
63. Sheps CG, Ibrahim MI, Leonard AH. *A Survey of the Teaching of Epidemiology to Students in North America.* Chapel Hill, NC: University of North Carolina, 1984 (unpublished).

64. Pemberton J. *Upgrading in Epidemiology: Report to the COMAC EPID, Director-ate-General for Science, Research and Development.* (Mimeographed). Brussels: Commission of the European Communities, 1985.
65. McKeown T. *The Role of Medicine: Dream, Mirage or Nemesis.* London: Nuffield Provincial Hospitals Trust, 1976.
66. Black DAK, Morris JN, Smith C, Townsend, P. *The Black Report.* London: Penguin, 1982.
67. Sagan LA. *The Health of Nations: True Causes of Sickness and Well-Being.* New York: Basic Books, 1987.
68. Vickers G. What sets the goals of public health? Lancet 1958:i:599-604.
69. Ibid, p. 599.
70. Ibid, p. 600.
71. Flexner A. *Medical Education in the United States and Canada. A Report to the Carnegie Foundation for the Advancement of Teaching.* Bull 4. New York: Carnegie Foundation for the Advancement of Teaching, 1910:26.

2
Redefining the Unacceptable

Measurement may not be the most important means of acquiring knowledge and wisdom, but it is essential for many forms of relatively objective comparison required to enhance understanding. Comparison, after all, provides the usual basis for "redefining the unacceptable." We conclude that some state of affairs is unacceptable when contrasted with what went before, what might be, or with conditions elsewhere. These conclusions motivate politicians, the public, and the medical profession to change priorities and practices. Sooner or later, recognition of unacceptable states drives most measures to improve the public's health.

Accordingly, this chapter traces the contributions of physicians and others to three central ideas responsible for developing the scientific means for identifying and controlling threats to the public's health. Appreciating the genesis of these ideas, especially the contributions of clinicians, provides the rationale for understanding the importance of contemporary opportunities for epidemiological concepts and methods to restore the common mission of medicine and public health.

Comparisons originally were based on gross observations; underlying limitations, influences, and biases of the observer often were ignored. But as differences become less and resources become scarcer, the choices become more difficult. At such times the questions asked are about the nature and extent of differences between one state and another. What is different and how different is it? What is the rate of change? And how do we know? Certainly, as Poincaré the mathematician observed, a difference that makes no difference is no difference at all![1]

At some point, precise knowledge in relation to the scope of a problem can best be obtained by measurement. That measurement may vary in its precision depending on the phenomenon being compared but it usually involves "the assignment of numerals to objects or events according to rules."[2] In most circumstances the process of measurement strives to provide a level of objectivity with which all can agree. We do not weigh cotton wool and battleships on the same scale; we do not equate a famine in the Sahel with bouts of "tennis elbow" in a suburb of Sydney.

The history of numeracy as applied to studies of man probably starts with the earliest censuses. Recruiting armies and levying taxes required estimates of the population and of other resources. The first censuses seem to have been taken in China during the Chou dynasty that ended in the third century B.C. The Jews,

Egyptians, Greeks, Romans, and Incas all undertook counts of their populations with varying degrees of thoroughness. The Doomsday Book enumerated the population of England in 1086, and a later census of sorts took place in 1374. Holland undertook a census in 1417, and the City of Nuremberg in 1449. The first census in what was to become the United States was taken in Virginia during 1614-1625.[3]

Counting the living was the first step. The next was to find out whether and by how much the population was changing. Marcus Aurelius (121-180 A.D.) introduced compulsory registration of births, but it was only in 1501 that the City of Augsburg, and later all other German cities, made the registration of baptisms (not births), marriages, and deaths compulsory. London introduced the same requirements in 1517, and from 1532 there was compiled a *Weekly Bills of Mortality*. The registration of vital events was decreed in France in 1539 and in Virginia a century later.[4]

The seventeenth century saw the dawn of the Enlightenment. Intellectual and scientific developments focused on ascertaining the size and weight of objects, on chemical analysis, and on mathematical calculation. The search began for fundamental and universal laws that governed the physical and natural worlds. A more rational approach to religious, social, economic, and political problems gradually emerged. It was the century of Galileo (1564-1642), the mathematician, who challenged ecclesiastical authority with a new dynamic view of the universe and living beings. For better or worse, his assertion that "the Book of Nature is written in mathematical characters" may have been one of the stimuli impelling scientific endeavors toward an ever more reductionist view of the human condition.

René Descartes (1596-1650), mathematician and philosopher, helped to overthrow scholasticism and advance science by asserting that there was a vast world, apart from human beings, that was amenable to observation, experimentation, and measurement. Although many of his ideas promoted enquiry at the time, their influence on medicine, on balance, has been negative. They artificially separated mind and body and fostered a dualism persisting to the present. His outmoded seventeenth century paradigm has severely constricted the application of medical and related knowledge for both individual and collective benefits (see Chapter 6).[5] Isaac Newton (1642-1727), the founder of prequantum physics, contributed substantially to the fields of optics, mechanics, astronomy, and mathematics. Francis Bacon (1561-1626), philosopher, essayist, and statesman, the most influential man of his day, published his *Advancement of Learning* in 1605 and fostered inductive reasoning as a major method for understanding man and nature. Unfortunately, in contrast to his theoretical insights, many of Bacon's first principles have not stood the test of time.

The work of these and other scholars contributed to the flowering of a powerful new intellectual and scientific climate, but their direct impact on medicine was limited. The hallmarks of the era were dramatic challenges to the received wisdom of the day, the introduction of new instruments for observing man and nature, and, above all, the use of mathematics to further comparisons and promote understanding.

Physicians played only limited roles in making these fundamental theoretical and methodological advances, but some did make important subsidiary contributions to understanding human physiology. Among them we recognize Sanctorius (1561-1636) of Padua, who invented, as well as other instruments, the thermometer, and Thomas Willis (1621-1675), Professor of Natural Philosophy at Oxford, who described the brain and its blood supply. Above all, there was William Harvey (1578-1657), Lumleian Lecturer on Anatomy and Surgery, who published in 1628 his revolutionary volume *On the Motion of the Heart and Blood in Animals.* By no means last was the greatest clinician of his century, Thomas Sydenham (1624-1689). He shook medicine free from the bonds of medieval scholasticism and might be considered the founder of modern clinical medicine. His was one of the earliest applications of epidemiological concepts to understanding clinical problems. Excelling in observation and meticulous descriptions of clinical entities, he pursued what he called "the natural history of disease." Although he argued in favor of unverified theories of disease, he was, above all, prepared to change his mind on the basis of evidence. Eschewing all but the simplest remedies, he favored those that had withstood the test of time and sought evidence of their relative efficacy. He decried idle speculation and emphasized the central importance of studying illness at the bedside.

From the intellectual and scientific ferment wrought by these and other eminent scholars of the day evolved the Royal Society (of London for the Improvement of Natural Knowledge). Started in 1645 as an informal group, soon to be known as the "Invisible College," it included several of the leading physicians of the day. A Royal Charter was received in 1645 and with the publication of the *Royal Society's Philosophical Transactions* 2 years later, this body was recognized as the center of European scientific knowledge; it was the cradle of modern science.[6,7]

Measurement and numeracy, together with instrumentation—technology, if you will—characterized advances made in the name of science and scholarship during this remarkable period. Many of the theories of the day have been superseded but, as a consequence of ideas and methods developed in the seventeenth century, observations and descriptions—the so-called facts—have come under ever more critical review to support or refute theories.

This brief historical review provides some insight into the intellectual and scientific climate within which matters bearing more directly on the public's health arose. The introduction of numerical methods into the study of health problems bolstered, if it did not initiate the capacity for redefining the unacceptable and prompted important advances during the following two centuries.[8]

John Graunt (1620-1674), as an apprentice to his tradesman father, studied Latin and French and became initially a "haberdasher of small wares" and later a textile merchant of some prominence in London. In addition he rose to the rank of major in the army, became a city councilman, a music teacher, and later Fellow of the Royal Society. Clearly a person of boundless energy and great learning, Graunt was typical of the commercial men of the day who mixed freely with statesmen, artists, and scientists. From his modest origins in Hampshire, Graunt, by the age of 31, had become a person of considerable importance in London. His claim to being the father of health statistics, however, arises from publication in 1662 of the remarkable treatise: *Natural and Political Observations Mentioned in a Following Index and Made Upon the Bills of Mortality.*

No longer did Graunt regard simple counts of the dead as adequate. Using empirical observations, astute assumptions, and mathematical calculations in analyzing the *Bills of Mortality*, he recognized sources of bias and questioned the validity of most of the labels attached to causes of death. As a cautious statistician he did not take mathematical manipulation to be a substitute for seeking credible data. But neither was he a pedant. As Major Greenwood puts it in a famous aphorism: "Making the best the enemy of the good is a sure way to hinder any statistical progress. The scientific purist who will wait for medical statistics until they are nosologically exact, is no wiser than Horace's rustic waiting for the river to flow away."[9]

From his analyses, Graunt demonstrated four important laws of large numbers. First, he recorded the regularity with which vital phenomena occur in populations in contrast to their apparent chance occurrences in individuals (at least according to our present level of understanding). Second, he was the first to remark on the excess of male births over female. Third, he showed the relatively high rate of mortality in early life, and fourth, he found the urban death rate to be higher than that in rural areas. He also produced a rudimentary life table and as such foreshadowed the development of actuarial science.

Graunt did not use the term statistics itself. The antecedent of that word, "statistik," was first applied in describing matters of statecraft by one of Graunt's contemporaries, Hermann Conring (1606-1681), a German physician who was also a professor of political theory. A century later Gottfried Achenwall (1719-1772) adopted this term for his work on constitutional history and elements of political economy; he did not recognize or use its numerical connotation. As such he is often regarded as the father of the term statistics in contrast to the quantitative concept that came to be more widely applied. Graunt, nevertheless, should be credited with pioneering the concept of "statistics" and the application of numerical methods to analyzing matters of state generally and health specifically.[10,11]

Graunt's close friend and physician colleague, William Petty (1623-1687), was at one time thought to have made substantial contributions to the *Bills of Mortality* volume. Neither Karl Pearson (1857-1936), Professor of Mathematical Statistics and Eugenics in the University of London, nor Greenwood believed this to be the case, although Graunt and Petty were close and undoubtedly exchanged ideas.[12,13] What Petty did contribute above all was an idea that enjoyed wide currency for more than a century: *Political Arithmetic.* More important than the term itself was his contribution to its intellectual substance, the first of the three central concepts used in "redefinings of the unacceptable."

Petty, like Graunt, was born in Hampshire, the son of a modest "clothier and dyer." He led a nomadic and impoverished early career in England, France, and Holland. Unusually bright, he supported himself as a minor trader, while rapidly acquiring a knowledge of Latin, Greek, mathematics, and, during a spell at sea, of navigation. At Caen, Utrecht, Leyden, Amsterdam, and later Paris, he studied medicine and obtained a Doctor of Physic degree at Oxford. After junior positions he was appointed Professor of Anatomy there at the age of 28. Many of his wide-ranging extracurricular activities were designed to enhance his straitened financial circumstances, a feat accomplished most successfully. He established a College for Tradesmen, served as Professor of Music at Gresham College and as Physician General to the Army, developed a pharmacopoeia, invented a copying machine, and spent 7 years in Ireland as a land surveyor. Petty was a friend of Milton and Sydenham, a founder of the Royal Society, and an adviser to Oliver Cromwell; he was knighted by Charles II.

In addition to his worldly accomplishments, Petty, at age 24, wrote a book on the *History of Trades*. In 1662 (at age 44), the same year Graunt published his volume on the *Bills of Mortality*, Petty published *A Treatise of Taxes and Contributions*. Both of Petty's books helped to establish his additional fame as one of the founders of economics. In his own *Observations upon the Dublin Bills of Mortality* (1681), Petty began by saying of Graunt's pioneering work, that "the observations upon the *London Bills of Mortality* have been a New light to the World." Later (1686) came Petty's *Essay Concerning the Multiplication of Mankind*, and published posthumously in 1692, *The Political Anatomy of Ireland* and its appendix *Verbum Sapienti*. In the latter volume Petty acknowledges his debt to Bacon and summarizes his own approach to elaborating what he called political arithmetic:

> Sir Francis Bacon, in his *Advancement of Learning*, hath made a judicious parallel in many particulars, between the body natural, and body politic, and between the arts of preserving both in health and strength: and it is as reasonable, that as anatomy is the best foundation of one, so also of the other; and that to practice upon the politick, without knowing the symmetry, fabrick, and proportion of it, is as casual as the practice of old-women and empyricks. Now, because anatomy is not only necessary in physicians, but laudable in every philosophical person whatsoever; I therefore have attempted the first essay of political anatomy.[14]

His posthumous work (1689), *Political Arithmetick*, is Petty's best known. Among the many contributions he made, one of great importance for our present deliberations is his recommendation that a central statistical office be created (and this some 150 years before the General Register Office was established in Britain). He saw the need to integrate not only vital records but also information about disease, occupation, education, income, housing, property ownership, manufacturing, trade, and other topics. Recognizing the breadth of factors impinging on societal well-being and their interrelatedness, Petty called for coordination of political, economic, social, and health surveys to inform public choices and collective action. His view of the broad sweep of "political arithmetick," as well as the need for precision, is captured in the following statement:

> The method I take is not yet very usual; for instead of using only comparative and superlative words, and intellectual arguments, I have taken the course [as a specimen of the political arithmetick I have long aimed at] to express myself in terms of number, weight, or measure; to use only arguments of sense, and to consider only such causes, as have visible foundations in nature; leaving those that depend upon the mutable

minds, opinions, appetites, and passions of particular men, to the consideration of others.[15]

Petty's refinements to data acquisition methods were numerous. For example, in urging that age at death be recorded, he wanted to determine "how many year's value the life of any person of any age is equivalent [to]..."[16] and, hence like Graunt, anticipated the later development of life tables and actuarial science. He used both Graunt's and his own methods to calculate from the available data the lifetime worth of an individual, the economic value of populations, and the losses sustained by "the Sword, Plague, Famine, Hardship and Banishment," thus advancing methods for redefining the unacceptable.

Perhaps of equal interest to epidemiologists, clinicians, and those concerned with the adequacy of health services was Petty's skepticism about the benefits of medicine. He challenged his colleagues in the Royal College of Physicians by asking:

> Whether they [*viz*. Fellows and Licentiates of the College of Physicians] take as much medicine and remedies as the like number of any other society.
> Whether of 1000 patients to the best physicians, aged of any decade, there do not die as many as out of the inhabitants of places where there dwell no physicians.
> Whether of 100 sick of acute diseases who use physicians, as many die and in misery, as where no art is used, or only chance.[17]

This early foray into "evaluative research," "quality assurance," "cost-benefit analysis," and other precursors of what is now called "cost containment" was not all. Petty also questioned the adequacy of the hospitals of the day, albeit with data and methods that left not a little to be desired by present-day standards. He wrote:

> That at London the Hospitals are better and more desirable than those of Paris, for that in the best at Paris there die 2 out of 15, whereas at London there die out of the worst scarce 2 out of 16, and yet but a fiftieth part of the whole die out of the Hospitals at London, and 2/5 or 20 times that proportion die out of the Paris Hospitals which are of the same kind; that is to say, the number of those at London who chuse [*sic*] to lie sick in Hospitals rather than in their own Houses, are to the like People of Paris as one to twenty; which shows the greater Poverty or want of Means in the People of Paris than those of London. We infer from the premisses, *viz*. the dying scarce 2 out of 16 out of the London Hospitals, and about 2 of 15 in the best of Paris (to say nothing of *l'hostel Dieu*) that either the Physicians and Chirugeons of London are better than those of Paris, or that the Air of London is more wholesome.[18]

From Petty's time on, the face of clinical medicine and public health was changed as, indeed, was the basis for making political choices bearing on health. Through his introduction of *political arithmetic,* and his advocacy of what he once called *political medicine*, Petty introduced quantification to link what later became three related branches of learning: economics, epidemiology, and political science. On his death, his friend Samuel Pepys found him "the most rational man that ever he heard speak with a tongue." Although Major Greenwood regarded Petty's work as flawed in many ways, he still had enormous admiration for his contributions. He wrote that "anybody who has felt the exhilaration...in the doing of sums concerning biological problems, feels his heart [was] warmed by the arithmetical knight errant who had so many statistical adventures."[19]

In Europe the need for adequate health statistics was given intellectual support from the great German mathematician, philosopher, and logician Gottfried Wilhelm von Leibniz (1646-1716). He published papers in the 1680s arguing that to cope with the population's health problems required not only the collection of appropriate statistics on its structure and on vital events but their critical analysis. Emphasizing the importance of birth and death registration, von Liebnitz urged that the latter include a record not only of the age and cause of death but also of the circumstances surrounding the fatal illness—a fundamental piece of information still missing from death certificates worldwide! In addition he seems to have been another early advocate for establishment of Health Councils to deal with these and related problems.[20]

Three other major streams of intellectual thought are associated with the original ideas advanced by Petty and Graunt. The first derived from primitive notions of actuarial science and the earliest life tables they conceived but that were developed more fully by Edmund Halley (1656-1742) the astronomer, another member of the Royal Society. Halley used registration data collected by Caspar Neumann (1648-1715), philosopher and theologian, and pastor of Breslau (now Wroclaw). Equally important, he used a second mainstream of intellectual thought—the theory of probability, first advanced by the French mathematician, Antoine-Nicholas Caritat de Condorcet (1743-1794). The third major stream focused on the collection and interpretation of observations from mass surveys, as well as those from registration and administrative sources. At first the methods for the latter were primitive, but from these early origins household- and population-based surveys have gradually become more sophisticated; they are now recognized as essential epidemiological and statistical instruments. Emergence of these ideas was a central prerequisite for applying Petty's and Graunt's concepts of political arithmetic more broadly. Their convergence marks the beginnings of a recognizable theoretical base for epidemiology and statistics, although it was not so identified at the time.

There were glimpses of statistical insight elsewhere. William (the elder) Heberden (1710-1801), a leading London clinician of his day, physician to King George III and to Samuel Johnson, is not usually thought of as an epidemiologist or medical statistician. In addition to his classical volume entitled *Commentaries* that provides precise descriptions of many clinical syndromes, he had an interest in the *Bills of Mortality*. His criticisms of them concerned both the accuracy of the numbers and the validity of the labels or "diagnoses." He went so far as to finance the publication of a volume containing the original data and various interpretative essays, including a preface in which he displayed his epidemiological insights and quantitative skills:

> The deaths imputed to the measles are very remarkably different in different years; and yet it is possible that this disease is not in reality so very irregularly epidemical or fatal, as by the bills it appears to be. The scarlet fever and malignant sore throat often occasion such appearances upon the skin, as may easily be mistaken for the measles by better judges than the mothers and nurses, who thinking themselves able to distinguish this distemper, and equal to the management of it, often call in no other

assistance. This mistake is well known to have been sometimes made within these few years, during which the scarlet fever and malignant sore throat have been so common. It may perhaps have happened in every year, in which an extraordinary number of deaths are charged to the measles: and consequently those two formidable distempers, (if they are two distinct distempers, and not one and the same) being disguised under the name of the measles, may have been older, and more general than is usually imagined.[21]

Thomas Short (1690-1772), a country practitioner, was more energetic than accurate in his pursuit of a better understanding of the impact of environmental factors on health and longevity. Two principal works suggest the breadth of his interests: *A General Chronological History of Air, Weather, Seasons, Meteors, etc*, published in 1749, and *New Observations, Natural, Moral, Civil, Political and Medical on City, Town and Country Bills of Mortality*, published a year later. Greenwood sums up Short's contributions by commenting that "...he did paint a vivid picture of the changing conditions of life as he saw it...Had [his works] been studied with more attention, had he been a leading London physician, instead of an obscure country practitioner, medical statistics would have progressed faster."[22] This must surely be one of the earliest examples of the need to couple the zeal of the social and environmental reformer, whether layperson or physician, with the quantitative measures of the epidemiologist and health statistician to influence political decisions aimed at redefining the unacceptable.

During this period both the theory and practice of statistics were evolving also in Europe. In 1798 a Scot, Sir John Sinclair (1754-1835), an agricultural economist and self-proclaimed "statistician," encountered the word "statistics" in Germany. He was apparently unaware of the political and governmental concepts with which the term, as noted earlier, was then associated after its introduction by Achenwall. Before that, however, in 1791, Sinclair had created a system of statistical accounts in Scotland based on organized inquiries made to each of the country's 850 parish clergy. Unwittingly, Sinclair seems to have further developed the concept and applied the term to it. He is thus credited with tying the concepts, methods, and term together in the usage we now recognize as statistics.[23]

So innovative was Sinclair's approach that word of his accomplishments spread to America. George Washington in a letter dated March 15, 1793 wrote him that:

> I cannot but express myself highly pleased with the undertaking in which you are engaged, and give my best wishes for its success. I am full persuaded, that when enlightened men will take the trouble to examine so minutely into the state of society, as your inquiries seem to go, it must result in greatly ameliorating the condition of the people, promoting the interests of civil society, and the happiness of mankind at large. These are objects truly worthy the attention of a great mind and every friend to the human race must readily lend his aid towards their accomplishment.[24]

The derivation of the word statistics itself from the German *Staat* emphasized the importance of data bearing on affairs of state. Information on such matters as population, natural resources, manufacturing, trade, education, military resources, and climate required for better governance was seen as the proper domain of statistics. Issues bearing on poverty, health, and the environment were of limited concern. Moreover, the task was seen primarily as one of aggregation and tabulation; mathematical maneuvers were employed to a very limited extent.[25]

In eighteenth-century France and Belgium, mathematicians were developing increasingly sophisticated methods of statistical analysis. Pierre-Simon Laplace (1749-1827), the French astronomer and mathematical genius, probably was influenced by Isaac Newton's (1642-1727) *Principia* and the earlier work of brilliant French mathematicians such as Condorcet and Joseph Louis Lagrange (1736-1813). Following several pioneering works on astronomy, Laplace elaborated the theory of probability in two classics: *Théorie Analytique de Probabilités* (1812) and *Essai Philosophique sur la Probabilité* (1814).

Most of Laplace's examples analyzed the distributions for large numbers of observations on a wide variety of natural phenomena such as droughts, floods, eclipses, population shifts, and a famous discourse on the probability of the sun rising tomorrow morning. He did, however, apply mortality tables to assess the effectiveness of inoculation and vaccination that he endorsed enthusiastically. He referred to several other medical applications of particular interest in the present context. The concepts of efficacy, case-control studies, and even randomization are presaged in the following observation:

> Thus, to recognize the best of the treatments for the cure of a malady, it suffices to prove each of them on the same number of sick individuals, all other circumstances being made alike; the superiority of the most advantageous treatment will manifest itself more and more as the number to whom it is applied increases, and the calculus will make known the probability corresponding to its advantage, and the ratio according to which it is superior to others.[26]

In a later section of the *Essai* Laplace discusses a statistical approach to estimating the veracity of the testimony from witnesses. He apparently failed, however, to make the connection between this application and the phenomena of observer error and observer variation—that was to come much later in the evolution of quantitative methods for analyzing medical matters. Nor does Laplace deal with such matters as poverty, malnutrition, ignorance, filth, and their bearing on the population's health. Karl Pearson provides an interesting explanation of the hesitancy, at least in France, to link statistical theory with social and political reality, as Petty had urged:

> [Laplace] was restrained [in his discussions of probability from 1783 to 1795] largely by the state of affairs in France. Probability has very mundane interests, and its results too often touch social and political institutions. Condorcet, the enemy of the Jacobins, had been driven to death in 1794, the year before Laplace lectured on probability. It was an unsafe topic, and all the men of science were under suspicion, especially those that dwelt on probability....It was far safer to deal with the Heavens, than with the more mundane scope of probability.[27]

At about the same time Carl Friedrich Gauss (1777-1855), another extraordinary mathematician and astronomer of the German school, also advanced the mathematical basis for probability theory; although he had little interest in matters political or medical, his ideas had profound implications for the future of both epidemiology and health statistics. Another prominent French contributor to statistical theory was the mathematician and physicist Siméon Denis Poisson (1781-1840) in his *Recherches sur la Probablités des Jugements* (1837). The statistical distribution named after him has wide applications to medical and population health phenomena, but it was his student, the physician Jules Gavarret (1809-1890), who made the medical community aware of its utility in his *Principes Généraux de Statistique Médicale, ou Dévelopment de Régles qui Doivent Présider à Son Emploi* (1840).

Lambert Adolph Jacques Quetelet (1796-1874), Belgian astronomer, mathematician, and social scientist, is another founding father of vital statistics. He contributed substantially to statistical theory by demonstrating the consistent distributions of natural, biological, and social phenomena in large populations. Through use of statistical variation as a basis for comparing populations, Quetelet provided a richer theoretical underpinning than had been available previously. He profoundly influenced both William Farr (1807-1883) and Florence Nightingale (1823-1910) and had long-standing friendships with both. During his attendance at the meeting of the British Association for the Advancement of Science in 1833, Quetelet encouraged his colleagues to found the Statistical Society of London. In other testimony given to a Select Parliamentary Committee on Parochial Registration he emphasized Europe's superiority compared to England's in the acquisition and use of vital statistics.[28]

The internalization of statistical concepts was signaled by formal substitution in the medical literature of the term medical statistics for political arithmetic. A German physician, Johann Ludwig Caspar (1796-1864), Professor of Public Medicine, expounded on the application of statistics to medicine in two volumes published between 1825 and 1835, and F. Bisset Hawkins (1796-1894), another physician, published in 1829 the first text on this new subject entitled *Elements of Medical (or Vital) Statistics*. Bisset defined the field as "the application of numbers to illustrate the natural history of man in health and disease." Perhaps an even greater contribution by Hawkins, however, was to have inserted into the first Registration Act of 1837 a requirement that the cause of death be recorded. On balance, however, Greenwood regards Hawkins as uncritical. "He had been diligent and brought together numerical data from all parts of the world and was certainly one of the first physicians to advocate a serious study of hospital records, but one can hardly say that, as a statistician, he was better equipped or more efficient than Dr. Short in 1750."[29]

Raymond Pearl (1879-1940), first Professor of Biology and Medical Statistics at The Johns Hopkins School of Hygiene and Public Health, considered the physician William Farr (1807-1883), as have many others, to be "the greatest *medical* statistician who ever lived."[30] It was Farr who established political arithmetic as an essential discipline for redefining the unacceptable in matters pertaining to health and disease. Building on Graunt's and Petty's original ideas, Farr can be credited with institutionalizing epidemiology.[31,32]

The General Register Office had been established by an Act of Parliament in 1837. Farr was first employed by Sir James Clark, a prominent clinician, to help in the preparation of a volume on *Consumption*. On the latter's recommendation and that of Sir Edwin Chadwick (1800-1890), the sanitary reformer discussed next, Farr was appointed to the new position of Compiler of Statistical Abstracts, or Chief Statistician, at the General Registry Office.[33,34]

Through the application of quantitative methods, Farr contributed dramatically to the evolution of concerns for the public's health. What distinguished Farr's approach was the increasingly precise quantification of the unacceptable. No longer was it sufficient to proclaim some state of affairs as intolerable. The questions now were refined to: "How intolerable?" and "Compared to what?"

The child of impoverished parents, Farr was adopted by an affluent neighbor who, in spite of his own indifferent early schooling, seems to have stimulated in the youngster a latent curiosity. Subsequently he was apprenticed to a neighborhood apothecary and became sufficiently intrigued by medicine that he sought further training in Paris and later in Switzerland. During 2 years in Paris he developed an interest in the then unpopular subjects of hygiene and medical statistics. From Gabriel Andral (1797-1876) he learned to question scholastic eccentricity in general and bloodletting in particular. He was exposed to Andral's precise, methodical methods, especially in the examination of blood and documentation of the natural history of disease. From Pierre-Charles-Alexandre Louis (1787-1872), to whom we return, he acquired his interest in *medical*, in contrast to *vital*, statistics. The principal message that Farr probably derived from Louis was an appreciation of the importance of descriptive and analytical studies, especially where experimentation is not possible.

On his return to England, Farr undertook hospital work as a locum tenens at which his performance was quite satisfactory. He lacked formal medical qualifications, however, and as a result failed to get a permanent appointment. Although probably a disappointment to Farr at the time, this episode deflected him from a rural practice to further study at University College and subsequent qualification as a Licentiate of the Apothecaries Hall.[35] After starting a none-too-successful medical practice in London, Farr turned to augmenting his income by teaching and writing articles on vital statistics for medical journals. He taught a subject labeled Hygiology—apparently a fancy word for what is now known as Public Health—but there were no takers. The subject was regarded as of slight importance by most of the medical leaders of the day, except Thomas Wakely, the founder and editor of the *Lancet*. Wakely recognized Farr's original talent and published a number of his early papers. These were followed by other articles on "vital and medical statistics." An unusually lucid, precisely written, and well-documented piece by this title published in 1837 in a volume entitled *An Account of the British Empire* seems to have established Farr as the leading authority on medical statistics, a field that had languished for several decades. That same year the registration of births, deaths, and marriages came into effect, and the newly appointed Registrar-General recognized the need for skilled scientific assistance in the compilation and analyses of the resultant statistics. This led to Farr's appointment there in 1839 and his 40-year career developing methods for studying the determinants and distribution of health and disease in populations.

Farr developed a system of vital statistics to inform more fully and accurately the tasks of political arithmetic, a system that would have delighted his predecessors John Graunt and William Petty as well as his mentors Andral and Louis. He created the system for England but it soon became the model adopted by the rest of the world.[36-38]

One example in particular is of direct concern in the context of this volume. As a clinician, albeit not for long since he forsook active practice on joining the General Register Office, Farr recognized both the fragility and critical importance of nosology and disease classification. Three articles published in 1837-1838 set forth his system of "nosometry" designed to facilitate the use of statistics for informing clinical judgment. In his first Annual Report he wrote that "nomenclature is of as much importance in this department of inquiry as weights and measures in physical sciences, and should be settled without delay." Out of the chaos of the times emerged what later became the International Classification of Diseases. Sir James Clarke, the eminent clinician who had recommended Farr for the job at the General Register Office, commenting on this aspect of his protegé's work wrote that its:

> ...indirect influence (an influence the source of which may not have been generally recognized) upon practical medicine must have been very great. The constant endeavour after exactness of diagnosis and precision of nomenclature is itself a wholesome discipline which reacts inevitably on treatment.[39]

Farr, a gentle, caring soul, was deeply concerned that his profession should respond to its full range of opportunities and challenges. He was not however above offering sharp and extensive criticisms that, a century and half later, have a contemporary ring:

> It has been shown that external agents have as great an influence on the frequency of sickness as on its fatality; the obvious corollary is, that man has as much power to prevent as to cure disease. That prevention is better than cure, is a proverb; that it is as easy, the facts we had advanced establish. Yet medical men, the guardians of public health, never have their attention called to the prevention of sickness; it forms no part of their education. To promote health is apparently contrary to their interests: the public do not seek the shield of medical art against disease, nor call the surgeon, till the arrows of death already rankle in the veins. **This may be corrected by modifying the present system of medical education, and the manner of remunerating medical men.**
>
> **Public health may be promoted by placing the medical institutions of the country on a liberal scientific basis; by medical societies co-operating to collect statistical observations; and by medical writers renouncing the notion that a science can be founded upon the limited experience of an individual** (emphasis added by KLW).[40]

Farr, a true genius, while working as a physician saw his pioneering work as part of medicine's collective task. Although he was never appointed Registrar General, he received many honors, including election to Fellowship in the Royal

Society. Perhaps none was more important than the Gold Medal awarded him in 1880 by the British Medical Association (BMA), in absentia because of poor health. The President of the BMA spoke of Farr's "labours which lie at the foundation of all researches in medical sciences." In receiving the award on behalf of Farr, Sir Henry Acland (1815-1900), another man of great learning, Fellow of the Royal Society and Regius Professor of Medicine at Oxford, said that the award "was the highest testimony which the profession could give of esteem and regard for the great services he had rendered to the profession and to the country; indeed, it must be said for services rendered to the world."[41]

If Farr was regarded as a preeminent figure within the English medical profession, he was held in even higher esteem in Europe and the United States. He is revered by medical statisticians, epidemiologists, and those concerned with the public's health throughout the world. Withal, Farr remains a physician, a venerated member of the profession who, self-taught for the most part, learned from his mathematical, statistical, and economist forebears. He revolutionized political arithmetic and transformed medical statistics by using census, registration, and administrative data, nosology, and probability theory to illuminate the problems of health and disease for populations and nations. He refined political arithmetic so that quantification supplanted the impressionistic and subjective approaches that were much in vogue for redefining the unacceptable.

The *sanitary idea* is the second central concept underlying efforts to modify conditions that influence the public's health. Debates about individual versus collective rights and the proper role of government had their origins with the ancients but they grew apace in the seventeenth and eighteenth centuries. Early in the eighteenth century, the Frenchman, Abbé Claude Fleury (1640-1723), a lawyer and ecclesiastical historian, argued with considerable specificity for expansion of government's role in human affairs. He provided great detail about the need for adequate provision of food, clothing, housing, and buildings, and the importance of an aesthetically pleasing appearance to the environment. In addition, he stressed that "care should be taken over cleanliness for health's sake; precaution against popular maladies; good air and good water supplies provided, all in abundance." Improving the lot of the entire population was the goal, not just clearing up the filth—almost the reverse of those then advocated.

Fleury believed that government should foster social cooperation for the common weal and, in the best tradition of the Greeks, help the population achieve its full potential. In this sense, redefining the unacceptable became a matter of reforming governments that were inept or worse and reordering society's collective priorities. Fleury may well have been the initiator of what came to be known as the social hygiene movement from whence evolved many philanthropic endeavors, food distribution arrangements, medical clinics for the poor, and eventually social insurance.[42] The medical profession tended to be observers and peripheral participants in these activities, not innovators or leaders.

In nineteenth century Europe, the poor were at first rejected as ignorant and slovenly and as a consequence prone to disease. The industrial revolution, however, brought urbanization, and home workplaces were replaced by factories. The health and hence the productivity of the labor force became an increasingly powerful economic and political concern to landlords, industrialists, and politicians. The need to increase the population, and with it consumption, trade, and military manpower, gradually came to dominate European political thought.

Progress in implementing these ideas was limited, however, by massive poverty, squalor, ignorance, and filth. Throughout the centuries the latter had been vaguely linked to disease but the notion of "miasma," that is, a local atmospheric state perhaps emanating from filth, as the cause of disease, was invoked widely in the eighteenth century. Initially this theory was used to explain the spread of malaria. Even Thomas Sydenham, critical clinician that he was, believed that effluvia from "certain hidden and inexplicable changes within the bowels of the earth" were associated with infections.[43] Sydenham also believed in the "epidemic constitution," a vestige of Hippocratic theories which held that variations in atmospheric and climatic conditions were important causes of many diseases or at least predisposed to them. A second contending theory of disease, "contagion," foreshadowed by Girolamo Fracastoro (1484-1553) a century earlier, held that diseases probably were spread from person to person by unseen "particles." These rival theories, miasma and contagion, contended for acceptance until they were supplanted by the "germ theory" in the latter part of the 19th century. At the other extreme was Rudolf Virchow (1821-1902), Germany's renowned pathologist and anthropologist, who later summed up succinctly the alternative approach in his famous aphorism: "Medicine is a social science and politics are nothing else than medicine on a large scale!"

The advocates of these diverse paradigms held strongly to their views, but both theories supported the practical utility of what came to be known as the sanitary idea. The notion that inadequate "sanitation" was a major contributor to the spread of disease, and to the increasingly virulent epidemics that beset Europe, gained ascendancy, in spite of the fact that there was no generally accepted theory of the mechanism by which diseases were spread or "caused." Useful action based on redefining the unacceptable, it was argued, did not have to await full understanding of the underlying disease processes.

Although the problems had been recognized for centuries, collective action to correct them was slow to emerge. Philosophers, lawyers, and political scientists increasingly became concerned in the eighteenth century about the responsibilities of monarchs and their bureaucratic minions for improving the populace's health and well-being. There was also a growing body of medical school teachers who were giving lectures on problems of the public's health.[44]

The first individual to set forth the full range of these problems and issues was the German physician Johann Peter Frank (1745-1821). His views were contained in a monumental medical compendium entitled *System einer Vollständigen Medizinischen Polizey* published over five decades. Frank is of special interest in connection with our present discussion since he was first and foremost a superb, indeed preeminent, clinician. Consulted by fellow practitioners and much sought after by the elite of Europe, he was the holder of professorial chairs in five universities, Dean of Medicine at Pavia, and one-time administrator of the great Wiener Allgemeines Krankenhaus. The breadth of his erudition and concerns makes him one of the principal figures who have argued forcefully for major economic, environmental, and social reforms to improve the health of populations.[45-47]

Frank's nine-volume treatise covered in enormous, one might say compulsive, detail the requirements for individual health from womb to tomb, as well as the legislative and regulatory requirements for the maintenance of a healthy community. Published during a period when mercantilism was in the ascendancy and absolute monarchs reigned, his prescription for what came to be called "police medicine" was received well in some quarters and not so well by those who sensed the early rumblings of the revolutions to come. The word police (*polizey,* in German) seems to have been confused with policy in the minds of many; a more complete term, *polizeiwessenschaft,* is best construed as the "science of management." This science was to instruct the citizens and their presumably enlightened rulers about the manner in which the state should be organized and administered to foster the welfare of all—not least that of the ruling elite. There is no denying Frank's authoritarian bent, as well as his authoritative (for those times) views. What he called for was much more vigorous control and supervision of the social and physical environment in which people lived, worked, became ill, and died.

To the title of Professor of Medicine he added, for several years starting in 1786, that of Director General of Public Health of Lombardy. He started with an extensive survey of his territory, calling on physicians, pharmacies, and hospitals, and talking to medical personnel at all levels. Visiting the population's homes and workplaces, he enquired about their health and living conditions. In an address entitled "The Peoples Misery: Mother of Disease," which Frank as Dean gave to the graduating class in medicine at the University of Pavia in 1790, he stated:

> Starvation and sickness are pictured in the face of the entire laboring class. You recognize it at first sight. And whoever has seen it will certainly not call any of these people a free man. The word has become meaningless. Before sunrise, after having eaten a little and always the same unfermented bread that appeases his hunger only half-way, the farmer gets ready for hard work. With emaciated body under the hot rays of the sun he plows a soil that is not his and cultivates a vine that for him alone has no reward. His arms fall down, his dry tongue sticks to his palate, hunger is consuming him. The poor man can look forward to only a few grains of rice and a few beans soaked in water. And to this he can add only very sparingly the condiments with which nature has provided mankind in such a liberal way.[48]

The medical historian Henry Sigerist, who had translated the address, read this passage to a seminar in the 1940s; his students thought Franklin D. Roosevelt had written it.

Frank followed up his first-hand enquiries by insisting that the causes of death, disease, and infertility be investigated through more extensive statistical (i.e., epidemiological) studies. He even saw the need for "small area" analyses, as suggested by the following example:

Philanthropic physicians should investigate the nature, situation and condition of the smallest village, its diseases and their causes, the ratio of the sexes, of the different classes of men, calculate the ratio of births and deaths, and thus produce a kind of geography of each district.[49]

Although not usually classified as an epidemiologist, Frank's concern with the use of evidence from population-based studies, added to his clinical observations, warrants that appellation. In addition to extensive instruction about personal hygiene, he placed great emphasis on improving sanitation, water supplies, sewerage systems, food supplies, and other sources of "contamination" associated with disease and death. The extent of his knowledge and the breadth of his interests were models for both his peers and his students. It is unfortunate, indeed, that his many contributions seem to have been overshadowed by critics who misconstrued his insistence on the promulgation of health "policies" as support for a narrowly defined and punitive "police" approach to their enforcement.

If Frank is a hero for the public health movement he must surely be embraced also as a hero for clinicians, epidemiologists, and health statisticians. He saw his individual patients as fellow citizens in the broader physical, social, and political environments that they shared. For him the clinician's responsibilities extended from the embryonic laboratories and the hospitals to the community and the population. "Was it not the physicians or their writings," he wrote, "which brought about the many excellent ordinances of enlightened governments that concerned public health and achieved such signal success?"[50]

Frank's students and adherents were many; numerous journals and textbooks by colleagues and students propagated his views. For example, one of the more widely used medical textbooks at the time encompassed "procreation, maternal and child welfare, recreation, occupation, accident prevention, control and prevention of epidemics, organization of the medical profession, provision of medical care, nursing the sick, and enlightenment of the public in health matters."[52]

Neighboring countries such as Denmark, Hungary, Russia, Switzerland, and especially Italy were also influenced by the thinking of Frank and his followers.[52] In Britain, his ideas were initially adopted at the University of Edinburgh where, separated from the social and absolutist philosophy of governments on the continent, lectures modeled after his *Medicinische Polizey* were presented to the medical students. At first the term medical police was used but it gradually gave way to public health and hygiene. This shift in terminology reflected fundamental changes in the concepts underlying the role of government in protecting and promoting individual and population health. A writer in 1842 complained that in England "people are apt to think...that medical police implies nothing more than the seizure of stinking fish or unsound meat; or at most a fear-spreading contrivance termed a Board of Health, and brought into action when cholera rages."[53]

Adoption of the sanitary idea in England had strong roots in the political and social philosophy that arose during the latter part of the seventeenth and early eighteenth centuries. Jeremy Bentham (1748-1832) and his Philosophical Radicals believed fervently that social problems could be solved by rational and scientific means. This hardy band of political philosophers cum social activists advocated a long list of reforms starting with parliamentary processes and proceeding through the law, education, trade, health, and extending to birth control.

One of their number, Edwin Chadwick (1800-1890), a lawyer and apostle of Bentham's, pushed to the forefront in matters of health. The mercantilists' concern for a healthy and productive labor force was hampered by ubiquitous poverty and the impotence of the justices of the peace to effect improvements in the lot of the poor. Since Elizabethan times the "locals" had run the social and support services at the parish level, a reasonably adequate arrangement for a predominantly rural society. Voluntary county hospitals started appearing in the late seventeenth and early eighteenth centuries. By the nineteenth century, however, these combined efforts were found wanting; new measures seemed essential, especially for the urban poor.

Although it was advocated as early as 1740, it was not until 1805 that a severe epidemic of yellow fever prompted the Privy Council to establish Britain's first Board of Health. Its tenure was short; when the epidemic waned a year later the Board was abolished. A quarter of a century later, a cholera plague resulted in the Board's reconstitution, but again for only a year. Both Boards included prominent physicians with the second one (a "Board of Physicians," the *Lancet* called it) meeting almost daily at the Royal College of Physicians. In 1832 the second Board was transformed briefly by the Privy Council into a full-time entity augmented by non-physician government officials. The creation of Boards of Health in all municipalities threatened by cholera was encouraged but there was no legislative mandate and no central financing. General practitioners perceived the "regula-tions" as threats and local politicians were reluctant to raise the necessary funds. It was unclear who was to be responsible for dealing with the poverty, social deprivation, and deplorable sanitary conditions that provided the nidus for the cholera plague.[54]

In 1832 Parliament established a Royal Commission to examine the workings of the Poor Laws. Chadwick, at first an Assistant to the Commission and later a Commissioner, played a major role in the Commission's Report and subsequent emergence of the Poor Law Amendment Act of 1834. Circumstances were right for the sweeping legislative changes in the nineteenth century that ushered in the sanitary revolution. The social and economic climate emphasized a free-market, laissez-faire system and some measure of governmental regulation, values that shaped the present-day public health movement in many Western industrialized countries.

Chadwick concluded from his work on the reform of the Poor Law that disease aggravated poverty and hence kept high the costs of supporting the poor. In turn he urged the adoption of measures to prevent disease, having concluded that it was the direct result of the physical and social environments in which people lived, an idea not far removed from views espoused by Petty and Frank. Chadwick even sought statistical confirmation of his observations, recommending the estab-lishment of a Bureau of Medical Statistics in the Poor Law Office. To control disease he seized on the idea of sanitation and the related problems of clean water and adequate sewerage.

Chadwick's next task was to complete one of public health's fundamental documents. In 1842, the *Report on an Inquiry into the Sanitary Condition of the Labouring Population of Great Britain* was published. Chadwick's unbending belief was that epidemic diseases were caused by "miasmas"; these, in turn, came from decayed waste of all types. In his opinion "the defects which are the most important and which come most immediately within practical legislation and administrative control, are those chiefly external to the dwellings of the population and principally arise from the neglect of drainage."[55] He turned the causes of contemporary disease into a set of engineering problems concerned with clean water, adequate drainage, garbage disposal, and effective sewerage, and a second set of architectural problems concerned with the design of better housing. Medical men might document the presence of disease, and statisticians might determine its extent, but engineers and architects were to fix the problems. Chadwick's low opinion of most of the medical profession was not helped by his aggressive, some have called it "demoniac," personality, nor by the crusading physicians with whom he associated. In Chadwick's view "the success of mere medicine" was much in question. The contributions to improvement of the public's health by the medical practitioner, trained in curative medicine, were modest indeed. Little could be expected from this source since in Chadwick's view disease was the product of injurious and unwholesome environments.[56,57]

Southwood Smith (1786-1861), a fellow Benthamite and Unitarian minister turned physician, was Chadwick's principal medical advisor. Although he wrote a well-received volume, *The Philosophy of Health*, with a physiological orientation towards personal hygiene, Smith was convinced that all disease stemmed from contagion and filth; he made few distinctions among diseases, especially those characterized by fever. Nor was he helped much by his fellow physicians who lined up, once again, in two camps, the "contagionists" and "miasmatists." Like Chadwick his metiér was reform, not science, and his arena was framed by social and political parameters that excluded biological and psychological influences. The environment was emphasized to the neglect of the host and agents.

Much good came of Chadwick's single-minded drive to reform the lot of the poor. In spite of being a vastly unpopular central figure among the humanists and social reformers, he successfully inveighed against political and economic corruption and incompetence. Chadwick's many contributions included fostering the legislation that created the General Board of Health in 1848. Without a doubt he placed "public health" on governmental agendas. But all this had many unanticipated negative consequences including, for what appears to be the first time, placing the medical profession in an adversarial position vis-a-vis the public's health—perhaps foreshadowing the schism yet to come.

Granted the profession in Great Britain may have been slow, even remiss, in not following the views espoused by Petty, Frank, and others, it is also true that physicians like Harvey, Edward Jenner (1749-1823), and Richard Bright (1789-1858) were starting to build the scientific infrastructure that was necessary, if not sufficient, for all future efforts to understand and control disease. The sanitary idea was completely compatible with the broader views of Petty and Frank emphasizing interactions between individuals and their living environments, as well as, in the case of Frank, their personal "lifestyles." Its aggressive pursuit, however, had important consequences for the relationships between public health and clinical medicine as well as for the capacity of each to move back and forth from the individual (micro) to the collective (macro) levels of research, education, and practice.

To his undying credit Chadwick recognized the importance of having full-time Medical Officers of Health. He saw to it that the positions, as well as the creation of local Boards of Health in "high-risk" municipalities, were mandated in the Public Health Act of 1948. Mere "training" was insufficient in Chadwick's view; the Medical Officer of Health "should have conducted some piece of successful research in the field of preventive medicine."[58] Unfortunately, the appointment of local Medical Officers proceeded sporadically. Two issues that heralded future problems, including the schism, characterized the debates surrounding individual appointments. The first had to do with the extent of the Health Officers' involvement in curative medicine. The Act stipulated that their "general duties...shall in no case comprehend treatment for the cure or alleviation of disease." At the same time, when it came to specific appointments, a significant impediment precluded the separation of curative medicine from public health work. Because only modest part-time stipends were offered, the abandonment of clinical practice for appointees was impractical. As a consequence the great majority of Medical Officers of Health were part-time practitioners.[59] Chadwick also argued strenuously that Boards of Health and their Medical Officers should submit, and publish, annual reports on the health status of their jurisdictions.

The Board of Health's militant crusade with Chadwick and Smith as members, supported by their fellow Benthamites, was brief; the General Board lasted only 7 years. It was widely condemned, and while local government was strengthened throughout Britain and much attention was paid to improvements in the water supply and sanitation, the formal advance of the "public health" cause was slowed. In 1854, Parliament, bowing to the opponents of the Board's inroads on vested interests and in the face of local apathy, did not renew the Act and Chadwick's official appointment was terminated. His fame rests less on his recognition of the importance of health statistics, or even the appointment of Medical Officers of Health, than on the clarity of his vision and his determination to fight vested interests—industrial, financial, bureaucratic, and medical—in the name of social justice and a better life for the oppressed.

Following the earlier appointment in Liverpool in 1847 of the first Medical Officer of Health, William Henry Duncan (1805-1863), John Simon (1816-1904), a surgeon at St. Thomas's Hospital, was appointed the first Medical Officer of Health to the City of London in 1848. Starting in 1855 the General Board of Health's tenure was renewed on an annual basis. Now under the aegis of the Privy Council, Simon served as its full-time salaried Medical Officer. His annual reports (1855-1871) documented the state of the nation's health and of particular diseases.

Above all he reaffirmed the importance of crowded housing, malnutrition, factory working conditions, and related unfavorable social conditions. With limited resources he made what progress seemed possible.

Simon's background, as well as his approach, is of special interest in connection with the present review. He made it a condition of his accepting the position of Medical Officer that he retain his clinical appointment at St. Thomas's. Throughout his career he maintained an interest in clinical medicine as well as public health. For example, he wrote a letter to the President of the Royal College of Surgeons on "Observations Regarding Medical Education." He traveled widely, was elected a Fellow of the Royal Society, and kept in close touch with the leaders of Britain's medical establishment. As a consequence he was able to involve many of that country's ablest clinicians in epidemiological research. Among these were William Augustus Guy (1810-1885), a pioneer in medical statistics and preventive medicine and one-time Dean of Medicine at King's College. Another was Edward Headlam Greenhow (1814-1888), a clinician, whose statistical and epidemiological prowess provided the basis for Simon's administrative reforms in public health. Greenhow, with an appointment at St. Thomas's arranged by Simon, became the first Lecturer in Public Health in Britain.

A third colleague was John Scott Burdon Sanderson (1828-1905), Oxford gold medalist, student of Claude Bernard (1813-1878), and faculty member at St. Mary's Hospital, whose appointment as Medical Officer of Health at Paddington brought him to Simon's attention. There followed a number of landmark epidemiological studies, especially of diphtheria and cholera. Sanderson too was elected Fellow of the Royal Society, appointed Regius Professor of Medicine at Oxford, and later Professor of Physiology at University College. There were many other colleagues and coworkers. Simon's reputation rests as much on his ability to integrate the population perspective with clinical medicine as it does on his accomplishments in improving the public's health.[60,61] A new Public Health Act was passed in 1875, placing health matters that impinged on the general population within the purview of local governments. The latter were given strong administrative bases and, henceforth, Medical Officers of Health were to be physicians.

The sanitary idea, with its broad view of the underlying problems that resulted in disease, gradually receded as a plausible all-purpose theory for improving the health status of the citizenry. In the face of growing evidence that many diseases were associated first with impure water and later with the spread of living organisms, more specific measures were needed. Sir John Simon, even before becoming Chief Medical Officer, had espoused this view.

The links between sanitation and microorganisms were strengthened by the observations of John Snow (1813-1858), clinician, anaesthetist, and "amateur" epidemiologist—also revered as one of the founders of modern epidemiology. Snow demonstrated the association between sewage-contaminated water supplies and outbreaks of cholera in 1854. His landmark studies of the circumstances surrounding the occurrence of this devastating disease introduced many of the central methods of modern field epidemiology. William Budd (1811-1880), a brilliant, well-educated country practitioner, was also a self-taught epidemiologist (there was then no other way). He independently advanced theories for the genesis of both cholera and typhoid that were similar to Snow's. In the case of typhoid he added the observation that disinfection of sewage and isolation of the sick were the most effective means of controlling its spread. Anticipating Robert Koch (1843-1910), Snow, as well as Budd and Farr, even predicted the existence of a specific microorganism.[62,63] When still a young country practitioner, in 1876 Koch identified the organism responsible for yet another major disease of the times, anthrax. He demonstrated the organism's specificity for that disease by means of exemplary experiments; later he did the same for tuberculosis and cholera. Koch's famous postulates of "proof," modified from those of his mentor Jacob Henle (1809-1895), became the gold standard for assessing scientific contributions to the understanding of contemporary notions about the "causes" of disease.

In 1820 an American physician, David Hosack (1769-1835), possibly taking his cue from Frank, had advanced his *Observations on the Means of Improving the Medical Police of the City of New York*. He urged modernization of the municipal water supply, improved housing for the poor, building a sewerage system, broadening the streets, prohibiting burials within the city, and the use of stone instead of wood in the construction of wharves and docks.[64] All were worthy objectives but also a far cry from Frank's views on the need to deal with the full panoply of factors influencing health and disease as well as a central part of clinical medicine's mission.

Word of the sanitary and Poor Law reforms under way in Britain traveled to the United States. If Chadwick became the hero of public health workers in Britain, Lemuel Shattuck (1793-1859), bookseller and publisher, has assumed a similar role in the United States. He brought yet another view of the human condition to his labors. Holding the strong moral conviction that inward virtue was linked to cleanliness and hence to health, Shattuck's reforming zeal was tempered by his awareness that changing the outward circumstances of their lives would enable the goodness within the poor to be revealed as improved health and well-being.

Shattuck developed an early interest in genealogy and vital events; from that experience he recognized the importance of recording, labeling, and classifying these events and illnesses accurately. His prowess in conducting detailed analyses of available vital and medical statistics brought wider recognition that quantitative approaches were essential for delineating the health status of populations and variations associated with social, economic, and environmental factors. He founded the American Statistical Association and corresponded with William Farr in Britain, later advocating adoption in the United States of the latter's system of nomenclature and disease classification. Shattuck's broad views on the origins of health and disease were reflected in his statement that it was inconsistent "with the present state of enlightened public opinion" not to collect statistics bearing on human life as it was influenced "by seasons, locality, disease and other circumstances that may exist."[65]

Shattuck's major contribution was his leadership in the conduct of the *Report of the Sanitary Commission of Massachusetts 1850*. With findings that paralleled many of those emerging in Britain and the Continent, the *Report* recommended the establishment of a decennial state census, a Board of Health to propose legislation for the prevention of disease, the promotion of health, the regulation of sanitary arrangements, and the promulgation of an annual report on the state's health status. Although Shattuck came to emphasize sanitation as a major responsibility of local government, and of greater importance than individual responsibility as he had argued in his earlier years, most of the Report's recommendations went unheeded for many decades. He receded into the background as a public figure and leader in public health reform. Shattuck, however, like Petty, Frank, and Simon, had recognized the broader context in which disease arose; others took up the cause.

Among the latter were leaders of the newly created American Medical Association (AMA), who, at its first meeting in Baltimore in 1848, established a Committee on Public Hygiene to report the following year on sanitary conditions in 10 major cities. Josiah Curtis (1816-1883), a Massachusetts physician, wrote the Committee's report which concluded that "certain causes were invariably in operation....[A]mong these [were] deficient drainage, street cleaning, supply of water and ventilation; together with improperly constructed houses and the various nuisances incident to populous places." In his view such matters ought to engage the medical profession actively. Individuals should be able to seek help with them from their physicians, and governments should heed the advice of the profession. By 1849 the AMA was on record as the caretaker of the people's overall health.[66]

In this early and high priority activity of "organized" American medicine we have a clear recognition that its mandate for improving the health of populations extended beyond the care of individual patients. Unfortunately this early organizational commitment was of relatively short duration. Faced with yellow fever and cholera epidemics, the option of quarantine (in contrast to sanitation) was seen as the best way to contain these scourges. Meetings during the 1850s that discussed the need for uniform quarantine laws were attended by delegates from the newly emerging Boards of Health, Boards of Trade, and the medical societies. The great majority of participants were physicians and "had it not been for the Civil War, [these meetings] might have led to a permanent public health organization."[67] In 1866 physicians played a major role in establishment of the Metropolitan Board of Health in New York City, bolstered by widespread support from a variety of citizens' groups.

Among these pioneering physicians was a surgeon, Stephen Smith (1823-1922), who in 1870 became the first president of the American Public Health Association (APHA), an organization that welcomed officials of health organizations and "citizens interested in sanitation." Indeed the principal objective of the APHA in 1872, as expressed in its Constitution, was "the advancement of sanitation science and the promotion of public hygiene." Many of the founders were again largely physicians, most of whom were members of their local medical societies and the AMA.[68]

One of the first initiatives of this new organization was to press for creation of a national health department. The United States Marine Hospital Service, however, saw its territory threatened, and when the state and local health officers fell back on the principle of states' rights to protect their interests, the move for the new department foundered. There were other contentious issues including the impact of national, state, and local quarantine laws on business and the ensuing lobbies to moderate their enforcement. A National Quarantine Board established in 1878 had its funds cut off in 1883. In spite of this there was active interest shown by many medical societies in supporting sanitary measures and quarantine regulations as well as creation of health departments at all levels of government. A major responsibility of the latter was conceived to be the maintenance of standards of practice through control of medical licensing. In their drive to raise professional standards, academic physicians were dominant in many of the medical societies advocating the creation of boards of health. Physicians who either were poorly trained or were "irregular" practitioners, and other healers of diverse types, were threatened by this incipient control and resisted strenuously.

In 1880 a major resolution to establish a National Board of Health put forward by the AMA's Section on State Medicine and Public Hygiene was vigorously attacked as a form of unnecessary centralized bureaucracy. From then on the medical societies seem to have engaged in a relentless retreat. Most of the early officers were characterized by humanitarian concerns, a broad view of the medical profession's responsibilities, and especially the new opportunities that laboratory medicine, as embodied in bacteriology, was opening up for the control of many diseases.[69]

There was more trouble ahead—financial trouble. The New York Academy of Medicine and academic physicians who recognized the need to provide free medical care for indigent groups in the larger cities urged establishment of hospital outpatient clinics and dispensaries. Again objections were raised, with the marginal practitioners, many barely making a living, leading the way. Other private practitioners were also threatened by health departments' calls for widespread immunization, and even by the control through sanitary measures of many diseases, that in turn might deprive these physicians of patients and their livelihoods. On top of this the provision of free bacteriological diagnostic tests to confirm diagnoses was claimed to be an unwarranted intrusion on private practice, particularly by those practitioners who had not yet accepted the "germ theory" of disease. Mandatory reporting of tuberculosis, and later of venereal diseases, further aggravated matters.

The AMA, however, continued to support public health measures well into the latter part of the nineteenth century. The institutionalization of the public health movement was supported also by those who saw themselves representing the underprivileged, disenfranchised, and neglected. As a consequence of such pressures, the AMA became an active proponent of Federal legislation to control the quality of foods and drugs, especially in view of the burgeoning market in proprietary medicines. The drug industry and members of the "unorganized" component of the medical profession opposed the legislation. Resistance to control was growing across the country, but a 1903 editorial in the *Journal of the American Medical Association* stated that a health department "should be a great aggressive organ of popular education regarding personal and public hygiene, and all that pertains to public health and physical well-being."[70]

Matters did not improve when one of public health's physician heroes, Hermann M. Biggs (1859-1923), first threw down the gauntlet to "organized" medicine. A clinician at heart, Biggs was creator of the New York City Health Department's enduring motto: "Human Lives Are Purchasable." He also started a war that he and his colleagues did not win. In an 1897 address, once again to the New York Academy of Medicine, he asserted that "the point of view of health departments and the profession are widely separated,...for health officials speak for the interests of the community whereas the physician speaks for the welfare of himself and his patient."[71] Advocacy for better care of mothers and children, the establishment of a Bureau of Child Hygiene in New York City, culminating later in passage of the Sheppard-Towner Act of 1921 providing Federal grants to the States for their care, further inflamed matters. Moves toward a system of compulsory national health insurance initially supported by the AMA added more fuel to the fire. Behind all this was the mushrooming American preoccupation with keeping government out of "business" and the cry that medicine was a form of "private enterprise." Containment of the public health movement—at all costs—became the watchword. Reorganization of the AMA at the turn of the century was an attempt to reflect more directly the views of state and local medical societies. The practicing profession required representation to battle an encroaching, and apparently threatening, government concerned with the public's health status.

Concurrently, the academic medical community was withdrawing into its research laboratories. This sector of the medical establishment's preoccupation with redefining the unacceptable focused on widespread professional ignorance about the underlying causes and mechanisms of disease. They too lost interest in embracing a wider role for medicine; this was to be somebody else's business, apart from clinical medicine. Perhaps it should be a concern for the evolving public health movement. Economic factors, if not pecuniary preoccupations, also separated the "practitioner" and the "academic" camps. The latter played an increasingly passive role with respect to public policy bearing on health in the decades to come. As academic physicians became further engrossed in ever more important laboratory research and in the reform of medical education, their influence in the AMA waned. Their concerns with the competence of the practicing profession and the distribution of physicians by specialties and geography and their interest in efforts of public health workers seemed to vanish. This withdrawal of the academic profession into its laboratories and its teaching hospitals presaged the schism still to come. Instead of cooperation and integration, divisiveness and conflict emerged.

For a time the AMA continued to press for a National Health Department but legislation was rejected by Congress in 1910 and again in 1911, largely for lack of public support. The cry was also raised that such legislation would strengthen the power of the AMA and lead to a medical monopoly. The AMA in turn became increasingly preoccupied with financial matters and the perceived encroachment of health departments on clinical practice. Next came the fight for national health insurance, led in large measure by prominent public health figures, further evidence that public health activities were perceived as dangerous for the practicing profession. "The physician who proclaimed in [1919] that the laws regulating drugs, venereal diseases, and so forth were suppressing 'Americanism' and making the physician 'little more than a stool pigeon, a clerk for the health boards,' may not have been typical, but he represented a large number of his colleagues."[72]

Divisiveness within the APHA is reflected in the protracted intellectual, political, and professional struggles surrounding the founding of its Medical Care Section.[73] Haven Emerson, a physician who headed the Department of Public Health at Columbia University, became the senior spokesman for a narrow interpretation of the role of the Health Officer. This group resisted all efforts to expand the APHA's mission beyond oversight of the community's sanitary measures and the provision of limited preventive services. Economic, political, social, and demographic shifts across the country were outrunning Emerson's limited vision with respect to the need for the provision and financing of personal health services. The arrangements his fellow Health Officers set forth "were no longer adequate to deal with current problems."[74] The contending forces included those who favored major reforms in the way America's fragmented medical services were organized, others who advocated compulsory national health insurance, and yet a third group who saw the need for much more research—research that eventually came to be known as health services research, technology assessment, health economics, decision analysis, critical appraisal, and what we now call clinical epidemiology. The Health Officers, however, saw their role restricted largely to matters related to environmental abuses and the most egregious forms of neglect with respect to personal hygiene and preventive services.

The Rockefeller Foundation played a major role in these debates. Starting in 1927 it contributed with other foundations to the work of the landmark Committee on the Costs of Medical Care, and in 1946 began annual support for the APHA's Subcommittee on Medical Care. Today the Medical Care Section of the APHA is by far its largest component.[75]

During the first two decades of the twentieth century, organized medicine had seized the initiative and defined "public health" ever more narrowly. In this it was aided and abetted by the APHA's limited delineation of its own mandate. Starting before the turn of the present century, this legacy persisted until comparatively recently when the AMA began to rethink its priorities and values. The organization's political and financial power had increased rapidly for 50 years, and for decades its control of legislators at all levels was awesome. "Public health," on the other hand, failing to define its mission broadly, drifted ever further away from medicine, especially from clinical medicine. Virtually its only political constituency consisted of the urban poor and society's downtrodden and abandoned, whose influence on legislators was at best minuscule.

Such was the public health enterprise's tenuous position vis à vis the public and its politicians that before acting its officials found themselves "clearing" everything with the leaders of the practicing profession. Political naiveté on the part of the former, and measures that smacked of medical terrorism on the part of the latter, characterized the two groups. Both defended their positions vehemently with little recourse to "facts" (i.e., numbers). "The net effect of the AMA's policy was to make public health officers cautious to the point of timidity. They dissociated themselves from major reforms and concentrated upon noncontroversial aspects of public health work."[76] In many jurisdictions, appointments of health officers had to be cleared with the state or local medical society. In the first two decades of the twentieth century, the formal schism yet to come was now appearing on both the political and operational fronts.

Petty, Frank, Snow, Farr, Simon, and others of their persuasion had tried to broaden both the medical profession's horizons and the politician's understanding. By contrast, the efforts of Chadwick, and to a lesser extent those of Shattuck, with their sanitary idea seemed to have had a constricting effect insofar as the medical profession was concerned. Indeed both Chadwick's and Shattuck's later public careers were foreshortened and their early efforts, while recognized and adopted in the long run, were of brief duration at the time. Given the period in which they worked, aggressive redefinition of the unacceptable was probably the only way to proceed. But by placing their approaches apart from the mainstream of contemporary medical thought, they may have contributed substantially to the emerging schism.

During the nineteenth century parallel efforts were afoot in France by yet another group of physicians to make medicine, and interventions directed at improving the public's health, more rational. The social reformers in Britain and the United States, supported by liberal political philosophies, focused on the environment as the major source of disease—the sanitary idea. Improved cleanliness of the environment, or hygiene as it was called on the continent, especially in France, became the main thrust of government action. Despite William Petty's early skepticism about the efficacy of clinical medicine, practitioners continued to use a host of remedies for which the underlying rationales were unexplored and the benefits unevaluated.

Efforts to develop greater numeracy in clinical medicine had started with the remarkable Bernouilli family of Basle who contributed at least four generations of physicians, mathematicians, physicists, painters, lawyers, and astronomers extending from the seventeenth century well into the nineteenth. They were both academicians and men (few if any women are mentioned) of action, occupying responsible governmental positions. The best known of the family was Daniel Bernouilli (1700-1782), who qualified as a physician and excelled in physics and mathematics.[77] This is not the place to dwell on his contributions to the latter two fields but rather to recall his interest in matters medical. Of these the most noteworthy was development of a formula for estimating the years of life added by vaccination against smallpox; the findings were not uncontested by his contemporaries. He went on to compare the benefits and risks of a medical intervention for a specific disease at both the individual and the population levels, surely another early example of cost-benefit analysis. Together with Pierre-Simon Laplace, the eighteenth-century mathematician mentioned earlier, Bernouilli made major contributions to the theory of probability.[78] His medical qualifications gave him a unique opportunity to influence clinical practice through the use of quantitative approaches.

Clinicians in France played major roles in research, the enactment of legislation, and the development of services such as those for pregnant women and children and for antimalarial drainage.[79] Distinguished academicians served on the famous Conseil de Salubrité. One of the best known was Michel Auguste Thouret (1748-1810), Dean of what was originally called the École de Santé but from 1796 was known as the École de Médicine. In his newly transformed school, Thouret took pride in the fact that, in addition to clinical medicine, subjects such as legal medicine, the history of medicine, hygiene, physics, animal chemistry, and natural history were taught.[80]

The shrill but fully justified cries for social and political reform in the middle decades of the nineteenth century were aided and abetted by the self-interests of a growing middle class whose commercial and industrial enterprises stood to gain substantially if an enlarging and increasingly healthy and productive work force could be assured. It was here that the statisticians, particularly those focusing on social and health statistics, exercised their influence. They described the extent and the locus of the problems and, not infrequently, the monetary costs of the prevalent diseases and the associated loss of productivity.

Louis René Villermé (1782-1863) is a notable example. Disenchanted by the futility of clinical practice as a military surgeon he switched his interests to hygiene, statistics, and epidemiology. As a result of his many achievements he was elected to the French Academy of Medicine and the Academy of Moral Sciences. Extensive research resulted in a volume entitled *The Physical and Mental Condition of French Textile Workers*. As a consequence new legislation was passed to counter the many abuses. Villermé "combined direct observation, statistics and reform proposals."[81]

Jules Gavarret's textbook on medical statistics, although an important innovation, did not attract much attention from clinicians. Quételet, the Belgian mathematician, astronomer, and statistician also mentioned earlier, was in frequent contact with statisticians and physicians in Paris. These brilliant pioneers in quantitative methods, however, had little impact on the practice of medicine or the development of health policy at the time. Insofar as they understood medicine, they seem to have been redefining the unacceptable by expressing a high level of skepticism about physicians' ministrations and by demanding greater precision to support claims of efficacy. Their ideas, however, were not yet internalized by most academic or practicing clinicians.[82]

Unequivocal commitment by a credible practicing clinician was required to demonstrate the utility of quantitative concepts and methods for the advancement of medicine. Pierre-Charles-Alexandre Louis (1787-1872) is the acknowledged founder of *the méthode numérique* in medicine. His use of this term to describe what were essentially statistical methods applied to clinical investigations is the third central concept that assisted in redefining the unacceptable. Louis had become disillusioned with the impotence of clinical medicine. Early in his career he was deeply influenced by a large diphtheria epidemic which, in spite of the broad armamentarium of medical interventions employed at the time, took a heavy death toll.

He concluded that much deeper study of the origins of disease was required before effective treatments could be developed, and further that a more critical approach to all manner of treatments was essential. Innate curiosity, skepticism towards the received wisdom handed down by academic authorities, and an inherent capacity for logical thinking set Louis apart from his colleagues. In 1825, with descriptions of tuberculosis (phthisis, in those days) based on two large series of clinical cases and autopsies, Louis provided new insights into the origins, as well as the clinical characteristics, of this disease. In a similar manner other acute observations enabled him to distinguish typhoid fever (to which he gave the name) as a distinct entity apart from typhus.[83]

Gabriel Andral questioned the efficacy of bloodletting but Louis demonstrated statistically, or provided "proof" as it was called at the time, that this treatment was not only useless but often harmful. The following quotation illustrates his conceptual approach to comparative studies and, parenthetically, records one of the first uses of the term "efficacious":

> In any epidemic, for instance, let us suppose 500 of the sick, *taken indiscriminately,* to be subjected to one kind of treatment, and 500 others, taken in the same manner, to be treated in a different mode; if the mortality is greater among the first, than among the second, must we not conclude that the treatment was less appropriate or less efficacious in the first class, than in the second?...that it is impossible to appreciate each case with mathematical exactness, and it is precisely on this account that enumeration becomes necessary; by so doing the errors (which are inevitable) being the same in both groups of patients subjected to different treatment, mutually compensate each other, and they may be disregarded without sensibly affecting the exactness of the results.[84]

Although Louis's study incurred the wrath of many fellow clinicians and its design by today's standards was flawed, he put numeracy on the clinical map. He challenged the notion that the experience of individual physicians with individual patients was a reliable guide to understanding the origins of disease or its prevention, diagnosis, and treatment. His use of the laws of large numbers to identify regularity in the patterns of diseases as well as to minimize observational error harked back to John Graunt and William Petty.

Louis probably influenced more medical men to undertake scientific investigations than any of his contemporaries. He had an enormous impact on clinical practice both in France and abroad.[85] Recourse to facts and figures in place of the vague theorizing that characterized most of medicine at the time was his epoch-making contribution.[86] Louis brought new intellectual life to the profession of which he was counted one of the leading clinical practitioners. Lack of an academic appointment in no way inhibited widespread respect for his work. A passage from his *Essay of Clinical Instruction* illustrates Louis's approach to sound clinical medicine:

> Whether we wish to make a summary of the facts observed during the course of clinical medicine, or to deduce general laws from those collected by the authors, we must, in the first place, assure ourselves of the exactness of the facts; remove from

our analysis all those which are not unimpeachable, and analyze the others *without distinction*; for the object is to arrive at exact results; and by proceeding in the manner pointed out, we make a complete enumeration, and thus take a sure means of avoiding great errors....In order then, that the results obtained...should be actually true, it is necessary that the facts on which they are based should be very exact; thus, among the cases where a symptom is wanting, we must not count those where it has not been noted, where no mention has been made of it, whatever may be the exactness of the observation in other respects....But to appreciate the value of a symptom in any disease whatever, we should not only know the proportion of the cases in which it presents itself, but also in what other affections it occurs, and in what proportion, in how many cases it is slight or severe....The numerical method is not less useful in the research of the causes of disease, whether in giving us the means of recognizing serious errors, or in enabling us to avoid them.[87]

It is hard to imagine a more apt statement for describing the fundamental building blocks of probabilistic thinking in clinical medicine and for observational studies of population-based phenomena bearing on health and disease.

As noted earlier, William Farr, one of Louis's best known students, spent some 2 years obtaining formal medical training in Paris, the mecca of clinical medicine at the time. Farr's quantitative turn of mind, including broad knowledge of work by his British statistical forebears, prepared him to be greatly influenced by his experiences in France. He was exposed to the superb clinicians of the day, including critical thinking about hygiene by the iconoclastic clinician, Andral, and to the teachings of French mathematicians. Farr spent most of his time, however, attending lectures and absorbing the statistical thinking of that preeminent clinician, Louis. The breadth of Louis's interests and thinking may be gauged by the fact that he was able to influence an epidemiologist/statistician like Farr as well as academic and practicing clinicians.

In addition to his paternal role in statistics, Farr is regarded as the father of *modern* epidemiology[*] when the term is narrowly construed by some epidemiologists to be based primarily on the analysis of vital and health events at the macro level. Louis, his mentor, also deserves to be recognized as a "father" of all epidemiology when it is construed to involve the accuracy and credibility of the initial clinical data and the logic governing their acquisition, collation, and analysis at the micro and the macro levels. Farr's deep interest in nosology, nomenclatures, and classifications may well have come from his exposure to Louis's ideas. The latter applied statistical thinking to clinical problems and in so doing insisted on the accuracy of labels employed for clinical entities; it is these labels that eventually find their way into aggregated vital and medical statistics, the raw material for many epidemiological studies. To this end he formulated what came to be known as Louis's rule: "Whenever practical, reduce observations to a numerical expression."[88]

---

[*] As well as earlier claims of paternity made on behalf of Hippocrates, Frascatori, and Petty.

Farr chose to focus his main interests at the macro level and the need for social reform and pursuit of the sanitary idea. Other physicians took from their experiences with Louis the application of his ideas at the micro level of clinical medicine. They recognized the power of quantitative thinking and analyses of group phenomena to advance medicine scientifically. One is not right or wrong, good or bad; both the individual and population perspectives are required. In no small measure, the work of Louis must be seen as central to the development of epidemiology, the evolution of clinical medicine, and the advancement of public health. He epitomized the *compleat epidemiologist* who can work readily at both the individual and population levels.

Louis was interested in preventive medicine and was a founder of the *Annales d'Hygiène,* the leading French journal dealing with this topic. He wrote widely for medical journals in other countries including the *Lancet* and the *American Journal of Medical Sciences.* Work as an investigator, clinician, teacher, and concerned citizen brought him a formidable reputation. The intellectual force of his ideas alone, not the implied endorsement of an institutional association, merited his prominence for, as observed earlier, Louis had no academic appointment.

The breadth of this remarkable physician's erudition and his impact on the profession are best documented by the range of brilliant students he attracted to Paris. In addition to his countryman Jules Gavarret, there was Josef Skoda (1805-1881), the tough-minded leading clinician of Vienna, whose constant doubts about the efficacy of available treatments undoubtedly influenced his Hungarian pupil Ignaz Philipp Semmelweis (1818-1865).

A plausible theory asserts that the conceptual basis for Louis's numerical method and what is now subsumed under the rubric clinical epidemiology, was in fact transmitted through the numerous British and American clinicians who studied with Louis and then returned to their native countries.[89-91] These students were a formidable group, many of whom provided vigorous scientific leadership for the medical profession. To some their efforts brought renown which seems even greater than that accorded Louis himself.

But Louis did more than lecture and give clinics. He supported his students in organizing a weekly self-learning tutorial, a virtual club, known as the Society for Medical Observation. An unidentified participant in an early exercise of what we now call "critical appraisal" gave this account:

> The members were arranged around a table that occupied three sides of the room, and each person had paper and pen or pencil before him. He was prepared...to note the most trivial omission or a too inconsiderate deduction made by the reader. Each subsequently criticized the paper from these notes. This was done in the keenest manner. Louis, as President, summed up the result of the meeting by not only criticizing the reader, but also his critics' remarks.[92]

This "new medicine" of which the hallmark was the numerical method was brought to Britain and America by Louis's students. Once home, their efforts, for the most part, were not limited to clinical teaching, research, and patient care. Many if not most of them seemed to have a much broader view of medicine and its responsibilities than was represented by the one-to-one encounters with patients, essential as those were. Perhaps they had recognized that groups of patients can be as instructive as individual patients. Many of these academic clinicians also supported movements for sanitary reform. They led in the creation of Boards of Health or Health Councils. They argued for improved nomenclatures, classifications, and recording of vital events, the promulgation of vital statistics, and the conduct of sickness surveys. Breadth of perspective and intensity of concern characterized much of the academic medical scene during the latter half of the nineteenth century. Experimental research in the laboratory was not their strong suit; observation, description, and analysis were their forte.[93]

Of the English students, three stand out. First there was, of course, William Farr. Second was William Budd, mentioned earlier, who is now regarded as a major figure in the early history of English epidemiology.[94] Although a country practitioner, Budd was a teacher at the University of Bristol's medical school and later a person of some substance in the medical world. Initially, however, his ideas were given short shrift, possibly because of the rural origins of his research.

William Augustus Guy, whom we also met earlier, was the third outstanding English student to propagate Louis's concepts and methods on returning home; he deserves to be better known, especially among clinicians. Guy, Professor of Forensic Medicine in the University of London as well as Dean of the Medical Faculty at King's College, was a Fellow of the Royal Society. An authority on occupational diseases, he was also a statistician of considerable note, being an active member of the Royal Statistical Society. He recognized the central importance of Louis's ideas for medicine's mission as suggested by the following quotation:

> Does not a single fact, that medicine required a Louis to teach the advantages of the "méthode numérique," and to set an example of its employment, so long after its introduction into the more advanced sciences, prove the necessity of making those sciences an example of our own.[95]

Guy also was active in the sanitary reform movement but at times, together with others, his enthusiasm for the cause outran the accuracy of his supporting evidence. As in the case of Louis's bloodletting studies, Guy's statistical analyses of the risks associated with various occupations were flawed. The importance of selective bias and the need for standardization were yet to be recognized. Although an acknowledged leader in statistics, Guy may have been less critical than many of his statistical colleagues.[96] He was, nevertheless, an important figure in disseminating epidemiological thinking in Britain, particularly to medical students.[97] Toward the end of a long career, Guy, the clinician, published in 1870, what may well have been the first textbook entitled *Public Health*. In this volume, he argued that epidemiological thinking should be extended from the clinical situation to the population perspective when he wrote:

> Of this numerical method which the French physician, Louis, so largely applied, and Gavarret so ably explained and illustrated, I have now to treat, as it lends itself to hygiene.[98]

On their return from France, Guy and Farr became actively involved in the Statistical Society of London. Founded in 1834, it was the precursor of the Royal Statistical Society. Among its broad range of interests, the Statistical Society included a component concerned with methodological problems in studies of health and disease. It was a beehive of activity for all those interested in statistical applications to medicine. The theories and applications discussed gradually permeated the medical establishment with epidemiological thinking, although the term had yet to be introduced.

At the time, cholera was, of course, the great concern not only of the public and its politicians but of the entire medical profession, especially those who called themselves "sanitary physicians." A variety of scientific papers using epidemiological tables and formats were presented by physicians, obstetricians, and surgeons to medical societies, most notably the Royal Medical and Chirurgical Society. The studies covered such topics as variations in hospital mortality, the efficacy of interventions, the impact of smallpox vaccination, and the health of Londoners. In Britain, by midcentury, epidemiological thinking was accepted by many as an important if not essential perspective within the prevailing medical paradigm. Epidemiological or statistical methods were employed widely for investigating many aspects of health and disease. Political arithmetic, the numerical method, and their newly designated analogs "vital statistics" and "medical and health statistics," had become internalized in the thinking of many academic medical faculty members. In addition to the more generalized epidemiological thinking, epidemiology was ready to emerge as a distinct discipline.[99,100]

There was, however, no forum, apart from the Statistical Society of London, in which intensive scientific discussions could take place not only about clinical and population-based problems but also about research methods in medicine. This was especially true for those concerned with the increasingly urgent drive to discover means for preventing the recurrent massive epidemics threatening Britain and the continent, to say nothing of the rest of the world, in 1848 and 1849.

The first move was made by one J. H. Tucker, who was probably a surgeon although he was not identified as a physician nor did he have an M.D. degree after his name. Under a pseudonym "Pater" he wrote letters to the *Lancet*, the first in 1848 and two more in 1849. Initially he urged the formation of a "society" to coordinate measures against cholera, then raging in Britain. The next two letters proposed first that the new organization be called the "Asiatic Cholera Medical Society" and then that the title should be the "Epidemic Medical Society." In yet another letter to the *Lancet*, Tucker identified himself and announced that a small group had been meeting and that the Epidemiological Society of London had been established on March 6, 1850.[101,102]

This was no tiny elitist organization open only to the properly anointed. Rather it was a broad-based initiative directed at informing the profession, the public, and the divided politicians about the life-threatening epidemics that were afflicting all citizens. The political response to Edwin Chadwick's 1842 *Report on the Sanitary Condition of the Labouring Population of Great Britain* had been mixed at best. One of his most prominent colleagues was the aristocratic landholder Anthony

Ashley-Cooper (1801-1885), later Earl of Shaftesbury. In spite of their different political persuasions Lord Ashley, as he was known at the time, embraced many of Chadwick's ideas. With great religious fervor and judicious political finesse, he was able to further passage of the Public Health Act of 1848 establishing the General Board of Health. Ashley served on that Board together with Chadwick and the latter's medical advisor Southwood Smith.

Ashley brought not only political (and social) credibility to the newly constituted Board but also enormous energy in pursuit of sanitary reform, especially in the face of the growing cholera epidemics facing the country.[103] So highly was he regarded by the scientific establishment, his fellow politicians, and the public generally, that he was asked to preside at the initial public meeting of the Epidemiological Society on July 30, 1850. Later he was made Honorary President and Chadwick was made Honorary Vice-President. This meeting was attended by about 200 people, many of whom may have been attracted as a result of the credibility provided by Ashley's leadership. Among those attending were prominent members of the medical profession, including distinguished academic clinicians such as Thomas Addison, the Society's first treasurer, and Richard Bright of Guy's Hospital Medical School; Sir Charles Hastings, founder of the British Medical Association; J. Haviland, Regius Professor of Physic (Medicine) at Cambridge; T. Clifford Allbutt, later also the Regius Professor of Physic at Cambridge; Southwood Smith, medical advisor to Chadwick; Sir John Simon, Medical Officer of Health for London; John Snow, anaesthetist; T. Spencer Wells, later Hunterian Professor of Surgery and Pathology; and William Budd, the country practitioner and Bristol medical school teacher.

Benjamin Guy Babington (1794-1866), a leading clinician, and Fellow of the Royal Society, gave his blessing to the organization by allowing himself to be elected the president at the Society's first formal meeting held not in some remote hall but in the quarters of the Medico-Chirurgical Society.[104,105] The gatherings of this Society were the birthplace of modern epidemiology as a central discipline in British medicine. The members included leading academic clinicians and scientists, as well as numerous miasmatists who spurned the contagion theory. Many can be numbered among the other clinical fathers of epidemiology; they, in turn, were descended from a long and distinguished line of grandfathers; Louis's spirit seems to have been present from the Society's inception.

At the Society's inaugural meeting, Babington set forth in his opening address the objectives of the new society. Its aims were:

> to endeavor by the light of modern science to review all those causes which result in the manifestation and spread of epidemic disease—to discover causes at present unknown, and investigate those which are ill understood; to collect together facts upon which scientific researches may be securely based; to remove errors which impede their progress; and thus, as far as we are able, having made ourselves thoroughly acquainted with the strongholds of our enemies and their modes of attack, to suggest those means by which their invasion may either be prevented: or if, in spite of our existence, they may have broken in upon us, to seek how they may be most effectually combated and expelled.[106]

A stronger manifesto for inspiring and guiding medical investigation would be hard to conceive; several elements are worth stressing. First, Babington referred to "all those causes," not just to "one" cause for each disease; the germ theory had not yet evolved and a monoetiological view of causation had not overshadowed the possibility of a broader view of medicine. Second, he put no restrictions on the source or characteristics of the "facts" on which to base scientific research. Third, he emphasized the need to guard against "errors." He stressed prevention as the top priority and commented that "statistics, too, have supplied us with a new and powerful means of testing medical truth, and we learn from the labours of the accurate Louis how appropriately they may be brought to bear upon the subject of epidemic disease."[107] "Legitimate" applications of epidemiological concepts and methods extended from the hospital to the population or community. The same statistical and epidemiological ideas could be used whenever and wherever appropriate for the investigation.

If the Society focused its efforts largely on communicable or contagious diseases, that was because those were the principal threats to the population's health at the time. The members recognized a much broader mandate, however, and pursued other problems as evidenced by the first committees appointed: Smallpox and Vaccination; Cholera; Epizootic; Hospitals; and Continued Fever. Two others were the "Committee Appointed to Inquire into the Diseases Appertaining to the Vegetable Kingdom" and the "Committee Appointed to Take into Consideration the Question of Supplying the Labouring Classes with Nurses in Epidemic and Other Diseases."[108]

The members were to examine a wide range of problems and issues; these embraced virtually all aspects of medicine and the public's health. Included were not only the contagious diseases but also the suggestion that the Society should pursue the investigation of chronic diseases through the "continued fever" committee, examine the adequacy of health services through the "hospitals" committee, and study health "manpower" supply through the "nurses" committee. They even discussed the provision of "home care" through the latter committee.

The leaders of this new organization included academicians and practitioners intent on addressing the full scope of their responsibilities. If membership did not include the Royal College of Physicians' (London) full roster, the heart of the medical establishment, many of its Fellows were participants. As a body the Society represented a cross section of Victorian medicine. Their greatest concerns were with cleaning up the environment and reforming the Poor Laws but they did not confine their interests to the sanitary idea, important as it was at the time, for controlling disease and improving the lot of the citizenry.

The Society's *Commemorative Volume* cites the work of the Committee on Smallpox and Vaccination as an example of its accomplishments. An exhaustive report on the subject was prepared with a title reflecting the dimensions of the Committee's concerns: *On the State of Smallpox in England and Wales and Other Countries, and of Compulsory Vaccination, with Tables and Appendix Presented to the President and Council of the Epidemiological Society by the Smallpox and Vaccination Committee, March 26th, 1855.* The Council delivered the Report to the Secretary of State for the Home Department who in turn presented it to Parliament. The result was a substantial modification of the legislation requiring compulsory vaccination.

Even this legislation, however, did not entirely satisfy the Committee on Smallpox and Vaccination or the Society's Council. A subsequent report was prepared on *The Prevention of Smallpox and the Extension of Vaccination*; this too was printed by order of the House of Commons. A deputation from the Society met with the Prime Minister, Lord Palmerston, and later with the First Lord of the Treasury to press for action. The members publicized their recommendations in the *Lancet* of April 24, 1858, under the heading: *The Humble Petition of the President and Council of the Epidemiological Society of London and the Honourable the House of Commons in Parliament Assembled*. The introduction to the *Commemorative Volume* concludes with this summary:

> The efforts of the Society in one or another direction had, by this time, been appreciated in all parts of the civilized world; and, as an instance of the esteem in which it was then held, it may be mentioned that the first edition of Hirsch's classical Handbook of Geographical and Historical Pathology, published in 1860, [was dedicated to the *Society*].[109]

The papers presented at the Society's monthly meetings were also well publicized. Abstracts and comments on its transactions were published in the major medical journals, the *Lancet, British Medical Journal*, and *Medical Times*. From 1855 to 1859 a portion of the *Journal of Public Health and Sanitary Review* was devoted to the proceedings of the Society, and from 1859 onwards the papers read before it were published in its own *Transactions* as well as in the major medical journals.[110] The interests of the membership were eclectic as suggested by the following titles:

- On the Geographical Distribution of Health and Disease, in Connection Chiefly with Natural Phenomena;
- A Sketch of the Principal Features of the Climate of the Crimea, and its Effects on Health, as Observed during the First Year of the Occupation by the Allied Forces;
- On the Difficulties of the Study of Prevailing Diseases;
- Suggestions for Utilizing the Statistics of disease among the Poor;
- Observations on the Climatology, Topography, and Diseases of Hong Kong and the Canton River Station;
- On the Diseases and Injuries of Artisans and Labourers, Traceable to their Respective Occupations;
- Vital Statistics of Tasmania in 1861;
- On the Present Position and Prospects of Epidemiological Science;
- On Scurvy in the Mercantile Marine;
- On the Prevention of Disease by the Reconstruction of the Dwellings of the Poor;

- On Errors in the Usual Methods of Investigating Epidemics;
- On Some Arithmetical Questions Involved in the Rise and Progress of Epidemics;
- On the Study of Medical Meteorology, Especially in its Relation to Epidemic Maladies;
- On Medical Statistics in the Public Health Section of the Ninth International Statistical Congress, held in Budapest, Hungary, in September 1876;
- Aids to Epidemiological Knowledge;
- The Prevention of Heat Apoplexy;
- On Beriberi;
- Famine: Its Effects and Relief;
- On the Study of Epidemiology;
- On the Comparative Mortality of English Districts.[111]

Nor were the concerns of the membership solely domestic; there were many papers presented about diseases in other countries such as the United States and those in Europe at similar stages of development to Britain. There were also numerous papers about medical problems in what are now referred to as the "developing countries" but what were then known as "the colonies." The following countries (represented by their names at that time) were involved in one or more papers presented at the Society's meetings:

Africa, China, East Africa, Egypt, Fiji, Formosa, Gold Coast, India, Jamaica, Malay, Mauritius, Mesopotamia, Persia, Peru, Polynesia, Syria, West Indies, and Zambesi.[112]

These details illustrate the breadth of scientific interest and professional commitment by many of medicine's academic leaders in Britain during the last half of the nineteenth century. A broad view of medicine's task and a broad paradigm to guide research and service prevailed, especially among the academic establishment. Both micro and macro interests were encouraged; studies extended from the individual to the population and from Britain to the developing world. Practitioners, especially those outside London, undoubtedly had narrower horizons and as is the case today were preoccupied with the care of their own patients, one by one. A substantial part of the medical profession's leadership, however, was united in its collective support for the use of epidemiological methods whenever suitable.

For 3 years (1850-1852), as a member of the Epidemiological Society, John Snow had listened to and participated in discussions of statistical methods applied to epidemiological problems. Following his earlier work on the transmission of cholera, he produced in 1853 a new and more extensive analysis of his observations in a paper presented to the Society on "The Comparative Mortality of Large Towns and Rural Districts, and the Causes by Which it is Influenced." His ideas may have been at variance with those of members who were miasmatists, but Snow at least had an important forum before which he could present his observations and theories about the origins and control of the cholera epidemic, especially that of 1853.

Benjamin Ward Richardson (1828-1896) was one of the early experimental physiologists in Britain, and as an inventor of a new general anaesthetic, became a close friend of Snow. The latter in turn seems to have introduced Richardson to the Epidemiological Society where he became an active member in 1852.[113,114] Subsequently Richardson supported Snow, as did Augustus Guy, in his theory that cholera was propagated by means of contaminated water, and he helped greatly in furthering acceptance of the theory by the medical profession.[115] Throughout most of his career Richardson was also in touch with Chadwick and Farr, and in time he became one of the acknowledged promoters of both the sanitary idea and the application of statistical and epidemiological methods to medicine.

In 1853 Richardson delivered to the Society what must be regarded as a pioneering paper entitled "The Investigation of Epidemics by Experiments." In it he advanced the following principles:

- That by certain experiment it might be ascertained in what excreta the poisons of certain of the epidemic diseases are located;

- By what surfaces of the body such poisons may be absorbed so as to produce their specific effects;

- Whether the virus in reproducing its disease in a healthy body, acts in the development of the phenomena by which the disease is typified primarily or secondarily—i.e., by its own reproduction and presence, or by the evolution of another principle or product;

- Whether climate, season, or other external influences modify the course of epidemics, by reproducing modifications of the epidemic poisons, or modifications in the system of persons exposed to the poisons.[116]

All this was set forth almost a quarter of a century before Koch promulgated his famous postulates, usually cited as marking the beginning of the "bacteriological era." They also antedated Louis Pasteur's (1822-1895) work inaugurating the study of immunology. In 1863 Richardson declared that epidemiology had come "into its own." "Let us then," he said, "as *scientific epidemiologists*, join hands with the sanitarian...."[117]

This pronouncement had far-reaching implications for two reasons. It was the first recorded reference to a new category of professionals—"epidemiologists."[118] As such the term defined a new medical discipline or specialty implicitly without describing the concepts and methods espoused or emphasizing their potential for contributing to the scientific progress of medicine. Second, Richardson, by specifically linking epidemiology and epidemiologists to the sanitary idea, strengthened the importance of both to clinical medicine. Unfortunately, he also may have been defining the field narrowly. Many enthusiasts for sanitary reform were often careless with their use of facts and even statistics. Richardson apparently wanted to introduce more science and critical thinking into the urgent task of cleaning up the environment. His views changed over the years; from work as an experimental physiologist expressing skepticism about the germ theory of disease he branched out to embrace broader concerns at the macro level. In 1855 he founded the *Journal of Public Health* and in so doing lent his support to spreading the gospel of public health. This journal was also used for disseminating the transactions of the Epidemiological Society until 1859 when it ceased publication for financial reasons.[119] Richardson was undoubtedly another founder of modern epidemiology and a primary promoter of its application to improving the public's health. He may inadvertently, however, also have laid some of the definitional groundwork for the schism to come through his attempts to restrict the applications of epidemiological concepts and methods. To his great credit throughout a productive career Richardson used science and scientific methods, including statistical and epidemiological methods, to help in redefining the unacceptable. Sir Arthur Newsholme paid tribute to him when he wrote:

> Richardson was a pathfinder...and he illuminated [many subjects] by research and advocacy, in writings which in eloquence and grace form a model for all medical authors. There ran through all Richardson's writings the unusual combination of suggestive research and of a powerful and vivid imagination, along with an always present desire to serve his fellow-men and to improve the conditions of life....[120]

The Society's first president, Benjamin Babington, died in 1866, as had most of the other founding members during the decade of the sixties. Toward the end of the century the Society met only for an annual dinner, the last being the Commemoration Dinner in 1900. Derived from seeds planted by Louis and his predecessors, a brief half century in the gestation of the epidemiological perspective drew to a close. Its influence continued on an even broader scale, however, as a founding body of the Royal Society of Medicine (RSM); it survives today as the RSM's Epidemiological Section (personal communication, Professor Roy M. Acheson, Cambridge University, March 12, 1990).

Louis's ideas traveled to the United States as well. Between 1820 and 1861 about 700 American physicians went to Paris for postgraduate studies; of these some 67 eventually became professors of medicine.[121] Although some studied pathology and many others clinical medicine, not a few were exposed to Louis's numerical method. Among the Americans who sat at Louis's feet were two of Boston's better known clinicians, both from influential families. First there was Oliver Wendell Holmes (1809-1894), with his unwelcome observations on the origins of puerperal fever. He also argued persistently against the use of popular nostrums, against quackery, and the lack of efficacy exhibited by most contemporary medical maneuvers. Holmes took considerable interest in the broader affairs of American medicine, attending one or more of the National Quarantine and Sanitary Conventions held at midcentury. He seems to have contributed little, however, to either the theory or applications of the numerical method. Nevertheless in the view of one authority, he should "be ranked as America's first outstanding epidemiologist."[122]

There was also Henry I. Bowditch (1808-1892), physician and physiologist, who developed a lifelong interest in public health. The field was referred to at the time in the United States as state medicine, following the publication in England of a volume with that name by Henry Wyldbare Rumsey (1809-1876) that was possibly based on the teachings of Johann Peter Frank. Bowditch thought little of Lemuel Shattuck's report, commenting that "it fell stillborn from the State printer's hands."[123] He pursued his concerns for broadening the horizons of medicine by advocating creation of state Boards of Health, having founded and chaired the first one in Massachusetts in 1869.[124]

Spreading Louis's ideas was accomplished less by Bowditch than by George C. Shattuck, Jr. (1813-1893), another Harvard physician. Like Bowditch, this Shattuck, in contrast to Lemuel, was from another prominent Boston family who at least interacted with, if he did not influence, his father George C. Shattuck, Sr. (1783-1854), also a physician on the Harvard faculty. But the father as well had statistical proclivities and served as the second president of the American Statistical Association his son had helped to found. Among others, the senior Shattuck seems to have inspired his student Edward Jarvis (1803-1883). The latter, one of the instigators of the United States federal census, was a keen student of vital statistics, a physician with serious doubts about the efficacy of most medical interventions, and an ardent sanitary reformer.[125] Even Lemuel Shattuck, however, the businessman, bookseller, and enthusiastic devotee of applied statistics, seems to have absorbed many of Louis's ideas through his associations with the younger George Shattuck and possibly Edward Jarvis.[126]

There was also a group of physicians from New York City who studied with Louis. The best known of these were Francis Delafield (1841-1915), author of a major pathology textbook, and Alonzo Clark (1807-1887), a pioneer in American medical education; both were on the faculty of New York's College of Physicians and Surgeons. Both also taught William Henry Welch (1850-1934), whom we encounter later. There are other linkages from Louis to major leaders of the American academic medical establishment and important figures in the development of improved public health practices. The former include William W. Gerhard (1809-1872), a prominent Philadelphia clinician, academician, and "perhaps the most brilliant American pupil of Louis."[127] William Pepper (1843-1898), also of Philadelphia and the University of Pennsylvania, was "editor of the first large American System of Medicine, leader in medical education and sometime provost of his university."[128] Others included Elisha Bartlett (1804-1855), who helped to elucidate the contagious character of typhus fever; Josiah Clark Nott (1804-1873), who proposed the "mosquito theory" for the transmission of yellow fever; and Alfred Stillé (1813-1900), who also contributed to distinguishing between typhus and typhoid fevers.[129,130]

Most of these physicians were academic clinicians as well as investigators and supporters, if not innovators, in the public health movement. The numerical method gave real impetus and growing credibility to the clinical research undertaken by this group of Louis's brilliant protegés. In addition, it gave authority to their documentation of hazardous health and environmental practices, contributions to redefining the unacceptable.

Such was the influence of Louis and his numerical method that in 1832 a group of the foremost American physicians who had studied in France formed an analog of his Parisian Society and the Epidemiological Society of London known as the Society for Medical Observation. This was long before the German-trained physicians in America, steeped in the emerging experimental laboratory methods, formed the American Society for Clinical Investigation in 1908. The earlier dominance of the French school in American medicine also may have accounted for the initial reluctance of its academic leaders to embrace the germ theory of disease initially.[131]

In the United States, observing the natural history of disease, classification, and measurement, together with critical appraisal of interventions through use of the numerical method, were not accomplished in the name of "epidemiology" or by professionals labeled "epidemiologists." But if the thinking of these physicians was not epidemiological in character it is difficult to know how to characterize it, and for this we have to credit Louis, his statistical forebears, and colleagues. To the seminal ideas of Petty, Graunt, Frank, and even Sydenham, we now must add those of Louis.

In spite of all this, Louis's influence among clinicians languished in France and the United States after his death in 1872. Almost a century later, however, in the 1963 James M. Anders Lecture entitled "The Numerical Method in Therapeutic Medicine," Michael B. Shimkin, Professor of Medicine at Temple University, traced the history of statistical applications in medicine from the days of Louis. In delivering this message to the College of Physicians of Philadelphia, Shimkin attempted to revive the interest of clinicians in these matters.[132]

Towards the end of the nineteenth century the bacteriological era began to eclipse the epidemiological perspective and even the work of epidemiologists. William Farr continued the practical application of those components of epidemiology represented by vital statistics and health statistics. Scientists with other statistical bents such as Francis Galton (1822-1911) and later Karl Pearson (1857-1936) were left to develop new methods and applications for epidemiological thinking. Interest diminished in epidemiology as a discipline and as a means of investigating the larger universe of factors that determine the manifestations of health, disease, health status, and the use of health services. The awesome power of bacteriology to determine the "cause" of each disease pushed other perspectives aside.

The decline of epidemiological thinking may be attributed, at least in part, to the lack of an effective vital statistics system in France and its delayed development in the United States. In spite of the work on probability theory by the French mathematicians and Louis's emphasis on accuracy of diagnosis, labeling, and recording, vital events were not adequately documented, collected, and tabulated until later in the nineteenth century. Similarly, in the United States, only at the end of that century were national tabulations of mortality statistics available.[133]

For epidemiology and epidemiological thinking to flourish throughout medicine five elements are required:

- An underlying philosophy (or in modern parlance, a conceptual paradigm) of epidemiology as a vital set of concepts and methods for scientific investigation. It needs to be fully understood and embraced throughout the health enterprise;
- Statistical theories and methods;

- Appropriate labeling and accurate recording of all clinical, vital, and administrative data (or in modern parlance, appropriate nomenclatures, terminology, and classification systems);
- Population-based sickness and health surveys, i.e., health statistics;
- Recognition of medicine's responsibility for "redefining the unacceptable" as reflected by the sanitary idea and the hygienic movement or in contemporary jargon, the environmental movement, and the drives for outcomes research, and cost containment.

By the end of the nineteenth century, all five elements had been introduced or developed to varying degrees by physicians, almost always clinicians. Of greater importance, they had been applied at the insistence and with the leadership of physicians, a great many of whom were associated with medical schools. To varying degrees, the professional associations of the day embraced these ideas. They were seen as fundamental components of the mission of medicine. Chadwick, Shattuck, and Shaftesbury, on the other hand, were the only laymen of importance in spurring the politicians to more effective action, largely in the interests of reducing poverty, improving the productivity of the workers, and cleaning up the filth associated with epidemics. These were worthy objectives and should be applauded, but as we have seen the influence of the nonphysicians on the medical profession—especially practitioners, their policies, and practices—was relatively modest compared to that of the clinicians who controlled the medical establishments and advised the politicians.

Towards the end of the twentieth century the principal focus for redefining the unacceptable, as in William Petty's era, has shifted once more to "value for money." The current labels are "cost containment," "cost-effectiveness," and "resource allocation." Concerns for the environment, for social justice (access to care and risk analysis), prevention, and, as in the days of Johan Peter Frank, health promotion. Clinicians are now finding that epidemiological concepts and methods provide the necessary but by no means sufficient means for accomplishing all these objectives.

The three central concepts—*political arithmetic, the sanitary idea, and the numerical method*—have had major impacts on the development of public health and clinical medicine throughout the Western world and, more recently, in the developing world. Epidemiology played a central role in the evolution of all three; an appreciation of their origins and influence over recent centuries should help to place more recent developments in perspective.

References

1. Poincaré H. *The Foundations of Science—Science and Hypothesis, Science and Method.* Halstead GB, transl. New York: Science Press, 1929.
2. Stevens SS. Mathematics, measurement and psychophysics. In: *Handbook of Experimental Psychology.* Stevens SS, ed. New York: Wiley, 1958:1-49.
3. Sand R. *The Advance to Social Medicine.* London: Staples Press, 1952:443-457.

4. Ibid.
5. Foss L, Rothenberg, K.: *The Second Medical Revolution: From Biomedicine to Infomedicine*. Boston: New Science Library, Shambhala, 1987.
6. Guthrie D. *A History of Medicine*. London: Nelson, 1945: Chapters VIII-XI.
7. Singer C, Underwood EA. *A Short History of Medicine*. New York: Oxford University Press, 1962: Chapter V.
8. Greenwood M. *Medical Statistics from Graunt to Farr*. Cambridge: Cambridge University Press, 1948:2.
9. Ibid, p. 28.
10. Ibid, pp. 27-35.
11. Pearl R. *Medical Biometry and Statistics*, 3d Ed. Philadelphia: Saunders, 1941: Chapter II.
12. Pearson ES, ed. *The History of Statistics in the 17th and 18th Centuries Against the Background of Intellectual, Scientific and Religious Thought: Lectures by Karl Pearson, 1921-23*. London: Charles Griffin, 1978:36-39.
13. Ibid, pp. 12-29.
14. Rosen G. *From Medical Police to Social Medicine*. New York: Science History, 1974:163.
15. Ibid.
16. Greenwood M. *Medical Statistics from Graunt to Farr*. Cambridge: Cambridge University Press, 1948:15.
17. Ibid, p. 16.
18. Ibid, p. 25.
19. Ibid, p. 27.
20. Rosen G. *From Medical Police to Social Medicine*, New York: Science History, 1974:127.
21. Greenwood M. *Medical Statistics from Graunt to Farr*. Cambridge: Cambridge University Press, 1948:50.
22. Ibid, p. 56.
23. Pearson ES, ed. *History of Statistics in the 17th and 18th Centuries Against the Background of Intellectual, Scientific and Religious Thought: Lectures by Karl Pearson, 1921-23*. London: Charles Griffin, 1978:126.
24. *The Correspondence of the Right Honorable Sir John Sinclair, Bart.*, Vol. I. London: Henry Colburn and Richard Bentley, 1831:230. Quoted by Theodore Woolsey, then Director of the U.S. National Center for Health Statistics, in a talk on June 28, 1973, at the Walter Reed Hospital, Bethesda, Maryland and provided in a personal communication to KLW.
25. Eyler JM. *Victorian Social Medicine: The Ideas and Methods of William Farr*. Baltimore: Johns Hopkins, 1979.
26. Laplace SP. *Essai Philosophiques sur les Probabilités* (p. lxxxv). Quoted by Karl Pearson in Pearson ES, ed. *History of Statistics in the 17th and 18th Centuries*, 1978, p.669.
27. Pearson ES, ed. *History of Statistics in the 17th and 18th Centuries Against the Background of Intellectual, Scientific and Religious Thought: Lectures by Karl Pearson, 1921-23*. London: Charles Griffin, 1978:651.
28. Rosen G. *From Medical Police to Social Medicine*. New York: Science History, 1974:42.
29. Greenwood M. *Medical Statistics from Graunt to Farr*. Cambridge: Cambridge University Press, 1948:69.
30. Pearl R. *Medical Biometry and Statistics*, 3d Ed. Philadelphia: Saunders, 1941:30.

31. Eyler JM. *Victorian Social Medicine: The Ideas and Methods of William Farr.* Baltimore: Johns Hopkins, 1979.
32. Eyler JM. The conceptual origins of William Farr's epidemiology: numerical methods and social thought in the 1830s. In: Lilienfeld AM, ed. *Times, Places and Persons: Aspects of the History of Epidemiology.* Baltimore: Johns Hopkins, 1980.
33. Humphreys NA, ed. *Vital Statistics: A Memorial Volume of Selections from the Reports and Writings of William Farr.* London: Edward Stanford, 1885. Republished for the New York Academy of Medicine with an Introduction by Mervyn Susser and Abraham Adelstein. Metuchen, New Jersey: Scarecrow Press, 1975.
34. Lewis RA. *Edwin Chadwick and the Public Health Movement: 1832-1854.* London: Longmans, Green, 1952:32.
35. Humphreys NA, ed. *Vital Statistics: A Memorial Volume of Selections from the Reports and Writings of William Farr.* London: Edward Stanford, 1885. Republished for the New York Academy of Medicine with an Introduction by Mervyn Susser and Abraham Adelstein. Metuchen, New Jersey: Scarecrow Press, 1975:xi.
36. Eyler JM. *Victorian Social Medicine: The Ideas and Methods of Wiliam Farr.* Baltimore: Johns Hopkins, 1979.
37. Eyler JM. Conceptual origins of William Farr's epidemiology. In: Lilienfeld AM, ed. *Times, Places, and Persons,* 1980.
38. Humphreys NA, ed. *Vital Statistics: A Memorial Volume of Selections from the Reports and Writings of William Farr.* London: Edward Stanford, 1885. Republished for the New York Academy of Medicine with an Introduction by Mervyn Susser and Abraham Adelstein. Metuchen, New Jersey: Scarecrow Press, 1975.
39. Ibid, p. xiv.
40. Greenwood M. *Medical Statistics from Graunt to Farr.* Cambridge: Cambridge University Press, 1948:71.
41. Humphreys NA, ed. *Vital Statistics: Memorial Volume of Selections from the Reports and Writings of William Farr.* London: Edward Stanford, 1885. Republished for the New York Academy of Medicine with an Introduction by Mervyn Susser and Abraham Adelstein. Metuchen, New Jersey: Scarecrow Press, 1975:xxi.
42. Sand R. *The Advance to Social Medicine.* London: Staples Press, 1952:187.
43. Wilcocks C. *Medical Advance, Public Health and Social Evolution.* London: Pergamon, 1965:119.
44. Rosen G. *From Medical Police to Social Medicine.* New York: Science History, 1974:137.
45. Lesky E, ed. *A System of Complete Medical Police: Selections from Johann Peter Frank.* Baltimore: Johns Hopkins, 1976.
46. Rosen G. *A History of Public Health.* New York: MD Publications, 1958.
47. Sand R. *The Advance to Social Medicine.* London: Staples Press, 1952.
48. Sigerist HE. *Landmarks in the History of Hygiene.* London: Oxford University Press, 1956:50-1.
49. Lesky E, ed. *A System of Medical Police: Selections from John Peter Frank.* Baltimore: Johns Hopkins, 1976:23.
50. Ibid, p. 291.
51. Rosen G. *From Medical Police to Social Medicine.* New York: Science History, 1974:145.
52. Ibid.
53. Ibid, p. 154.
54. Brockington CF. *Public Health in the Nineteenth Century.* Edinburgh: Livingstone, 1965: Chapters 1 and 2.

55. Ibid, p. 195.
56. Brockington FC. *Public Health in the Nineteenth Century*. Edinburgh: Livingstone, 1965: Chapter 3.
57. Lewis RA. *Edwin Chadwick and the Public Health Movement: 1832-1854*. London: Longmans, Green, 1952:194-5.
58. Ibid, p. 79.
59. Brockington FC. *Public Health in the Nineteenth Century*. Edinburgh: Livingstone, 1965: Chapter 3.
60. Ibid.
61. Simon J. *English Sanitary Institutions*. London: Cassell, 1890.
62. JHT. William Budd—General practitioner and epidemiologist (editorial). JAMA 1962;182:180-181.
63. Eyler JM. *Victorian Social Medicine: The Ideas and Methods of William Farr*. Baltimore: Johns Hopkins, 1979:105.
64. Ibid, p. 154.
65. Rosenkrantz BG. *Public Health and the State: Changing Views in Massachusetts, 1842-1936*. Cambridge: Harvard University Press, 1972:22.
66. Ibid, p. 25-27.
67. Duffy J. The American medical profession and public health: from support to ambivalence. Bull Hist Med 1979;53:1-22.
68. Ibid, p. 3.
69. Ibid, p. 8.
70. Ibid, p. 13.
71. Ibid, p. 16.
72. Ibid, pp. 19-20.
73. Viseltear AJ. Emergence of the Medical Care Section of the American Public Health Association, 1926-1948. Am J Public Health 1973;63:986-1007.
74. Rosen G. Historical trends and future prospects. In: McLachlan G, McKeown T, eds. *Medical History and Medical Care*. London: Nuffield Provincial Hospitals Trust and Oxford University Press, 1971:76.
75. Viseltear AJ. Emergence of the Medical Care Section of the American Public Association, 1926-1948. Am J Public Health 1973;63:1004.
76. Duffy J. The American medical profession and public health: from support to ambivalence. Bull Hist Med 1979;53:1-22.
77. Pearson ES, ed. *The History of Statistics in the 17th and 18th Centuries Against the Changing Background of Intellectual, Scientific and Religious Thought: Lectures by Karl Pearson, 1921-23*. London: Griffin, 1978:222 *et seq.*
78. Ibid, pp. 556, 560, 660.
79. Ackerknecht EH. *Medicine at the Paris Hospital: 1794-1848*. Baltimore: Johns Hopkins, 1967:149-160.
80. Ibid, pp. 34-38.
81. Ibid, pp. 153-154.
82. Rosen G. *A History of Public Health*. New York: MD Publications, 1958:261-3.
83. Garrison FH. *An Introduction to the History of Medicine*, 4th Ed. Philadelphia: Saunders, 1929:410-411.
84. Louis PCA. *Researches on the Effects of Bloodletting in Some Inflammatory Diseases and on the Influence of Tartarized Antimony and Vesication in Pneumonitis*. (CG Putnam, trans.) Boston: Hilliard, Gray, 1836. Quoted by Lilienfeld DE, Lilienfeld AM. The French influence on the development of epidemiology. In: Lilienfeld AM,

ed. *Times, Places and Persons: Aspects of the History of Epidemiology*. Baltimore: Johns Hopkins, 1980:30.

85. Feinstein AR. *Clinical Epidemiology: The Architecture of Clinical Research*. Philadelphia: Saunders, 1985:410.
86. Sand R. *The Advance to Social Medicine*. London: Staples Press, 1952:446.
87. Louis PCA. *An Essay on Clinical Instruction* (P Martin, trans.). London: S. Highley, 1834:27. Quoted by Lilienfeld DE, Lilienfeld AM. The French influence on the development of epidemiology. In Lilienfeld AM, ed. *Times, Places and Persons: Aspects of the History of Epidemiology*. Baltimore: Johns Hopkins, 1980:32.
88. Newsholme A. *Fifty Years in Public Health: A Personal Narrative with Comments*. London: Allen & Unwin, 1935:37.
89. Lilienfeld DE. "The greening of epidemiology": sanitary physicians and the London Epidemiological Society (1830-1870). Bull Hist Med 1979;52:503-528.
90. Lilienfeld AM, Lilienfeld DE. What else is new? Am J Epidemiol 1977;105:169-179.
91. Lilienfeld DE, Lilienfeld AM. The french influence on the development of epidemiology. In Lilienfeld AM. *Times, Places and Persons: Aspects of the History of Epidemiology*. Baltimore: Johns Hopkins, 1980.
92. Atwater EC. Touching the patient: the teaching of internal medicine in America. In Leavitt JW, Numbers RL, eds. *Sickness and Health in America: Readings in the History of Medicine and Public Health* (2d Ed.). Madison: University of Wisconsin Press, 1985:131.
93. Ludmerer KM. *Learning to Heal: The Development of American Medical Education*. New York: Basic Books, 1985:22.
94. Ibid, p. 33.
95. Lilienfeld DE. "The greening of epidemiology": sanitary physicians and the London Epidemiological Society (1830-1870). Bull Hist Med 1979;52:511.
96. Rosen G. *A History of Public Health*. New York: MD Publications, 1958:260-261.
97. Lilienfeld DE. "The greening of epidemiology": sanitary physicians and the London Epidemiological Society (1830-1870). Bull Hist Med 1979;52:513.
98. Ibid, p. 511.
99. Ibid, p. 517.
100. Brockington FC. *Public Health in the Nineteenth Century*. Edinburgh: Livingstone, 1965.
101. Ibid, p. 520.
102. Epidemiological Society of London. *The Commemoration Volume: Containing An Account of the Foundation of the Society and an Index of the Papers Read at Its Meetings Between 1855-1900*. London: Shaw, 1901:4.
103. Battiscombe G. *Shaftesbury: A Biography of the Seventh Earl, 1801-1885*. London: Constable, 1974:222.
104. Ibid, p. 223.
105. Epidemiological Society of London. *The Commemoration Volume: Containing An Account of the Foundation of the Society and an Index of the Papers Read at Its Meetings Between 1855-1900*. London: Shaw, 1901:4.
106. Ibid, p. 7.
107. Lilienfeld DE. "The greening of epidemiology": sanitary physicians and the London Epidemiological Society (1830-1870). Bull Hist Med 1979;52:521.
108. Epidemiological Society of London. *The Commemoration Volume: Containing An Account of the Foundation of the Society and an Index of the Papers Read at Its Meetings Between 1855-1900*. London: Shaw, 1901:10.
109. Ibid, p. 12.

110. Ibid, p. 54.
111. Ibid, pp. 55-79.
112. Ibid.
113. Lilienfeld DE. "The greening of epidemiology": sanitary physicians and the London Epidemiological Society (1830-1870). Bull Hist Med 1979;52:525.
114. Newsholme A. *Fifty Years in Public Health: A Personal Narrative With Comments.* London: Allen & Unwin, 1935:104-105.
115. Lilienfeld DE. "The greening of epidemiology": sanitary physicians and the London Epidemiological Society (1830-1870). Bull Hist Med 1979;52:525.
116. Ibid, pp. 525-526.
117. Ibid, p. 526.
118. Ibid.
119. Ibid.
120. Newsholme A. *Fifty Years in Public Health: A Personal Narrative with Comments.* London: Allen & Unwin, 1935:105.
121. Ludmerer KM. *Learning to Heal: The Development of American Medical Education.* New York: Basic Books, 1985:18.
122. Smillie WG. *Public Health: Its Promise for the Future.* New York: Macmillan, 1955:160.
123. Rosen G. *A History of Public Health.* New York: MD Publications, 1958:242.
124. Ibid, p. 303.
125. Rosenkrantz BG. *Public Health and the State: Changing Views in Massachusetts, 1842-1936.* Cambridge: Harvard University Press, 1972:40-44.
126. Smillie WG. *Public Health: Its Promise for the Future.* New York: Macmillan, 1955:253.
127. Garrison FH. *An Introduction to the History of Medicine.* 4th Ed. Philadelphia: Saunders, 1929:440.
128. Ibid, p. 633.
129. Lilienfeld DE, Lilienfeld AM. The French influence on the development of epidemiology. In: Lilienfeld AM. *Times, Places and Persons: Aspects of the History of Epidemiology.* Baltimore: Johns Hopkins, 1980:35.
130. Atwater EC. Touching the patient: the teaching of internal medicine in America. In: Leavitt JW, Numbers RL, eds. *Sickness and Health in America: Readings in the History of Medicine and Public Health* (2d Ed.). Madison: University of Wisconsin Press, 1985:131.
131. Ludmerer KM. *Learning to Heal: The Development of American Medical Education.* New York: Basic Books, 1985:23.
132. Shimkin MB. The numerical method in therapeutic medicine. Public Health Rep 1964;79:1-12.
133. Pearl R. *Introduction to Medical Biometry and Statistics*, 3d Ed. Philadelphia: Saunders, 1941:23.

3
Changing Paradigms

The usual account has *Hygieia*, the Greek goddess of health, as the daughter of *Æsculapius*; others place her as the latter's wife. The Encyclopedia Britannica, however, states that "[t]he oldest traces of her cult...are to be found at Titane...where she was worshiped together with Æsculapius, to whom she appears completely assimilated, not an independent personality." From that perspective medicine should embrace not only prevention and treatment but what we now refer to as health promotion and health maintenance. Until comparatively recently they were all part of a whole; they were all part of the mission of those endowed with the appellation "physician."

Led by Claude Bernard, interest in experimental physiology emerged during the last half of the nineteenth century. Bernard kept his laboratory close to patients, showed little interest in the work of the French hygienists, and hoped to influence the progress of clinical medicine over the long haul with improved understanding of the *milieu interieur*. New discoveries changed all that.

Others had previously suspected the existence of microorganisms, but Antonj van Leeuwenhoek (1632-1723), one-time city hall janitor, amateur naturalist, and later member of the Royal Society, is generally credited with providing the first detailed descriptions of microorganisms by means of his invention, the microscope. He did not, however, associate them with disease or ascribe particular significance to them. Several eighteenth-century physicians in Britain identified the infectious nature of puerperal fever, and in 1843 Harvard's Oliver Wendell Holmes argued that it could be prevented by regular handwashing on the part of birth attendants. These messages went unheeded until Ignaz Philipp Semmelweis (1818-1865), a Hungarian working as a junior physician in Vienna, demonstrated in 1849 by a carefully constructed comparative study the infectious nature of the disease, the source of the infection, the mode of transmission, and the means of prevention.

Many of his younger colleagues accepted the implications of Semmelweiss's findings, but his senior colleagues failed to understand them. Their fierce opposition has also been attributed to Semmelweiss's participation in the political events in Vienna of 1848. Liberal views resulted in his being denied a university appointment initially. Humiliated professionally, he grew disenchanted with Vienna and moved back to Budapest where in 1850 he became Professor of Obstetrics. A decade later, however, the hygienic practices he advocated for physicians were codified in law. As the sanitary idea was gaining momentum, the *bacteriological era* started in earnest. It was Semmelweis's pioneering application of epidemiological methods to the analysis of a clinical problem that helped to demonstrate their practical utility. He too can be counted as one of the early epidemiologists whose work influenced both medical practice and public policy.

In the midst of the multiple arenas in which medicine was advancing, the French chemist Louis Pasteur emerged. A brilliant scientist by any standard, he was initially a crystallographer and developed the field of stereochemistry. Moving on to the study of fermentation and subsequently to the study of microorganisms, he gave expanded credibility to the field of bacteriology. Others had preceded him, and his contemporaries were far from idle, but Pasteur's work set a new tone, standards, and aspirations for medical science. His epoch-making discoveries helped to precipitate a major paradigm shift for medicine; the shift was to last a century or more—it was a prelude to the schism. Pasteur was largely responsible for enunciating the "germ theory" of disease and legitimizing the bacteriological era. To Pasteur, "germs" were not "good" or "bad"; they existed and required investigation. A scientist characterized by boundless curiosity, enormous energy, and great compassion, his interests were in the unexplored worlds of the endless new species of microorganisms he and his colleagues were describing. Meticulous investigations led to identification of the physical characteristics, the means of propagation, and the relationships of these new "populations" that inhabited worldly space with humans. His findings were applicable both to commercial processes, Pasteur's initial arena of inquiry, and to diseases afflicting his fellow citizens. Pasteur increased the precision with which specific microorganisms were associated with infectivity. But infectivity is not synonymous with either ill-health or disease, and not all diseases, then or now, involve microorganisms.

Interest in immunity was initiated by Edward Jenner, another country practitioner, as a result of his experiments with cowpox and the derivative practice of vaccination. Jenner embraced a broad ecological paradigm. He was as much concerned with the host's experiences with disease and the resultant responses as he was with a presumed disease agent itself. The same was true for a number of Pasteur's colleagues 75 years later. For example, Ilya Metchnikoff (1845-1916) argued strenuously for assigning as much importance to the body's reactions to the microbes as to the microbes themselves (the phagocytic theory of immunity), and Alexandre Yersin (1863-1943) stressed the importance of toxins and antitoxins in producing the manifestations of disease (the humoral theory of immunity). In spite of the advances made by bacteriology, William Osler (1849-1919) never stopped reminding us that: "It is as important to know what kind of a man has the disease, as it is to know what kind of a disease has the man!" Almost two centuries after Jenner's observations, there is now greatly renewed interest in the importance of immunity in health and disease, especially in the new field of psychoneuroimmunology (see Chapter 6).

The advent of the bacteriological era did more than overshadow concern for the host's role in the genesis of disease. The ecological paradigm that emphasized the

importance of individuals interacting with one another and with their "environments" to create healthy or unhealthy states—the sanitary idea—while helped
scientifically was also adumbrated as the model for medical research. The
power of the earlier paradigm had already been demonstrated by John Snow's
identification of water systems contaminated with sewage as the medium by
which cholera was spread. Flight of the population from the lethal environment
and removal of the handle on the Broad Street pump had promptly ameliorated
the epidemic without benefit of the germ theory; the prevailing ecological
theory had been adequate for effective action. Epidemiological thinking applied
by Snow, a prominent clinician, had shown the way. Now a different, much
more restrictive, but at the same time highly productive paradigm evolved.
Henceforward, the way medicine perceived the origins, prevention, and treatment of disease was to be different. The search for specific organisms was to
provide the framework for deploying society's intellectual and material resources to advance medical research, guiding medical education, organizing its
personal health services, and implementing new knowledge directed at improving the public's health.

This is not the place to recount once more the scientific miracles wrought by
Pasteur and his followers. Formerly dreaded diseases that killed millions have been
eliminated or brought under control—yellow fever, typhus, typhoid, diphtheria,
poliomyelitis, rabies, scarlet fever, and smallpox are only the more obvious. Other
potentially noxious organisms have been identified, and efficacious immunization,
vaccination, control measures, and treatments developed. There is no question that
his contributions had a fundamental impact on the course of medicine and public
health for many decades and that much permanent good flowed from his work.
What concerns us here is the massive shift in priorities, sites, and emphases in
medical research occasioned by his work; the impact of these sea changes cannot
be overemphasized.

The first victims of the bacteriological era were the hygienists and their movement. If diseases could result from almost any noxious, even untoward, interaction,
then where should one begin the search for methods of intervention? For example,
in 1876 the matters under discussion by the hygienists included "water, lifesavers,
gymnastics, women's work, 'methods of developing among the laboring classes a
spirit of thrift and saving habit,' alcoholism, and working-class housing."[1] The
prospect of narrowing the "search" implied by the prospect of a single "germ" as
the cause of disease was almost irresistible in the face of all the nebulous and
daunting alternatives. But much might have been accomplished had the hygienists
prevailed. As the French sociologist Bruno Latour observes:

> [W]ithout the microbe, without vaccine, even without the doctrine of contagion or
> variation in virulence, everything that was done [after Pasteur's discoveries] could
> have been done: cleaning up the towns; digging drains; demanding running water,
> light, air and heat. Pettenkofer who swallowed cholera bacilli without becoming ill
> but made Munich a healthy city through large-scale public works, is for everyone the
> eponym of this attitude in history.[2]

It is the hygienist movement that defined what was at stake, prescribed the aims, posed the problems, demanded that others should solve them, distributed praise or blame, and laid down priorities.[3]

The germ theory offered a "quick fix" for the epidemic diseases of the times. This allowed politicians, industrialists, landowners, and even the medical profession to avoid the hygienists' and the social reformers' message, a message that was bound to engender vehement opposition from many vested interests. Speedy results without social and political upheaval were promised by the advent of the germ theory.

If the hygienists were the Pasteurians' strongest allies, they were also the greatest casualties of "pasteurization." They were taken over by the bacteriologists; they lost their own identity and with it much of their power and influence. Gradually their interests shifted from microbe hunting to preoccupation with processes and implementation of measures to contain bacteria. The *Revue Scientifique* published fewer and fewer scientific articles but more and more about professional sanitary organizations, methods of water purification, ways to set up bacteriological monitoring stations, and methods for "policing" the environment. The public was to be informed, educated, and retrained with new habits. "If we are beginning to get the disinfection of hotel rooms implemented...it is thanks to the publicity already given by the newspapers to the contagiousness of tuberculosis, which is making new arrivals demand guarantees."[4] The drive was on to influence the public who in turn coerced the innkeepers to disinfect the premises to drive out the tubercle bacillus.

Controversies originally promoted by the hygienists about the role of "scientific medicine" in the improvement of health continued over the next century. Like Chadwick and Shattuck and, in the twentieth century, René Dubos, Ivan Illich, and the late Thomas McKeown (1913-1988), they argued that most of the improvement in the public's health can be attributed to better nutrition, housing, working conditions, sanitation and, more recently, population control.[5-7]

Vital and health statistics had to some extent quantified the temporal and human dimensions of epidemics. The apparently erratic character and distribution of epidemics was reflected in the crude nature of the available data. Mortality statistics suggested *what* the problems were but less frequently *where* they were and, until Snow's work, with what other conditions or circumstances they were associated. The hygienists and the political reformers were in the ascendancy and experimental physiology was proceeding slowly, but there were no dramatic breakthroughs. Skepticism about the efficacy of clinical medicine supported by Louis's numerical method was making inroads against the tenuous basis for clinical practice. Into this environment Pasteur stepped and perhaps unwittingly, seized the initiative from the other players. Latour observes that:

...[I]n 1880 there was *no connection* between an infectious disease and a laboratory....At the time, a disease was something idiosyncratic, which could be understood only on its own ground and in terms of circumstances. This could not be put inside the walls of a laboratory.[8]

What Pasteur and his colleagues did was to connect "diseases" and "laboratories." "They were to succeed by moving diseases on to the terrain of the laboratory where they, the Pasteurians, had the upper hand. They therefore forced all those groups interested in infectious diseases, but who expected nothing of consequence to emerge from the laboratory, to become interested in those laboratories."[9] The experimental physiologists, medical "numeracists," emerging epidemiologists, medical statisticians, hygienists, and social reformers were suddenly all complementary to Pasteur's innovations. The earlier ascendancy of the hygienists and of *hygiène publique*, or public health as it came to be known was halted.

Pasteur also used statistical methods in designing his experiments and simulating epidemics. "With laboratory-made statistics he counted the sick and the dead, and those that underwent spontaneous cure. He performed on dogs, chickens, sheep, what the hygienists did with the help of nationally made statistics on real populations."[10] The statisticians could scarcely complain that such a meticulous investigator as Pasteur was ignoring their concepts and methods.

The laboratory—and it rapidly became a highly focused type of bench laboratory—was to be the center of most medical progress for a century; medical research became synonymous with bacteriology and, more specifically, the bacteriological laboratory. From this quite reasonable, virtually imperative, development great benefits flowed, but in its wake many other potentially fruitful arenas for research were placed in limbo.

The Pasteurians reformulated not only the answers but also the questions. By focusing on microorganisms they did not even embrace the whole of pathology but only those aspects relating to the symptoms of the disease under study, the reverse of the clinical situation. Pasteurians asked: "What 'bug' is associated with this 'disease'?" Clinicians asked: "What 'disease' is associated with this 'symptom'?" Similarly those "bug hunters" who embraced epidemiological methods did not have to cover the whole broad range of epidemiological evidence but restricted themselves to studying the epidemiology of microbes.

What Pasteur and his colleagues did was to demonstrate and then reify the link from the disease to the microbe while virtually excluding all other predisposing, proximate, precipitating, and perpetuating links or causes as they now began to be referred to in medical circles. For example, the words anthrax bacillus became a code term for all those other characteristics that were formerly subsumed under the term anthrax. A single "cause" was substituted for either a "causal chain" or a "web of causality." As Latour points out: "Without this link and translation, Pasteur would have had a microbe that performed certain things *in* the laboratory and a disease left to itself *outside* the laboratory with endless talk filling the gap."[11]

Pasteur employed clear-cut dichotomies in his investigations: present or absent; before or after; pure or impure; living or dead. Scientists and laymen alike could understand this language. Better still he demonstrated quantitatively and graphically at the population level, in both the scientific literature and to interested audiences, the impact of such findings as those resulting from the use of Anthrax vaccine and the reduction in the mortality of huge livestock herds from 9 to 0.65.

Not only was France "pasteurized" but so was much of Europe, including Britain, where Lord Lister (1827-1912) revolutionized surgery by the extension of Pasteur's concepts to antisepsis. A complete Pasteurian takeover of medicine was in prospect. The end of curative medicine was predicted, and preventive medicine was seen as the wave of the future. "Pasteur alone...has made more progress in medicine than have 10,000 practitioners more competent than he in medical science."[12] The physicians of the day faced the prospect of becoming obsolete according to this scenario.

With Pasteur and the bacteriologists in the ascendancy they proceeded to redefine not only the doctors but also the hygienists and even the sciences, at least the natural sciences. For the ecological, even "holistic," paradigm that had guided the medical and health enterprises heretofore, there was substituted a massive search-and-destroy mission directed at *the* causal agent associated with each disease. The prior theories of disease causation with their appeals to assorted deities, evil spirits, miasma, and "spontaneous generation" were banished. The emerging fields of experimental physiology, natural selection, and later cell biology were at best implicit rather than explicit influences on research and practice. Whatever the limitations of each (and there were obviously many), they had the great merit of leaving open the possibilities for new and broader theories and explanations of variations in the human condition we refer to as diseases. The core ideas in the theory of miasma might have become, in the long run, as powerful as those embodied in the theory of contagion. The former theory (miasma) was inclusive, even holistic, and epidemiological in its concepts and even its methods; it was in many ways closely related to the concepts embraced by Johann Peter Frank. The latter theory (contagion) was reductionist and exclusionary.[13] A mono-etiological concept of causality ensued and was, of course, strongly supported by the expanding identification of ever more microorganisms.

The advent of the Pasteurian revolution made many of those possibilities seem remote and even absurd; no respectable physician, scientist, or hygienist would consider tackling them. Contagion became the received wisdom; the place to look was wherever microorganisms might be thought to lurk. The site for research was to be the laboratory, especially the bacteriology laboratory. The place to care for the bulk of patients was in the infectious disease hospital. And the way to improve health was through controlling the quality of the water and food supply, and ensuring safe sanitation; all useful interventions. But what mattered most for medicine was pursuit of the "big bug hunt." The population and the environment in which people were born, worked, lived, and died (along with the bugs, parasites, and other unknown entities that also inhabited the planet) were less and less seen as the arenas of observation and the objects of investigation.

None of this should diminish our gratitude for the extraordinary benefits to all mankind stemming from the work of Pasteur and his followers. Nor is it fruitful to speculate about what might have evolved had microorganisms never been discovered and had vaccines never been developed. What should be noted, however, is the way in which the bacteriological era and the accompanying monoetiological paradigm overshadowed, even shut out, other theories of health and disease, other approaches to improving health or containing risks, and other modes of clinical practice. Scientific and clinical myopia gradually came to characterize the work of all those concerned with the health and medical enterprises.

The obsession with pasteurization and disinfection spread to the United States; it is still a dominant cultural theme. An address to the New York Academy of Medicine during this period was entitled "Bacteriomania." The speaker warned the profession not to rely on a single theory of causation to explain all the complexities of etiology, pathology, and therapeutics. "If the bacteriomania of modern time has not been accepted uniformly as the universal gospel of modern pathology," the speaker observed, "that merit...belongs to a great extent to Virchow."[14] At the very first meeting of the American Public Health Association a paper on "Disinfection and Disinfectants" was presented; this was followed by a discussion of the "Germ Theory of Disease and its Relation to Hygiene" by the then president of Columbia University. Tests of efficacy focused on the power of disinfectants rather than on drugs and other patient-oriented interventions.[15] Occupational hazards, overcrowding, malnutrition, alcoholism, poverty, and the stress and strain of attempting to survive were neglected as disinfection dominated public efforts to control disease. "[T]he poor were the ones who were now besieged by the hygienists, the biologists, the public authorities, the physicians, the surgeons, the midwives, the prefects, the mayors, the disinfection services, the teachers, the army doctors."[16]

For clinical medicine, the relative impotence of physicians was exposed for all to see as the focus shifted from the patient and the disease to the microorganism. Physicians were enlisted, even coerced, through quarantine laws and the promotion of sanitation, into participating in the endless search for microbes as *the* causes of disease. Later the use of serum for treatment provided a modicum of efficacy to the physician's limited armamentarium. The notion that there might be other approaches to health and healing came to be regarded as charlatanism; bacteriological orthodoxy became the dominating paradigm.

The ideas and methods of Louis, and his patient-oriented efforts to assess the efficacy of clinical interventions, receded in the face of the Pasteurian revolution. His influence waned in the face of the successes wrought by the microbe hunters in demonstrating the presence of causal agents, but not necessarily in successfully treating patients. This era may have been responsible for introducing into medical education and practice the quaint notion that accurate diagnosis is more important than efficacious treatment and management of the patient's problem.

If Pasteur's genius established the experimental and theoretical basis for the germ theory of disease, Robert Koch provided the exquisite methods and techniques that firmly established the field as a distinct scientific discipline. He was "unquestionably the greatest bacteriologist the world has seen."[17] Research proceeded apace not only to establish the causal microbes associated with domestic epidemics but also for those plaguing the tropics and frequently decimating the colonial populations on which commerce and trade depended. Bacteria were frequently replaced by parasites and insects but the paradigm was the same; these were *the* causes of the diseases. Microbes were henceforth to be viewed as both necessary and sufficient factors in the genesis of disease.

Max von Pettenkofer (1818-1901), chemist, pharmacist, physiologist, physician, and founder of experimental hygiene, however, took exception to Koch's theory
that a bacillus was the cause of cholera.[18] Pettenkofer held that for a patient to become
ill with cholera four conditions were essential: (1) a specific microorganism; (2) certain
local conditions; (3) certain seasonal conditions; and (4) certain individual conditions.[19]
At the age of 74 he put his doubts about Koch's hypothesis to the test. Together with
an assistant who repeated the experiment, von Pettenkofer swallowed a vial of cholera
vibrio supplied by Professor George Gaffky (1850-1918) of Koch's laboratory. Both
men lived to tell the tale. This story, often repeated, has two versions. One states that
the culture received from Gaffky was obtained from the watery stools of a patient
dying of cholera in the epidemic then ravaging Hamburg.[20] Another version states
that Koch's laboratory sent von Pettenkofer a weakly virulent culture of the
bacteria.[21] Nevertheless he and his assistant seem to have made the point that, in
addition to a microorganism associated with a high mortality rate, a susceptible
host and an inhospitable environment are required before clinical manifestations
appear. The presence of an infectious agent is not the same as the occurrence of
disease—relationships still not fully appreciated by all members of the medical
profession or the public.

The field of immunology advanced, but largely from the point of view of the
microbe, not from that of the patient or the population. The natural history, the
habitat, and the life cycle of the microorganism became the centers of attention.
There was diminishing interest in the natural history of the patient's illness and
domestic, occupational, and social habitats and the life cycle of the individual's
encounters with family, friends, and community. There had been a massive shift
in the balance of forces comprising the armies of investigators, teachers, practitioners, and administrators concerned with medicine and health. Pasteurians
"were able to renew medicine *without ever taking disease as an object of study* and
to renew politics *without ever taking the poor or the social outcast as a unit of
analysis.*"[22] The common enemy was the microbe and the language of medicine
became the language of bacteriology. The search was on for a single cause for each
disease, and for a "magic bullet" to demolish it. Microbes even seemed to join
people and property as the principal components of society. Extraordinary benefits
ensued from the declaration that "bugs are the enemy" but there were equally great
costs.

Among the latter, as suggested earlier, was the co-opting of epidemiology by
bacteriology and the germ theory. John Snow's insights into the distribution
patterns of disease and the presence of pockets of extreme virulence and others of
relative safety, the ecological relationship between the sources and the consumption of water, the geographic patterns of sewage disposal and water intake and,
most importantly, the requirements for control of the epidemic, all seem to have
been minimized during the ensuing 50 years or more. Exceptions in Europe and
the United States were numerous epidemiological investigations of contagious
diseases conducted without knowledge of either the presence or characteristics of
so-called etiological agents.[23] These descriptive studies might have led to a wide
variety of causal hypotheses were it not for the all-powerful impact of bacteriology.[24]

Using epidemiological concepts, observational methods, and a primitive clinical trial, clinicians such as James Lind (1716-1794) had demonstrated the importance of citrus fruits in the prevention of scurvy.[25] A retired country practitioner, Sir George Baker (1722-1809), using similar inductive and epidemiological reasoning, demonstrated in 1767 that the drinking of cider contaminated with lead was associated with the Devonshire Colic, characterized by abdominal pain and "palsy" of the wrists and arms—lead poisoning.[26] Sir Percival Pott (1714-1788), a renowned surgeon, recognized in 1775 that cancer of the scrotum was an occupational hazard of chimney sweeps.[27] Building on the pioneering work of Bernardo Ramazzini (1683-1714), the father of industrial hygiene, or occupational medicine as it came to be called, clinicians such as Charles Turner Thackrah (1795-1833), a surgeon in Leeds and founder of that city's medical school, published a volume on *The Effects of Arts, Trades and Professions on Health and Longevity* in 1835. Thackrah documented the deleterious impact of contemporary working conditions on health with resulting incapacity, permanent disabilities, and premature death. Among the noxious influences he associated with a wide range of accidents, diseases, and disabilities were dust and other atmospheric pollutants, unnatural body postures, excessive muscular effort, "close work" affecting vision, high temperature, "anxiety and mental worry," and "low, varied, and uncertain wages."[28] More recently (1887) Baron T. Kanehiro Takaki (1858-1920) found that a diet of polished rice was associated with the onset of beriberi and that adding fish, meat, and vegetables virtually eliminated the disease.[29] Somewhat later (1926), Joseph Goldberger's (1874-1929) classic experiments demonstrated that pellagra was associated with dietary deficiency of a factor in vitamin B, subsequently determined to be nicotinic acid; it was not an infectious disease as many had thought.[30]

With the onset of the germ theory, the prospect of describing a single, necessary, and tangible factor took precedence over searching for many other factors that might prove more amenable to elimination or modification than any microorganism—again, not an unreasonable strategy given the state of knowledge at the time. But the medical detective work required to determine the relative importance of dietary, occupational, and environmental factors associated with other diseases was given increasingly short shrift.

In Britain, Sir John Simon, the enormously creative Medical Officer to the General Board of Health, sought to develop the scientific underpinnings of public health. He describes the two major categories of research pursued in the Board's laboratories: Infectious Processes—Acute and Chronic, and Organic Chemistry. "[T]ill 1883, both these lines of work were followed; but from 1883, when the more physiological study was brought to a close, the investigations have found sufficient subject-matter in questions of *Infection* and *Disinfection*, including the intimate special pathology of various *Infective Diseases*, and of late much particular study relating to questions of *Prophylaxis*."[31]

In the United States as well, control of environmental pollutants and of what came to be called communicable diseases merged. The bacteriology laboratory became the final arbiter of causation for the hygienists, and also for the new public health movement, as Health Departments, starting with Rhode Island and Michigan in 1888 and followed by New York in 1892, opened what were essentially bacteriology laboratories. The privately owned Hoagland Laboratory in Brooklyn seems to have been the first used to teach bacteriology to medical students. Not only had epidemiology become virtually synonymous with bacteriology but so had medical research.[32] In spite of the messages brought back by Louis's students, "[e]pidemiology, as a science, got a halting start in America and did not get into its stride until after World War I. [Charles V.] Chapin's productive studies in Providence, relating to the epidemiology of communicable diseases of childhood, and the work of Lumsden, Frost, Rosenau, and Carter of the United States Public Health Service stand out as oases in a great desert of unproductive efforts."[33]

The influence of various movements and forces—social, political, and scientific—on the evolution of both the paradigms and the institutions that attempt to address society's problems of health and disease is well illustrated by the bacteriological takeover. If Hygieia and Æsculapius were as closely bound in spirit and action as some accounts would have us believe, by the end of the nineteenth century they were drifting apart, a prelude to the schism yet to come. Perhaps this drift strengthened the version that had Hygieia, the daughter of Æsculapius, as his mate and not an integral part of the total persona.

Society benefited in ways heretofore undreamed of from the combined efforts of the Pasteurians and the social reformers. Each contributed massively to redefining the unacceptable. The cost was great, however. And we have not seen the end, as the technological era is superimposed on the bacteriological era. In Europe and America the implications for medical education and the attitudes and priorities of the medical profession were enormous. Today many leaders of academic medicine, public health, and the medical establishment have grown up believing that bugs are the principal problems; in many settings specialists in infectious diseases continue to hold positions of great power and influence.

The genesis of this state of affairs merits brief review. The earliest initiatives in both Britain and the United States to standardize medical credentials and raise educational standards lost opportunities to broaden the perspective of physicians. In England, Sir John Simon described medicine's status 10 years after enactment of the first Public Health Act and just before the passage of the Medical Act of 1858. He wrote:

> The legal titles of medical practitioners were as varied as the names of snuffs or sauces. Twenty-one disconnected corporate authorities within the United Kingdom were issuing their heterogeneous credentials of qualification (more or less) for responsibilities in Medicine. The authorities were mainly of medieval root; some in trade-guild sort, some in sorts ecclesiastical. From an authority of the former sort, a man might hold a license to practice medical or surgical business within particular boundaries; or from an authority of the other sort (perhaps deriving primarily from the pope) he might be certified to the world at large as an orthodox teacher of medicine, who, if competent to teach, was inferentially also competent to practice: but the licenses and degrees did not secure anything like a professional preserve to those who held them;

for though in some cases poachers were threatened, there was in effect almost no restriction on practice, and any one who chose might entitle himself *surgeon* or *doctor*....[34]

....Against this disorderly state of things, public-spirited members of the profession had long, but vainly, protested: urging that the various medical titles ought to be brought to have real significance; ought, all of them, to guarantee the possession of professional skill and knowledge according to some one common standard of minimum-qualification, and ought, under that condition, to carry equal privilege in all parts of the Kingdom. Legislation for purposes such as these could scarcely have been opposed on any reasonable ground; but whenever it had been attempted, the intricacies of parts of the matter, and the antagonisms and jealousies of so many conflicting jurisdictions and interests, had shown a chaos which statesmen in general could only regard with despair.[35]

And so began the formal organization of medicine's practicing and academic branches as state-sanctioned enterprises in Britain. The Act created the General Medical Council, a body apart from the professional organizations (i.e., the Royal Colleges and the embryonic British Medical Association) and the universities. The Council had two principal functions. The first was responsibility for maintaining one central register on which all authorized medical practitioners would be listed. The second was responsibility for approving and overseeing all medical education throughout the country, a matter of interest in connection with the theme of this volume.

With this power over the broad contents of the medical curriculum came opportunities to guide, and influence, the overall paradigm within which medical education was conducted. Here, indeed, was a golden opportunity to reinforce the advances already made in improving the public's health, to make certain that medical students were exposed to discussions of the full spectrum of factors that were believed to influence health and disease, and to discuss the clinician's responsibility for preventing disease as well as for treating it. But little was done to include such instruction in the medical curriculum, to say nothing of requiring the professors to set examples of disease prevention through their own practices, or demonstrate their concern for the public's health.

For the bottom-up or population-based approaches advocated by Petty, Frank, and Virchow, and the population-based research of the early epidemiologists, a top-down—many would say elitist—ivory-tower perspective was substituted. This was no deliberate decision; nor was the subtle shift in interests and priorities accomplished from any but the highest motives. The professors gradually restricted their concerns to hospitals and adjacent bacteriology laboratories; as a consequence their own exposure to the population's health problems became ever more constricted. Again, the prospect that for the first time laboratory research could yield at least better understanding of some diseases, if not improved therapies, was a thoroughly reasonable basis for assigning it top priority.

The health needs of the public, however, could not be ignored. Instead of broadening the General Medical Council's mandate with respect to the content of undergraduate medical education, the British Parliament in 1886 passed an amending act giving the General Medical Council power to establish a postgraduate Diploma in Public Health. This was to certify competence in "sanitary science" for medical graduates who wished to become Medical Officers of Health as recommended by the Royal Sanitary Commission (1869-1871) and instituted by the Public Health Act of 1875.[36] To their great credit, the academicians of the day did see the importance of physicians to the public health enterprise. What they did not perceive was the creeping impact of reductionism on medicine's intellectual paradigm, the so-called *medical model*, as it came to be called. This process initiated and energized by the advances in bacteriology constrained the vision of academic medicine for a century.

The work of the social reformers and the impact of the sanitary idea were making a substantial difference. Because sanitation was rapidly becoming the handmaiden of bacteriology, the professors had no reason to question these initiatives, but practical implementation was another matter. By the last quarter of the nineteenth century, Britain had been divided into several thousand sanitary areas each presided over by a District Medical Officer who was usually a part-time local practitioner. Within the next few decades additional part-time practitioners were appointed as "factory surgeons" overseeing compliance with the Factory and Workshop Acts of 1878. Later came School Doctors, and then Maternity and Child Doctors, followed by others responsible for providing public services to patients with tuberculosis, venereal diseases, and mental deficiency. The gradual accretion of categorical approaches to discrete diseases was to characterize the public health movement for decades to come (see Chapter 1). For every "disease" or health problem there was to be a separate vertical "program" or cadre of health workers.[37] This fractionated solution foreshadowed the schism's emergence.

The state was pressing the profession aggressively by redefining the unacceptable through legislation. There was little evidence in Britain, however, that the practicing medical profession at the individual or micro level was responding. The medical education of undergraduates failed to provide them with an understanding of strategies for prevention or for improving the public's health. As a consequence "between 1874 and 1930 Parliament imposed statutory duties of a *preventive* kind upon *every registered medical practitioner*."[38] These draconian measures achieved only limited success with the core of the academic medical profession and the practitioners who had been their students. Prevention may have been the political watchword at the time, but the excitement associated with the new advances in bacteriology was determining the educational and research priorities for the academicians. Curative medicine was still relatively impotent but it dominated medical education and practice; public health and preventive medicine soon were to evolve in a world of their own.

In 1875 a distinguished Professor of Surgery, first at Zürich and later at Vienna, Theodor Billroth (1829-1894), published a classic volume on the evolution of medical education in the German states.[39] His extensive historical and substantive review provides a second example of the gradual but unrelenting separation of clinical medicine from public health. Billroth described the evolution of medical education in the German-speaking countries and their intellectual and scientific posture towards the end of the nineteenth century. The academic establishment in collaboration with the state asserted leadership and shaped the paradigm within which medical research would be pursued and the education of physicians conducted.[40]

The Prussian state qualifying examinations gradually were expanded with respect to content and extended geographically to cover the North German Federation. Both moves led to formal promulgation in 1869 of more extensive rules governing all state examinations for medical licensure. In turn this dictated what was to be emphasized in teaching and examinations conducted by the country's universities. An even more important issue was determination of the examiners. Were they to be university professors or practitioners? Billroth had no doubts; he believed the academicians should establish and control the standards. Their perspectives, values, and experience should determine the content of medical education.[41]

Nothing is said about "prevention" or "preventive medicine" in Billroth's treatise. He points out that "public health" was included in the curricula of all German medical schools and was taught as the three fields of medical jurisprudence, public sanitation, and hygiene.[42] In spite of the efforts of statisticians, the practitioners of the numerical method, and the epidemiologists, Billroth's views seem to embody the priorities of the entrenched professors of the day:

> From a scientific point of view it would be possible **to oppose the claims of all these subjects to be taught at the university**, for in teaching them we are not concerned with the investigation of scientific questions outside the sphere of chemistry, anatomy, physiology, pathological anatomy, general pathology and etiology, toxicology, practical medicine, surgery, ophthalmology and obstetrics—sciences that are already represented—but with the application of these sciences to quite definite unfortunate and harmful social conditions. They, like political economy, are still struggling for their separate scientific existence (emphasis added by KLW).[43]

He went on to affirm, sarcastically:

> ...The physician, as one of the most important members of the community, is expected not only to help in cases of individual sickness, but in community diseases as well. He is even expected to do his part in curing the stupidity and indifference of humanity. A beautiful task, but one that can be accomplished only by many generations of physicians, and then only imperfectly!...The fanatical champions of public health are fighting for a goal that is too high for my myopic vision. I can admire the struggle, but I cannot become interested in it.[44]

This pronouncement is surely another herald of the schism, now emerging. Billroth argues for a substantial shift in the interests, values, and priorities of academic medicine, certainly in Germany. The ideas and ideals of Frank and Virchow were to be abandoned; the laboratory, driven by the "big bug hunt" was to take precedence over the population and the environment as the locus for research and intervention. Promulgation of such notions had reverberations throughout Europe and America that continue to this day. Billroth's account of medical education in the Germanic countries is replete with great detail about the structure, organization, staffing, and equipping of the medical schools. Much is also written about the curriculum, costs, tuition, the examiners, and the examinations. By contrast there is little or nothing said about the mission of the profession, the objectives of medical education, or the underlying paradigm that was to guide the whole endeavor. Process took precedence over purpose.

In spite of his new priorities Billroth evinced great respect for Frank. It was as an inspirational teacher, however, that he revered him, rather than as someone with important ideas about the origins of disease and what medicine as a profession serving society might do about them. In Billroth's view the individual patient should be the focus of the medical profession's ministrations; the precursors of illness and the state of the population's health were not concerns for the medical faculty.[45] Today these views still dominate discussions about the missions of most contemporary medical schools.

On the one hand, we see the gradual denigration of public health throughout the medical curriculum by the leading medical academicians. On the other, we observe rejection of the broader paradigm espoused by Frank. There is no mention by Billroth of epidemiology or of the numerical method in the curricula of the Germanic schools. At best the problems of safe water supplies and adequate sanitation were seen as municipal problems to be left to the District Physicians, first introduced by Prussia in 1825 and formalized by Ministerial Order in 1873.

Two emerging conflicts were represented by Billroth's expressions of values and priorities. First was the issue of the balance in the content of medical education between the viewpoints, interests, and priorities of the two major branches of the profession—the academic faculties and the practitioners in the community. Should medical education be based on the academicians' limited clinical experiences as hospital-based consultants? Should it be based on the experiences of the communities' practitioners in their day-to-day encounters with unselected patients? Or should both perspectives and experiences be weighted in some way? Second was the conflict over the scientific content of the educational experience. Should it be based largely on the current research interests of the professors, or should it reflect all the concerns of society that center on health and disease? In the Germanic universities the first viewpoints apparently prevailed in both instances; they became sufficiently rooted in the academic culture to dominate the entire medical enterprise. There was apparently no contest; Billroth and his contemporaries had seized control. The schism was now almost inevitable.

In the United States recognition of the need for regulating practice and awareness of the power associated with that authority resulted in a rather different process but a similar outcome. During the nineteenth century state medical societies and schools of medicine were vying with one another in setting standards and in seeking authority to license practitioners. Given the strong "states rights" traditions underlying the nation's origins, it was to be expected that a system would emerge for regulating medical practice by which state legislatures would grant authority to their own state medical societies to license practitioners. The first site for these enactments was New York in 1760; many other states followed shortly thereafter.

In the middle of the nineteenth century, while England was preparing to pass the Medical (Practice) Act of 1858, the United States rejected, as an elitist idea, the notion that all practitioners should be required to meet uniform, albeit only basic—even rudimentary—national standards.

Following the Civil War, however, there was a resurgence of interest in licensure at the state level, never at the federal level, and all the states gradually enacted licensing acts that essentially vested authority in the state medical societies to license and monitor physicians and their practices. This pluralism in regulation was further complicated by the assumption of internship control by the hospitals and the later advent of specialty organizations with their associated residency programs, and of boards that examined and certified their own candidates.

Dispersion of power undoubtedly had advantages in encouraging diversity but it also resulted in wide variations in standards across the country. For an emerging profession with little in the way of a scientific base or of traditions for performance and behavior, the content of medical education was left largely in the hands of the individual medical schools—both those that were university based and the numerous proprietary ones—and within the schools to the individual departments. By the first decades of the twentieth century, the American Medical Association's Council on Medical Education, the Association of American Medical Colleges, and the voluntary National Board of Medical Examiners were all in a position to influence the content and balance in medical education both directly and indirectly. The representatives of these bodies were, of course, primarily academicians. Their views and priorities prevailed.[46]

The foray into matters concerning the public's health by the American Medical Association described in Chapter 2 was short lived. Neither the practicing profession nor the emerging academic branch of the medical establishment showed much interest in prevention or public health; medical curricula reflected little emphasis on either. The two great European traditions in France and Germany that had advanced medical science engendered only a modest influence on American academic medicine and clinical practice. In spite of the exposure of many postgraduate medical students during the first three quarters of the nineteenth century to the French observational and quantitative methods, and of many others during the last third, to the Germanic experimental method, American medicine was slow to develop a tradition of medical research or to enunciate a guiding framework for medical education.[47]

Change began in 1871 with the drastic reform of medical education imposed on the Harvard medical faculty by Charles W. Eliot (1864-1926), the university's new president. Eliot, a chemist who had studied in both France and Germany and observed their systems of medical education, had concluded that the future of medicine lay through strengthening the "basic sciences," the "hard sciences." He decided that these had been neglected by the French clinicians in their pursuit of clinical acumen bolstered by application of the numerical method and that, in fact, French medicine was "decadent." Bitter faculty warfare ensued at Harvard.

The conflict was not, as in Germany, between the elite academicians and the practicing profession, but between two groups of academic elitists. Oliver Wendell

Holmes, a formidable figure in medical, literary, and social circles, and it will be recalled a student of Louis, was among the senior clinicians who opposed the plan advanced by Eliot and supported by several of the younger faculty trained in Germany or Austria. The educational reforms advocated and implemented "because," asserted Eliot, "there is a new President," gave much greater emphasis to laboratory medicine and much less to clinical experience.

There were other issues such as assumption of full control of the medical school by the university and the substitution of full-time salaries for the current practice of dividing up fee collections among the faculty, but laboratory medicine versus clinical skills dominated the debates. There seems little question, however, that Eliot's insistence on giving primacy to the laboratories and the basic sciences as the means for advancing all aspects of medical knowledge and as providing the underpinning for all medical education marked a turning point in American medicine. Clinical skills, the numeric method, and the population perspective were assigned second place. They were supplanted rapidly as arenas for serious concern by the truly remarkable advances in biomedical research that soon ensued.[48]

Experimentation was seen as superior to observation when it came to unravelling the mysteries of health and disease. The laboratory superseded the clinic and the bedside as the site for investigations. Concern for the community with its social and environmental influences on health and disease was largely disregarded. Research priorities, based principally on experiences with horizontal patients cared for in university teaching hospitals, dominated medical education. The German tradition of relating the problems of health and disease ever more closely to what were at first called the "natural sciences" soon gave way to a narrower spectrum of disciplines, employing the mechanistic model of the contemporary physical sciences, all to be studied in the hospital-based laboratory. The logic of this seems questionable since the principal "enemies" for the foreseeable future were proclaimed to be the microbes—biological organisms. The perspectives of the critical clinical observer using the model of the naturalist, the biologist, or the botanist observing phenomena in their natural habitats were replaced by those of the narrowly focused laboratory investigator using the model of Newtonian physics and chemistry and the reductionist model favored by the bacteriologists.

The patient and the community were not viewed as important sources of information for understanding the genesis, natural history, and management of disease at either the individual or population levels. All truly useful information was to come from study of the pathophysiological processes governing the anatomical and clinical manifestations and the course of disease. Effective preventive and therapeutic interventions, it was argued, were most apt to stem from laboratory investigations. The observational contributions of Petty, Graunt, Frank, Pettenkofer, Semmelweiss, Louis, Snow, and Farr, to recall some of those mentioned earlier, were of relatively minor import compared to the power of experimental laboratory methods.

Similarly the social reformers in England, Europe, and America—Chadwick, Shaftesbury, Virchow, Shattuck, and even the early leaders of the American Medical Association—were seen as a breed apart. By redefining the unacceptable in concrete terms these pioneers argued for improvements in housing, working conditions, and the urban infrastructure. As a consequence, they were viewed as threats to the property owners, newly emerging industrialists, and all others with a vested interest in maintaining the status quo; that is, so long as deterioration of the environment did not promote or perpetuate epidemics that decimated rich and poor alike. Virchow's aphorism went by the board.

The deprecating attitude toward "public health" espoused by medical academicians and unreservedly endorsed by leaders such as Billroth, and indirectly by President Eliot, represented the thin edge of the wedge. Germanic values and priorities in medical research and education were carried back to the United States by the tens of thousands of Americans who studied, even briefly, in German and Austrian universities during the last third of the nineteenth century and who continued to flock there until the beginning of World War I. Much good came of all this but there were also losses.

Not everyone accepted the prevailing viewpoint in Germany. William H. Welch (1850-1934), German-trained Professor of Pathology and Dean of The Johns Hopkins Medical School, wrote an Introduction to the 1924 English translation of Billroth's volume on medical education in Germany.[49] Welch himself had been a beneficiary of extensive indoctrination into scientific medicine as epitomized by laboratory experimentation, especially in the bacteriology laboratory, in contrast to clinical observation and therefore was fully aware of the potential of this new application of science to medicine. But Welch also recognized the narrowness of the paradigm Billroth and his peers were employing. Their denigration of a broader view of the population's health did not escape him. He wrote:

> Even more startling at the present time is Billroth's confession to a lack of interest—a "myopia" he calls it—in respect to public health and the diseases of the community, as distinct from those of the individual. With the immense progress since his day in the prevention of disease and the protection of health so frank a confession would not now be expected, but there is reason to believe that the vision of not a few members of the profession in matters of public health remains today as short-sighted as that of Billroth. Still in his [list] of the nine professors who should constitute the inner or restricted medical faculty is included, as the ninth, the chair of "social medicine" (medical jurisprudence, public health, hygiene).[50]

The stage was set during the first quarter of the twentieth century for a reassessment of the respective roles of clinical medicine and public health. Was the task of medicine and the health enterprise to be determined by the top-down view of the cloistered academicians, sequestered but nonetheless exceedingly productive in their laboratories, or was it to be determined from a bottom-up view as experienced by the population who did the suffering and paid the bills? Could a rational balance be achieved between the laboratory, the clinical, and the population perspectives? The earlier themes of political arithmetic, the sanitary idea, and the numerical method, as well as Frank's views, waned. They had guided enquiries into the origins of disease, and the political and social pressures were reflected in legislation, but they were supplanted by the dramatic impact of bacteriology and the "big bug hunt." The unquestioned message, that for each disease there was a single cause and that for most known diseases there was probably a single microbe, had changed the entire landscape for medical education, research, and practice. Laboratories were in, patients and populations were out; a new paradigm was guiding the medical enterprise. The outlines of the fundamental realignment of the ideas about the nature and genesis of disease were now apparent; their formal separation is the subject of the next chapter.

References

1. Latour B. *The Pasteurization of France*. (Sheridan A, Law J, transl.). Cambridge: Harvard University Press, 1988:20.
2. Ibid, p. 23.
3. Ibid, p. 25.
4. Armaingaud of Bordeaux. La tuberculose. Rev Scient 1893;14:33-42. (Quoted by Latour B. *The Pasteurization of France*. (Sheridan A, Law J, transl.). Cambridge: Harvard University Press, 1988:139.
5. Dubos R, Dubos J. *The White Plague: Tuberculosis, Man and Society*. London: Victor Gollancz, 1953.
6. Illich I. *Limits of Medicine: Medical Nemesis: The Expropriation of Health*. Harmondsworth: Penguin, 1981.
7. McKeown T. *The Role of Medicine: Dream, Mirage or Nemesis*. London: Nuffield Provincial Hospitals Trust, 1976.
8. Latour B. *The Pasteurization of France*. (Sheridan A, Law J, transl.). Cambridge: Harvard University Press, 1988:20.
9. Ibid, p. 62.
10. Ibid, p. 63.
11. Ibid, p. 85.
12. Jousett de B, Richet C. Polémique avec la rédaction. Rev Scient 1882;22:509-510. (Quoted by Latour B. *The Pasteurization of France*. Cambridge: Harvard University Press, 1988:122).
13. Vandenbroucke JP. Is 'The causes of cancer' a miasma theory for the end of the twentieth century? Int J Epidemiol 1988;17:708-709.
14. Warner JH. *The Therapeutic Perspective: Medical Practice, Knowledge, and Identity in America 1820-1885*. Cambridge: Harvard University Press, 1986:281-282.
15. Smillie WG. *Public Health: Its Promise for the Future*. New York: Macmillan, 1955:364.
16. Latour B. *The Pasteurization of France*. (Sheridan A, Law J, transl.). Cambridge: Harvard University Press, 1988:139-40.
17. Singer C, Underwood EA. *A Short History of Medicine*. New York: Oxford University Press, 1962:341.
18. Sigerist HE. *The Value of Health to a City*. (Two lectures delivered in 1873 by Max von Pettenkofer and translated by Henry E. Sigerist). Baltimore: Johns Hopkins, 1941.
19. Hume ED. *Max von Pettenkofer: His Theory of the Etiology of Cholera, Typhoid Fever & Other Intestinal Diseases—A Review of His Arguments and the Evidence*. New York: Paul B. Hoeber, 1927:45.
20. Ibid, p. 55.

21. Breger M. *Max von Pettenkofer*. Leipzig: S. Hirzel, 1980:207-208.
22. Latour B. *The Pasteurization of France*. (Sheridan A, Law, J, transl.). Cambridge: Harvard University Press, 1988:104.
23. Smillie WG. *Public Health: Its Promise for the Future*. New York: Macmillan, 1955:378-384.
24. Richmond PA. The germ theory of disease. In: Lilienfeld AM, ed. *Times, Places and Persons: Aspects of the History of Epidemiology*. Baltimore: Johns Hopkins, 1980:84-93.
25. Stewart CP, Guthrie D, eds. *Lind's Treatise on Scurvy*. Edinburgh: University Press, 1953.
26. Baker G. *An Essay Concerning the Cause of Endemical Colic of Devonshire*. London: J. Hughes, 1767. (Reprinted by the Delta Omega Society, 1958.)
27. Singer C, Underwood EA. *A Short History of Medicine*. New York: Oxford University Press, 1962:179.
28. Newman G. *The Rise of Preventive Medicine*. London: Oxford University Press, 1932:172-173.
29. Singer C, Underwood EA. *A Short History of Medicine*. New York: Oxford University Press, 1962:611.
30. Terris M, ed. *Goldberger on Pellagra*. Baton Rouge: Louisiana State University Press, 1964.
31. Simon J. *English Sanitary Institutions: Reviewed in Their Course of Development, and in Some of Their Political and Social Relations*. London: Cassell, 1890:413.
32. Smillie WG. *Public Health: Its Promise for the Future*. New York: Macmillan, 1955:391.
33. Ibid, p. 385.
34. Simon J. *English Sanitary Institutions: Reviewed in Their Course of Development, and in Some of Their Political and Social Relations*. London: Cassell, 1890:268.
35. Ibid, p. 269.
36. Ibid, pp. 332-352.
37. Newman G. *The Rise of Preventive Medicine*. London: Oxford University Press, 1932:253-254.
38. Ibid, p. 254.
39. Billroth T. *The Medical Sciences in the German Universities: A Study in the History of Civilization*. (Translated from the German with an Introduction by William H. Welch). New York: Macmillan, 1924.
40. Ibid, p. 112.
41. Ibid, p. 119.
42. Ibid, p. 89.
43. Ibid, p. 89.
44. Ibid, p. 90.
45. Ibid, p. 248.
46. Stevens R. *American Medicine and the Public Interest*. New Haven: Yale University Press, 1971:73.
47. Ludmerer KM. *Learning to Heal*. New York: Basic Books, 1985:9-28.
48. Ibid, pp. 47-52.
49. Billroth T. *The Medical Sciences in the German Universities: A Study in the History of Civilization*. (Translated from the German with an Introduction by William H. Welch). New York: Macmillan, 1924, p. x.
50. Ibid, p. x.

4
Institutionalizing the Schism

Following initiatives in 1794 by the Écoles de Santé (formerly schools of medicine) in Paris, Montpelier, and Strasbourg, other European medical schools began establishing departments and chairs of hygiene. These were concerned largely with occupational diseases, industrial hazards, and environmental sanitation—an indication that medical faculties were aware of the importance of their understanding for disease prevention. Possibly as a result of Johan Peter Frank's push for legislative enforcement to further his precepts, hygiene was linked to the teaching of medical jurisprudence, as recounted in Chapter 3. At the other extreme, because occupational risks were frequently chemical in nature, many of the early professors of hygiene were physicians with additional training in chemistry or were chemists; later bacteriologists predominated.

In the event, much of the activity in public health and hygiene on the continent and in Great Britain was found in the medical schools, especially at the postgraduate level. This was considered part of their academic mission, albeit often peripheral. Their initiatives were sustained by enactment of assorted statutes about public health matters, especially the creation of Boards of Health during the latter half of the nineteenth century.

In 1865 an Institute of Hygiene was created for the renowned physician and chemist Max von Pettenkofer (see chapter 3). Although somewhat apart from the rest of academic medicine, the new Institute was essentially a department within the Faculty of Medicine; it was not a separate "school." The Institute's establishment marked the formal academic institutionalization of a tradition of research as a basis for public health practice; initially at least, its interests were broad.

> Pettenkofer devoted great attention to social and psychological factors in public health; he was well aware of the environmental factors which made for the good life and did not confine himself to the narrower aspects of hygiene. Much of his teaching showed that there was no magic formula for improving the health of the people, and he rendered a great service in opening up the channels of experimental medicine based on bacteriology. In fact he drew a splendid picture of the modern public health programme: a careful survey of existing conditions; intelligent planning based on scientific investigations; and, above all, patient and continuous pressure on public opinion.[1]

A century after Frank, Pettenkofer was espousing an approach not too different from that of the "father of public health." Scientific advances were supporting the measures he advocated for improving the public's health and enhancing the education of physicians. This trend was strengthened when in 1885 the University of Berlin also created an Institute of Hygiene. Robert Koch was appointed Professor of Hygiene, a move that further strengthened bacteriology as the premiere basic science of medicine; new rigor and specificity were brought to the investigation of disease.[2]

The creation of separate Institutes of Hygiene, first in Germany and then gradually throughout most of central Europe, gave new prominence to the leaders of these Institutes in the academic hierarchy and brought more generous financial support. In addition the Institutes, still within the ambit of the medical schools, were responding to growing legislative requirements that the vocational training of Medical Officers of Health be improved and made more appropriate to the demands of their jobs. Many of these measures required that Medical Officers of Health—by definition physicians—complete specified courses of postgraduate training and, in the case of Britain as observed earlier, acquire a Diploma of Public Health through examination. This move had the unfortunate effect of separating undergraduate from postgraduate education in public health. Undergraduates learn (in contrast to being "taught") attitudes, concepts, values, priorities, and behavior, as well as "facts" and methods, from their peers and those preceding them along the educational ladder. Under the new arrangements undergraduate medical students were isolated increasingly from those who understood the importance of public health. There were few opportunities for them to consider health and disease at the population level where many problems were most amenable to investigation and understanding. The sequence population-patient-laboratory was replaced by the sequence laboratory-patient, in that order; the population was to become an entity apart from clinical medicine.

The institutionalizing of public health apart from medicine can be traced to yet another extremely important set of observations and circumstances. Most of the influences and events discussed so far have occurred in the temperate regions of the world. Earlier, however, we saw something of broader interests in the medical problems of the tropics expressed by members of the London Epidemiological Society. Hindu and Roman physicians in the first century A.D. had concluded that malaria—a disease that then, as now, killed tens of thousands—was spread by mosquitoes. Others in the eighteenth and early nineteenth century shared this view, but it was only in 1879 that Sir Patrick Manson (1844-1922), renowned as "the father of tropical medicine," described the tiny parasitic worms, filaria, that are transmitted by mosquitoes. Two decades later, in 1897, Sir Ronald Ross (1857-1932) showed that the Anopheles mosquito was the specific culprit. Many others serving in colonial armies of occupation and in government health services in the tropics contributed to our understanding of a whole spectrum of diseases differing largely in their mode of transmission and the environmental circumstances in which they ravaged populations.[3]

The need to investigate these diseases to further the economic interests of the merchant colonizers was as great a stimulus as any humanitarian concern. After a period of research in Britain, Manson returned to the Far East and in 1886 established in Hong Kong what was to be the world's first School of Tropical Medicine. He left China 4 years later and in 1898 was instrumental in starting the London School of Tropical Medicine.[4] Manson was, for the most part, a clinician with unbounded curiosity. He used both observational and experimental methods to productively investigate a group of diseases indigenous to another part of the world from that where he grew up. As in the case of hygiene, Manson unwittingly may have contributed to further separation of medicine and public health by fostering yet another institution apart from the mainstream of medicine. Obviously, not all physicians should undertake careers in tropical medicine. Nevertheless, the prospect of attracting at least a few young physicians to tackle these "great neglected diseases" of the tropics is most likely to be fostered when medical students rub shoulders with practitioners and investigators who are knowledgeable role models.

Public health, linked to legislative mandates and statutory educational standards, was drawing further and further away from clinical medicine. Hygiene was linked largely to the health of urban dwellers; there were limited applications to factories and working conditions, and in some settings industrial hygiene was emphasized. Bacteriology, then parasitology, and the germ theory, however, continued to reinforce the notion of "single causes." Epidemiology, as observed earlier, had now become linked almost exclusively to bacteriology and infectious diseases; its broader uses were overlooked. Although Manson used statistical methods in his research, and William Farr had developed the vital statistics system in Britain to the point where it was of modest value for guiding health policy such as it was and for investigating epidemics, Louis's numerical method was not in vogue for most clinicians. First in Europe and later in America, public health and hygiene, and the remnants of clinical medicine's interests in the population's health, were moving away from scientific developments in medicine, apart from their mutual involvement in bacteriology.

The shift was far from complete, however. Two examples illustrate the attitudes of the leading clinician's of the day. The fourth edition, published at the turn of the century, of William Osler's *The Principles and Practice of Medicine*—undoubtedly the leading medical textbook of the period—maintained a relatively broad approach in discussing the causes, distribution, diagnosis, prevention, and treatment of disease.[5] Most of the descriptions of disease had an introductory section on "etiology" and many of these included discussions of the epidemiological distributions of the problem. Of special note was Osler's emphasis on the global and historical manifestations of many diseases, including considerable attention to those found in the tropics. Cushing's biography of Osler is replete with numerous references to his long-standing interest in public health and his broad view of medicine's responsibilities.

From Osler's earliest days at McGill (1881) he served on various public health boards investigating disease outbreaks, especially of typhoid fever.[6] His interest and influence beyond the bedside continued during his tenure at the Johns Hopkins. Cushing observed that:

...like Virchow, whom he so much admired, he became the champion of improved public health measures, national and local; and though unlike Virchow, he never held public office, his time, and his pen, and his great personal influence had almost as much to do with the modern sanitary improvements which Baltimore has come to enjoy, as Virchow's influence had to do with those instituted during the 1880s in Berlin.[7]

And later that:

...the influence which, first and last, Osler exercised as a national and civic sanitary propagandist has been too little emphasized.[8]

There is little doubt that Osler enthusiastically embraced the germ theory and the growing power of bacteriology as the dominant scientific discipline for medicine, but his vision of the factors engendering disease and of medicine's mission encompassed much more.

Osler's clinical and public health crusades directed at the abolition of typhoid, malaria, and tuberculosis were distinguished as much by his holistic approach as by his interest in their morphological characteristics. At a meeting in Dublin in 1907 he began his remarks by saying:

It may not be known to many, or to any of you, that it was in this city that a strong public health movement was first inaugurated by that remarkable man, Sir William Petty, whose studies on the public health of Dublin I commend to all who are interested in the question or in antiquarian research.[9]

From his knowledge of the origins of Anglo-Saxon measures to improve the population's health, Osler's cosmopolitan interests expanded to embrace, as noted above, medicine and health in the tropics. In 1909 he eloquently addressed the tenth opening session of the London School of Tropical Medicine on the subject of "The Nation and the Tropics":

It is no light burden for the white man to administer this vast trust. It is indeed a heavy task, but the responsibility of Empire has been the making of the race. In dealing with subject nations there are only two problems of the first rank—order and health. The first of these may be said to be a specialty of the Anglo-Saxon...[B]ut you will, I think, agree that the second great function of the nation is to give to the inhabitants of the dependencies, Europeans or natives, good health—a freedom from plague, pestilence and famine. And this brings me to the main subject of my address, the control of the tropics by sanitation....Quietly and surely this great work has been accomplished by a group of patient investigators, many of whom have sacrificed health and life in their endeavors. Let us pause for a moment to pay a tribute of gratitude to these saviours of humanity who have made a new mission possible—to Pasteur, to Koch, to Laveran, to Reed and his fellows, to Ross, Manson and Bruce.[10]

Osler was also a strong proponent of government intervention and "the administrative control of disease." In 1918 he participated in an important meeting of the Royal Society of Medicine on "the future of the Medical profession under a Ministry of National Health." In speaking on "Research and the State," he said:

....A strong Ministry of Health backed by a united profession, could initiate important reforms which seem at present hopeless. The reconstruction of our medical schools, the destruction, preliminary to re-arrangement, of the curriculum, the establishment in our hospitals of up-to-date cliniques (*sic*), a degree for London students...some at least of these reforms a strong central organization could force through the blind opposition of vested interests.[11]

Osler's discussions of treatment were more tainted with certainty and dogmatism than Louis or his disciples would have sanctioned with their numerical method. Such blemishes may be forgiven readily when contrasted with the breadth of this remarkable clinician's vision and influence. Osler carried his attitudes, values, and priorities from Montreal to Philadelphia, Baltimore, and Oxford, to say nothing of profoundly influencing several generations of medical students through his textbook and bountiful other writings.

Sir James Mackenzie (1853-1925), the father of modern cardiology and a hero the world over to family and general physicians, provided yet another model for clinicians during the early decades of the twentieth century. Although two excellent biographies of Mackenzie are available, he is not as well known to contemporary medical academicians as Osler.[12,13] The highlights of his life's work epitomize the effort of yet another distinguished clinician to bridge the gap between medicine's responsibily for individuals and for populations. This gap was heading the profession toward ever narrower interpretations of its mission.

Mackenzie was an indifferent student at the University of Edinburgh and entered general practice in the small town of Burnley, Lancashire. Here he began his lifelong practice of careful history-taking, meticulous observation, and detailed notekeeping. As a family physician through long periods (i.e., 10, 20 years, and more) of "wait-and-see" observation, Mackenzie was able to document the benign nature of many cardiac murmurs and arrhythmias. In later life he moved to Harley Street, became the leading cardiac consultant of his generation, wrote numerous classic textbooks, and was knighted. Never forsaking his view that many of the problems of health and disease could be understood only by careful observation of the earliest onset of symptoms and their natural progression over time, Mackenzie gave up a lucrative, demanding, and prestigious position in 1918 and left London for the university town of St. Andrews, Scotland. Here he established what later became The James Mackenzie Institute for Medical Research. Its staff was to study disease as naturalists would; the investigators were to start with the earliest manifestations of ill health and follow them until the patient recovered or died. It was to be a population-based or bottom-up approach, not a top-down, tertiary care approach. From a symptom's origins in the patient's natural habitat, an ecological viewpoint was to prevail. The long-range objective was, above all, the prevention of disease. The more specific goals of Mackenzie's Institute were to:

- Investigate disease before the occurrence of any structural change in any
  organ of the body, with the view of providing a diagnosis at a period earlier

than is possible by the methods now in use, and in order to obtain a knowledge of the circumstances that favor the onset of disease.

- Investigate minor symptoms and maladies which interfere with efficiency or comfort, with the object of determining:
  -the mechanism of their production;
  -their bearing upon the future health of the patient.
- Study the conditions under which the patient lives (food, work, surroundings, etc.).
- Record all cases and keep in touch with patients who have been seen, with the aim of discovering the relation between environment, ailments, and subsequent disease.
- Follow-up patients in order to observe the outcome of complaints...
- Provide postgraduate courses of instruction for the training of general practitioners in methods of clinical research, which they may employ in their practices.
- Train general practitioners to undertake research, in collaboration with specialists in charge of departments for Bacteriology, Chemistry, Radiology, etc.[14]

Here we have Mackenzie delineating, from the perspective of the micro level, the ecological approach espoused by those concerned with hygiene and interested in improving the public's health at the macro level. He did not disregard the now-dominant field of bacteriology, but he saw it as an ancillary source of information and knowledge about disease—certainly not the sole or even the major source.

His biographers provide no evidence that Mackenzie was influenced by Johann Peter Frank's views about the best means for understanding the vagaries of health and disease. Apart from Frank's proposals for harsh legislative sanctions, however, these two remarkably farsighted clinicians seem to have had much in common. Not only were they both concerned with prevention but they also recognized the importance of investigating the full range of circumstances in which disease arises. Mackenzie may have been less of a social reformer than Frank, but he was certainly an innovator when it came to medical research, practice, and education.[15]

Mackenzie's view of the patterns of medical education emerging in the United States in the early decades of the twentieth century are worth noting. They have important implications for understanding aspects of the schism's genesis. In 1918, at the request of the British Government, Mackenzie made his second visit to the United States as a participant in the Annual Meeting of the American Medical Association in Chicago. This pilgrimage took him to a number of the country's principal medical centers. He singled out one visit for special mention:

> From Cincinnati we went to Baltimore, and were shown over the Johns Hopkins Hospital. It was reckoned to be in the very forefront of medical schools, having enormous endowments, so that medicine is broken up into a great number of specialties, and the students have to learn an enormous number of different methods, but in conversation with the authorities, I never was more surprised to find such a

stupid outlook as they possessed. I could say with confidence, that we were far better taught in our student days than the men (*sic*) are today in such places. But what struck me above all, was their absolute conceit and complacence, and when we discussed certain phases of medicine in which they pretended to being the most up-to-date, I found them extraordinarily superficial. So far as my own work is concerned, they had not even realized the elementary principles necessary to guide them in understanding the meaning of the symptoms which their numerous methods revealed.[16]

The differences were striking between Mackenzie's approach to clinical medicine and that at the Johns Hopkins which, since the advent of the Abraham Flexner's (1866-1959) landmark Report on *Medical Education in the United States and Canada*, had become the model for all American medical education.[17] A reductionist, experimental, laboratory-oriented set of values and interests took precedence over an observational, analytical, and ecological set. Although they were making extraordinary strides in understanding disease mechanisms, the clinical faculty in Mackenzie's view, had lost touch with the population it was established to serve.

Mackenzie, the consummate clinician, world-renowned investigator, inventor of the polygraph, highly regarded Harley Street and London Hospital consultant physician, and Fellow of the Royal Society, foretold the future development of epidemiology. I have found no evidence in either of his two biographies that Mackenzie had any association with The London Epidemiological Society apart from one meeting about 1905 with a Dr. Ewart, a prominent London consultant, who may have been Sir Joseph Ewart, one of its Vice-Presidents. At any rate, Mackenzie was no stranger to the concepts and methods of epidemiology. He understood that just as it was important to make and record observations at the individual level so was it also important for generating a different type of knowledge to study groups of patients. Of particular interest in connection with the present treatise is his description, and coining of the term, "the new epidemiology."

From about 1914 to 1920 Mackenzie carried on a lively correspondence with a young cousin, Andrew Garvie, who was entering general practice. Garvie had a mathematical and engineering background and in that sense was competent with numbers and accustomed to handling aggregated data. Here are excerpts from their exchanges:

Mackenzie to Garvie, 1915:

...[P]ay attention to your patients and note the conditions you are ignorant of and after a year's observation...work out a plan of campaign for the future....[18]

Mackenzie to Garvie, 1918:

Let me have your records, imperfect as they are, as soon as you can. I'll compare them with mine; I want the facts broadly. You should continue your observation, and try to compare your results with those of the hospital statistics and death statistics with much greater minuteness than I am doing; the object is to call attention to the great differences between the statistics of death and those of diseases which impair the community.

There is an attempt, I suspect, to get up clinics in the state medical service with 'consultants' reared in hospitals and laboratories. I want to point out from these statistics that the 'consultant' should come from the general practitioners, and if you get on with this work I can foresee a great field for you.[19]

There follows an extended correspondence with numerous suggestions for choosing research topics carefully, focusing the questions, and refining methods of observation and recording. Garvie completed a thesis for the M.D. degree on *Pandemic of Influenza 1918-1919 as it Affected an Industrial Area* and in 1920 sent it to Mackenzie for comment. Although Garvie's examiners had been less than enthusiastic, Mackenzie thought highly of the research and in 1920 wrote him that:

...[I]t has put you upon a line of observation which is much required, and by similar observations on other diseases you will throw a flood of light in dark fields.
If you continue this line of work, in five years' time you will have done more for epidemiology than any other living man, **and you need not limit your observations to epidemic diseases** (emphasis added by KLW).

Do you know my latest craze? The creation of Panel Doctor Specialists![*] The hospital specialist sees disease only when it has damaged the body—the Panel Specialist sees it through its whole life history. You will become **the first Panel Epidemiological Specialist if you care** (emphasis added by KLW).[20]

Epidemic diseases at the time, in spite of the work of Lind and Baker, meant measles, scarlet fever, chickenpox, tuberculosis, and perhaps diseases that by then were more prevalent afar such as cholera, malaria, and yellow fever. Mackenzie clearly was referring to the epidemiology of noninfectious diseases and the role of practicing clinicians—especially family and general physicians—and their unrivaled opportunity and responsibility for studying them.

Mackenzie's time in St. Andrews, marred by personal illness, was all too short. He developed angina pectoris (about which he wrote a classic volume) and succumbed to an untimely death in 1925.

Osler and Mackenzie enjoyed a prolonged friendship starting when the former first visited his general practitioner colleague at Burnley. On balance these two eminent clinicians and investigators of the early twentieth century conducted their professional lives on the premise that medicine was a broadly based profession. For them, as for Frank and Virchow, the great questions of health and disease involved personal, environmental, social, and political considerations; much more than microbes were involved. They recognized no dichotomies between the micro and macro levels, between the individual and the population levels, between what could be learned from the observation of individual patients one by one, and what could be learned by observing groups of patients. They learned much from meticulous observation, precise notekeeping, counting, and measuring. They were the true "generalists"—role models for the renaissance of general or family

---

[*] General practitioners with special clinical interests who were not hospital-based.

medicine under today's rubric of "primary care." In spite of such leaders, however, the climate in academic medicine after the turn of the twentieth century was changing. The schism was dividing the profession into those who care for individuals, and those who care for populations (made up, one should add, of individuals!).

The Rockefeller Foundation was founded in 1913, and its early history, including the perceived motivations and values of those responsible for making the initial decisions, has been well reported elsewhere.[21-25] The initial Rockefeller philanthropies starting with the General Education Board in 1902 were all characterized by four major themes. First was great religious fervor and a conviction on the part of both John D. Rockefeller (1839-1937) and his principal advisor, Frederick T. Gates (1853-1929), an ordained Baptist minister and erstwhile Administrative Head of the Baptist Education Society, that their mission was and that they were "doing good" of a most fundamental kind. Second was the conviction, as John D. Rockefeller himself put it, that "[t]he best philanthropy involves a search for cause, an attempt to cure evils at their source"—the "root causes" approach, as it came to be known within the Foundation and elsewhere. Third was the conviction that the germ theory provided the supporting paradigm for the entire edifice of medical education, practice, and research directed at improvement of the population's health.[26] Fourth was Gates's deep distrust of the social sciences. He persuaded the Board not to support them, convinced as he was that medical science alone was the key to furthering "the well-being of mankind throughout the world."[27] This formidable mixture of unchallenged assumptions bolstered by the Rockefeller largesse was to shape much of American, even world, medicine for generations to come. Redefining the unacceptable was seen almost exclusively in terms of "the big bug hunt." The root problem was the ubiquitous presence of microbes and their biological cousins, parasites. If these could be eliminated the health of both individuals and populations would be improved dramatically. However, the same could be said of poverty, economic exploitation, malnutrition, and filth.

In 1897 Gates, having read William Osler's *Principles and Practice of Medicine,* became imbued with the idea that medical research was the means for doing something substantial for his fellow humans and that distribution of Mr. Rockefeller's fortune was the way to help. Seized by the importance of the germ theory, he explained to Rockefeller that:

> Nearly all disease is caused by living germs, animal and vegetable, which finding lodgement in the human body, under favorable conditions multiply with enormous rapidity until they interfere with functions of the organs which they attack and either they or their products poison the fountains of life.[28]

Later he wrote:

> I brought my Osler [text] into my office...and there I dictated for Mr. Rockefeller's eye a memorandum in which I aimed to show to him the actual condition of medicine in the United States and the world as disclosed by Dr. Osler's book. I enumerated the infectious diseases and pointed out how few of the germs had yet been discovered

and how great the field of discovery; how few specifics had yet been found and how appalling was the unremedied suffering.[29]

In fact, Osler's textbook ran to 1150 pages of which 379 deal directly with infectious and parasitic diseases, and about a quarter of the remaining pages were partially related to infection; at least half the text and the larger portion of all the diseases described by Osler were non-infectious in origin and many were chronic.[30]

Given Gates's endorsement of the then current dominance of bacteriology and its unquestioned successes in identifying assorted microorganisms associated with a wide variety of infectious diseases, the priorities chosen by Rockefeller and his advisers were thoroughly reasonable. Certainly the thrust to improve the scientific basis of medical practice was of unquestionable benefit. Unfortunately, the broader ecological views espoused by Petty, Frank, Sydenham, von Pettenkofer, Virchow, Mackenzie, and even Osler himself seem to have played little or no role in the early deliberations of those directing the original Rockefeller philanthropies. Chadwick's and Shattuck's dedication to establishing the role of poverty and accompanying filth seems to have been overshadowed by the general notion that "bugs" were where the action was to be. There were few, if any, doubts at the Rockefeller Foundation about what needed to be done.

The earliest efforts of these innovative philanthropists to improve health stemmed from the work of the General Education Board and the Rockefeller Sanitary Commission for the Eradication of Hookworm Disease spawned by the former in 1909. The sequence of events leading to the establishment of the Commission is worth recounting. A Professor of Zoology, Charles Wardell Stiles (1867-1941), was committed to improving the lot of poor southerners, and at the time was working in the Hygienic Laboratory of the U.S. Public Health and Marine Hospital Service. He convinced Wallace Buttrick (1853-1926), another clergyman and then secretary of the General Education Board, that the ravages of hookworm, known by the lay term "ground itch," fully justified an aggressive campaign to eliminate it. Buttrick in turn persuaded Gates, then Chairman of the General Education Board, of the problem's importance. They then enlisted the help of Simon Flexner (1863-1946), a former professor of pathology at the University of Pennsylvania who was by that time Director of the Rockefeller Institute, to conduct a 1-year study of the feasibility of launching a massive hookworm eradication program. From this exercise sprang the Rockefeller Sanitary Commission with Professor Wickliffe Rose as Director. The latter was a brilliant authority on Kant and Hegel, Chairman of the Department of Philosophy and Dean at Peabody College, Nashville, Tennessee, and by 1908 an officer of the Peabody Education Fund. These were the men (the whole enterprise was peopled only by men in those days) who started the Rockefeller Foundation on its path toward improving the health of the people. As far as I can determine no clinicians were involved or consulted about any of the strategies or decisions taken.

Although hookworm disease could be treated with a drug combination of thymol capsules and epsom salts developed in Italy, it was, more importantly, preventable through provision of sanitary latrines and wearing shoes to avoid contact with the contaminated soil. The campaign, staffed largely by Sanitary Inspectors, also required substantial local initiative by practicing physicians and others concerned with public health. With the establishment of the Rockefeller Foundation in 1913, the Sanitary Commission was transferred to the Foundation and renamed, first the International Health Commission (1913-1916), then the International Health Board, and finally in 1927 the International Health Division. I refer to it by the latter term throughout the balance of this account.[31]

For a decade Wickliffe Rose was the director of the Foundation's work in public health. Experience with the hookworm eradication programs shaped the Foundation's approach to public health and to education for work in public health throughout his tenure. The hookworm disease campaign met with considerable success. Rose, however, was disappointed by the reaction of the practicing medical profession (largely the general practitioners) and disturbed by both the poor quality and scarcity of health officers available to cooperate with the Commission's large staff. He saw the lack of trained health officers as the central problem. Deficiencies in medical education or inadequate postgraduate training of general or family physicians were not identified as major impediments to the further success of his campaign in particular or to the improvement of the public's health in general. In Rose's view health officers should focus primarily on public education, sanitary inspection, surveys, and enforcement.

From these beginnings, Rose, in partnership with Gates, moved on to a global view of what might be accomplished to improve the public's health. If the hookworm eradication program was to be a success on the scale required by the surveys that had been conducted widely in tropical and subtropical countries, appropriately trained personnel would be required. This was not just an American problem; it was a global problem. The emphasis was to be on sanitation. The sanitary idea became synonymous with the germ theory, and the big bug and worm hunts assumed global dimensions.

Clinicians were no longer in the picture. William Welch, the principal medical advisor to the Rockefeller Foundation, was not a clinician and, despite his renowned administrative and organizational capacities and his unquestioned abilities as a medical statesman of the first order, his record as an investigator was modest. The other major advisor to the Foundation, by this time Assistant Secretary of the General Education Board, was of course Abraham Flexner (1866-1959). In Osler's opinion, Flexner despite his landmark critique of North American medical education, Flexner did not understand clinical medicine.[32] At the apex of this power pyramid was Frederick Gates whose dedication to matters medical was, as observed earlier, largely stimulated by his reading during the summer vacation in 1897 of Osler's entire textbook of medicine.

Osler left the Johns Hopkins in 1904, in the midst of a battle royal within the faculty about the establishment of full-time clinical chairs and departments, although his departure was not necessarily because of it.[33] The full-time idea, that had originated in Germany, prevailed under the leadership of Welch, the pathologist and microbiologist, and Franklin Paine Mall (1862-1917), Professor of Anatomy. Laboratory research was to dominate the interests of the faculty. Broader concerns for patient care and the provision of services to improve the population's health were gradually relegated to secondary importance. The resultant perspective, as James Mackenzie had observed during his visit to Hopkins in 1918, was a set of attitudes, priorities, and practices permeating the entire School of Medicine. Could there be little doubt that the practicing profession was increasingly suspicious of academic medicine's growing power? Like Mackenzie, Osler saw the need for medicine, and especially clinical medicine, not only to embrace its new scientific base but to do this within a broad ecological paradigm. Yet the leaders of the Rockefeller philanthropies, advised by Welch—the only physician, a pathologist and bacteriologist, not a clinician—saw matters differently.

In 1914, at the instigation of Rose the General Education Board assigned Abraham Flexner, by then its Secretary, to investigate possible sites for endowing an institution to train health officers. Two distinct issues immediately arose; an appreciation of them is central to an understanding of the formal *institutionalization of the schism*. The manner in which these two issues were resolved marks the almost total abrogation by clinical medicine, and for that matter by academic medicine, of overall responsibility for the public's health.

First was the nature of the task itself. Milton J. Rosenau (1869-1946), a physician and Professor of Preventive Medicine at Harvard, wrote Flexner that "public health is a distinct profession, separate from the practice of medicine....In fact it is often difficult to bend the doctor into a sanitarian."[34] Charles-Edward Amory Winslow (1877-1957), not a physician but a graduate of Professor William T. Sedgwick's (1855-1921) program in sanitary engineering at the Massachusetts Institute of Technology (M.I.T.), was a statesman, man of action, and educator.[35] Although he contributed little original to the discipline, he used epidemiological principles soundly and his comprehension of the discipline's power helped make him a vigorous promoter of public health as a distinct profession. He wrote Flexner that "public health is not a branch of medicine or engineering....The ideal school of public health should train all the various grades of sanitary workers from the highest to the lowest. Public health nurses, sanitary inspectors, and health officers for small towns are far more urgently needed than highly-trained medical officers of health."[36]

Winslow's mentor Sedgwick, after embarking on the study of medicine, shifted to biology and became Professor of Biology at M.I.T.; he had a different view. He saw the need for at least a substantial biological, if not clinical, background for the public health worker. Sedgwick devised a "Y-plan"[*] with the help of George C. Whipple (1866-1929), Professor of Engineering and Statistics at M.I.T., Milton J. Rosenau (1869-1946), Professor of Preventive Medicine, and Richard P. Strong (1872-1948), a distinguished parasitologist with his own School of Tropical Medicine, all of Harvard. This formidable array of academic talent was backed by leaders in the Medical School including Walter B. Cannon (1871-1945), the

---

[*] A similar plan was advanced independently by a Professor Ruzicka in the first number of the *Czech Journal of Public Health*, Prague, March 1921.

creative physiologist, who was expanding medicine's paradigm to include the influence of emotional and cultural factors in the genesis of disease; Ida Cannon (1877-1960), the first Social Worker to be attached to a medical school; and Richard C. Cabot (1868-1939), arguably the most innovative professor of medicine in the country at that time. The Y-plan had substantial support from the Harvard Medical School's clinical faculty; the same could not be said of the Johns Hopkins arrangements. The former plan was to have involved an initial 2 years at Harvard studying anatomy, physiology, bacteriology, pathology, etc. This phase was to be followed by one arm consisting of 2 years' clinical training leading to the Doctor of Medicine degree and a second arm of 2 years leading to a Doctor of Public Health. Since 1913 a joint Harvard-M.I.T. School for Health Officers (forerunner of the Harvard School of Public Health) had offered a 1-year certificate course; it would be abolished under Sedgwick's plan. Events overtook the planners and the plan was never fully promulgated.

Of even greater interest in the present context, however, was Sedgwick's view of the problem surrounding public health education. In a 1921 speech describing his Y-plan, Sedgwick, the biologist, stated that:

> The medical man (*sic*) without further training, has been tried and found wanting, and it is for this reason that special Schools of Hygiene and Public Health have sprung up here and there. These, however, are and long will be wholly inadequate to supply the needs of the time, and our only hope at present for any adequate relief is that the medical schools of the land shall seize the opportunity that is theirs, to divert into the public health channels with proper preparation, some of the talent now going into medicine.[37]

For most of the twentieth century the debate has never stopped: Who should provide leadership for public health? What should they do and how should they be trained? Certainly the initial emphasis was almost entirely on sanitation and the eradication of microbes and parasites. Sedgwick, the biologist, seems to have been the only person both to draw a distinction with his Y-plan between the environmental and personal health services and to ensure that those concerned with these two aspects of society's health problems had at least some of their educational background in common.

William Welch was to retire as Dean of the Johns Hopkins Medical School in 1914. He considered that public health required physicians with a broad education in the basic (i.e., primarily physical) sciences as well as clinical experience, including an internship, followed by 2 additional years training "that would make him a doctor of public health." "The rest is application....[I]t requires specialized training, but it almost takes care of itself, and it is easily supplied."[38] He further emphasized the importance of public health by advocating an advanced degree, equivalent to the Ph.D. degree.

The second major issue, put in the boldest terms, concerned the quality and motivation of the physicians who were to be attracted to a career in public health. Earlier, Rose had noted that:

At present the county health officer in most counties is a practicing physician; he is paid an insignificant sum [and] must depend for the support of himself and his family on his private practice; it is not his fault that the service is ineffective....

As Greer Williams, a student of these matters, observed:

Rose did not mention that it was a matter of common knowledge that the private physician who took the public health job was often the least competent physician in town, sometimes less interested in saving lives from filth-borne diseases than playing politics with county commissioners and making a few hundred dollars a year. Not infrequently, the part-time health superintendent was a relative of the chairman of the county board.[39]

At one point during the subsequent meeting in 1914 to discuss the funding of Schools of Public Health, Gates asked:

...[I]sn't it true that...many men (*sic*) who are practicing physicians, who have all the necessary qualifications...are not successful in practice, who have certain peculiarities of manner or lack of the graces...which 'ring the doorbell' and bring them full practice, and yet they are very able?
Now, why cannot there be a career for just such men right here, large numbers of them, too...Let these men...come to [a school of public health] for a more or less short time and fit themselves in the special services...and from those failures in practice draw your health officers?[40]

To which Hermann M. Biggs (1859-1923) responded: "I think that is what actually will happen."[41] Williams comments:

Strangely, no one thought to observe that, if public health was to be simply a haven for clinical medicine's misfits rather than stand on its own feet as a prideful profession, its attractiveness to a medical graduate seeking his niche would be about equal to that of a junk pile.[42]

Nor did anyone seem to recognize that if the nascent field of public health were to recruit an adequate share of the best minds in medicine, as much or more attention had to be given to the selection of undergraduate medical students and the content of their education, as to the postgraduate training of Medical Officers of Health. Neglect of this vital matter of recruitment has been central to the plight of public health ever since.

During debates on the best way to advance educational strategies to meet the urgent needs for public health personnel, Rose suggested that someone should visit Europe and review experiences there.[43] By the summer of 1914, World War I had intervened and the trip was never made. That is unfortunate because the experience might have been helpful to Rose and other Foundation officials. In Great Britain the professors of medicine had taken the lead in developing both courses and degrees for what was initially referred to as "state medicine." This initiative stemmed from the requirement under the Medical Act of 1886 that the General Medical Council approve the qualifying examinations for Medical Officers of Health.

A central figure in espousing the establishment of academic public health in Britain was Sir Henry Acland (1815-1901), Regius Professor of Medicine at Oxford, and a Vice President of the London Epidemiological Society. Acland was supported in this crusade by two other distinguished physicians, Sir George Paget (1809-1892), Regius Professor of Medicine at Cambridge, and William Stokes (1804-78) an eminent clinician of Trinity College, Dublin. All three were strongly influenced by the volume written in 1856 by Henry Wyldbore Rumsey (1809-1876), a General Practitioner from Gloucester, entitled *Essays in State Medicine*. At his personal expense Rumsey had 100 copies printed for members of the London Epidemiological Society. By his own admission, Rumsey's views were strongly influenced by the German "medical police" model, all harking back to the works of Johann Peter Frank. But Rumsey also embraced Frank's larger paradigm for medicine.[44]

In 1867 at a meeting of the British Medical Association where proposals for developing teaching in public health were the principal matters to be discussed, Rumsey advocated for this endeavor that "the cooperation and support of the National Association for the Promotion of Social Science be obtained." The BMA enthusiastically agreed.[45] Acland, Paget, and Stokes, three distinguished academic clinicians, agreed on the need and worked together, against considerable opposition especially for Acland at Oxford, toward eventual establishment of curricula leading to university conferred Diplomas in Public Health in accordance with standards promulgated by the General Medical Council.[46]

At Edinburgh developments took a somewhat different course with the science faculty having a majority influence on the curriculum. Led by Sir Robert Christison (1797-1882), Professor of Medical Jurisprudence and Dean of Edinburgh's Faculty of Medicine, a curriculum leading to the Diploma in Public Health was eventually introduced. The arrangements there were also modeled on the German pattern.

Substantial differences existed between the approaches in England and the United States. In the former leadership was taken by clinicians, professors of medicine—and the leading ones at that—whereas in the United States it was taken largely by nonphysicians, advised by nonclinicians—albeit prominent figures such as William Welch. The British group encountered increasing opposition to both the importance of their ideas and the need for formal training. For many decades, however, much of the limited undergraduate and postgraduate training in public health was kept under the umbrella of the medical schools. Advocates in both countries agreed that physicians were to be the principal recruits for postgraduate training in public health.

In the United States Welch initially argued strongly for developing public health training within the medical school, similar to the conclusion Sedgwick reached. Eventually Welch altered his position in the face of mounting opposition from within the medical faculty. "Welch insisted that public health work would be as attractive to medical men as the inducements of practice. He further asserted that many physicians would be eager for graduate training in public health and would see it as a 'splendid opportunity.'"[47] Welch seems to have taken the easier course once he retired from the deanship of the Medical School in 1914; he then opted for establishment of a separate School of Public Health.

We come now to the famous Welch-Rose Report of 1915.[48] It ended discussions over the previous 3 years about the nature and locus of training for public health. The Report has been described as "the Declaration of Independence by which American Schools of Public Health sought to differentiate themselves as training and research institutions while pledging allegiance to the university and avowing a close alliance with the medical school."[49] Welch even argued that education in hygiene should be part of the education of all physicians planning to enter clinical practice. "The mission of the practicing physician is in many respects changing, and there can be no doubt that a year or more of graduate work in hygiene would be eagerly sought by many physicians...if the proper opportunities for such work were provided."[50] Greer Williams comments that Welch "appeared to have lost his license to practice as a prophet. Such an eagerness never emerged. On the contrary, clinical training discouraged it."[51]

The academic struggles between Harvard and the Johns Hopkins for primacy in this Rockefeller venture and the power struggles within the Rockefeller philanthropies have been explored fully elsewhere.[52-55] The strange assumptions, scant documentation, and weak justification for the decisions taken are, however, of interest in light of the Foundation's emerging reputation for tackling the root causes of problems. A single 1-day summit meeting was held in New York by the General Education Board on October 16, 1914, to consider what should be done about public health education. Not one clinician was present; the participants were bacteriologists, pathologists, sanitary engineers, and laymen.

Notably absent from the meeting was the preeminent epidemiologist of his times—albeit a Professor of Biology—William T. Sedgwick, who had developed the Harvard-M.I.T. Y-plan. From his writings and speeches, it is clear that Sedgwick was one of the best informed and most constructive commentators on public health training, and yet he was not invited to the meeting. My point is not to suggest that the Harvard-M.I.T. group should necessarily have prevailed over the supporters of Hopkins; rather, it is to emphasize that influential faculty members at Harvard seem to have had an unusually broad outlook on the task of preparing professionals for work in public health. Although William Welch at first argued strongly for the teaching of hygiene and public health within a department of the medical school, he was not supported by his medical faculty. Eventually of course he acceded to the more limited institutional arrangement that was eventually embraced by the Foundation.

In addition to Sedgwick, other notable leaders of the public health movement were absent from the October 16th meeting. These included Victor C. Vaughan (1851-1929), a student of Robert Koch, founder of the Michigan State Hygienic Laboratory with its emphasis on water purification and Professor of Medical Chemistry at the University of Michigan; Watson S. Rankin (1879-1976), a pioneer in the creation of state and county health departments in North Carolina; and Charles V. Chapin (1856-1941) of Rhode Island, probably the country's leading municipal Health Officer. Also excluded from the gathering was Edwin Seligman

(1861-1939), a political scientist at Columbia University who headed a 12-person committee that advanced a plan for a school of public health based on a balanced program combining medical, engineering, and social science courses. Seligman forwarded a letter from E.H. Lewinski-Corwin proposing, that public health be regarded as a social science. In Lewinski-Corwin's view, most public health problems were much less medical or technical than social and political:

> Congestion of population in cities, the condition of tenement houses, the elimination of slums, recreation centers, alcoholism, prostitution, the standard of living, social insurance, the saving of human wear and tear in industry, the elimination of the insane and feeble minded, and many other similar problems affect the public health as much as the sewerage system, food inspection, and the quarantine of measles.[56]

If the meeting was not "rigged" it certainly had the appearance of concentrating the advisory talent in the fields of bacteriology, chemistry, and sanitary engineering; no clinicians, no social scientists, and no political economists were present, despite intimate involvement by the forerunners of these disciplines in the problems of population health since the days of William Petty.

Selection of the participants for the Conference might have been understandable had the meeting produced a carefully reasoned document weighing the alternatives and providing a clear rationale for the establishment of schools of public health separate from the medical schools. Did Rose, propelled by Welch and Flexner, recognize that the Foundation was about to institutionalize the schism? That was the result of their decision.

Two versions of the Report, the first having been prepared by Rose and the second, generally regarded as the "official" version, almost completely rewritten by Welch and co-signed by Rose, failed to define the problems being addressed to say nothing of their root causes, except in the most general terms. There are in fact two quite different views expressed about the type of educational innovation required to improve the population's health. Rose's version described the need for a national system whereby public health workers would be deployed in health departments at the several governmental levels: federal, state, county, and municipal. Public health would be based on a "science of hygiene." The leaders would be trained and the fundamental research would be conducted in one or two central institutions serving the entire country. The other personnel, including nurses, supervisors of state laboratories, technicians, inspectors, and extension workers would be trained in a much larger number of state centers blanketing the country.

The model to be employed was that of the Land Grant Colleges and the Agricultural Extension Agents that had done so much to improve farming in the United States. In addition Rose, the philosopher, was adamant that "the proposed central school will contribute toward the creation of a science of hygiene; and toward the establishment of a public health service as a distinct profession."[57]

> It is frequently said that there is no science of hygiene; that we have a science of chemistry, a science of physics, a science of biology, etc., and that we make application of these several sciences in hygienic living,—but a science of hygiene? There is none.

But the fact remains that in these separate sciences we have now an important body of facts which if assembled, organized, and focused on the one point, would enable us to prolong human life and to increase human efficiency....And in the sense that science is organized knowledge this would be an important contribution towards a science of hygiene....The work of assembling and organizing what is known on the subject of hygiene will offer both stimulus and clews (*sic*) to the discovery of new knowledge.[58]

This exercise in tautology may have been useful at the time but would hardly be convincing today. There were, however, other aspirations:

...[H]and in hand with this creating of a science of hygiene will go the work of establishing the service which applies this science to community living as a distinct profession offering to young men of ability a worthy career. The medical school embodies our highest achievements in relieving the sick; it has contributed and is contributing toward a science of medicine; it has made medical practice a distinct and honorable profession. The school of public health will be the embodiment of our highest reach in protecting the well; it will focus public attention as perhaps no other agency can focus it on the fact that the science of protection is quite distinct from the science of cure; and that the administration of public health calls for a preparation and an inspiring and guiding purpose all its own.[59]

Rose emphasized the importance of having the new school of public health and its institute of hygiene "related to a medical school," of having a "university connection," but he also argued that it "must maintain its separate identity."

[T]his school of public health should be established on its own foundation, and should preserve and emphasize its own identity as a separate institution devoted exclusively to the science and service of public health; it should have its own buildings, and its own grounds, its own governing board, its own corps of instructors and adequate provision of its own for instruction and research.[60]

Discussions of process and organization continued to take precedence over those of recruitment and curriculum. Rose detailed the extent to which the school could draw on the resources of the rest of the university, including its schools of medicine and engineering. The central idea was to refocus the separate disciplines and professions on measures for improving the population's health. In spite of his circumlocutions, Rose provided no adequate definition of "hygiene," no definition of "public health," no description of the responsibilities of a health officer—only a list of their bureaucratic titles. There was no documentation of the several reputed deficiencies, and no evidence that earlier efforts to improve the public's health had been examined.

The second version of the Report, rewritten by Welch and presented by Rose, was now entitled *Institute of Hygiene*. It became the official version, adopted by the General Education Board on May 17, 1915 and published in the 1916 Annual Report of the Rockefeller Foundation.[61] The prevailing situation was described as follows:

In this country we are woefully lacking both in laboratories of hygiene and in opportunities for training in public health work. Three or four medical schools have hygienic laboratories, but none is complete, and adequately equipped and supported. Still other schools attempt something in the way of instruction in this subject, but it is all inadequate and unsatisfactory.

The need for supplying these deficiencies is at present the most urgent one in medical education (*sic*) and in public health work, and is recognized on all sides. The cry comes loudest from public health officials, social workers and others interested in public health administration, national, state, municipal and rural, who realize the lack of trained leaders and trained workers in all grades of the services. Here with the rapidly growing appreciation of efficient public health organization new and promising careers of useful service are opening for those who are qualified by ability, character and training. Scarcely less important is it for medical students and physicians who engage in practice to be well grounded in the principles of hygiene and of preventive medicine. Furthermore the advancement of knowledge in this field, the cultivation of hygiene as a science, is one of the great needs of this country and should be a fundamental aim of an institute of hygiene.[62]

This statement places much greater emphasis on medical education (presumably undergraduate education) than the previous document, but it fails to discuss how this is to be accomplished. Welch's optimism about the attractiveness of public health education to young physicians was not reflected in the remarkable retreat from his original position that hygiene and public health should be located organizationally and taught regularly within the medical school proper. As observed earlier, there was little support for his views within the Hopkins medical faculty, especially from the clinical departments. Perhaps Welch also experienced academic battle fatigue from the "full-time faculty" wars that had consumed considerable administrative energy for much of the previous decade.[63]

The problems of recruitment to careers in public health was not of much concern to Welch, as I noted; he thought the prospects of a career in public health would readily attract first-rate medical graduates. Welch's experience in Pettenkofer's laboratory 30 years earlier undoubtedly influenced his views. As Welch is said to have expressed it at the October 1914 Conference, "the only solution to the difficulty of finding public health personnel was a university department of hygiene on the German model...everybody knows the risk of starting men too soon in technical training without a good knowledge of general principles."[64] Rose's first version, however, acknowledged the difficulties when he observed that the preparation of "health officers of the second rank" (i.e.,to serve in smaller towns and at county level) "should be as thorough and almost as comprehensive as that of health officers of the first rank. But under the present conditions this is not to be expected; the compensation these positions offer does not attract men of the highest qualifications."[65] There were other anomalies: statisticians were to be medically qualified and like epidemiologists were classified as "higher technical officials without administrative functions." Rose's version also had this to say:

The school will undertake to select its student body. This will be done not so much by excluding the unfit as by providing a plan for systematically discovering and bringing in the fit. In carrying out the work outlined above the school will keep in intimate touch with the public health work and workers in all states; it will use this net-work of acquaintances and official relations to discover the young men (*sic*) in the ranks who have shown by their energy, their ability, their qualities of leadership and devotion to the service that they are coming men, the men who are going to shape the policies and direct the work in the public health service of their states.[66]

This was strange reasoning in the light of the October 1914 meeting's discussion about the dearth of talent in public health and even the earlier comment on the poor quality of Health Officers at lower levels. The possibility that a Gresham's law of talent was operating did not seem to cross the minds of these eminent scholars. If one wanted to attract first-rate young talent to the vitally important task of working for the improvement of the population's health, would one really start this way?

Welch, in contrast to Rose, did have recourse to European experiences. He observed that "in Germany every university has its Department or Institute of Hygiene, conducted by a professor and a corps of assistants, where the subject is represented broadly in all its varied aspects, etc."[67] He omitted to say that these Departments and Institutes were all integral parts of medical schools. By way of contrast he observed that "[i]n England...the important hygienic laboratories are few and mostly governmental or independent. For training the emphasis is laid upon public health administration, in which respect Great Britain leads the world. Those desiring to qualify as medical officers of health must possess the diploma in public health....It seems obvious that lessons are to be learned from both the German and the English systems, and that the ideal plan will give due weight to both the scientific and the practical aspects of hygiene and public health."[68] That may well have been true for the educational content of the proposed school but it failed to deal with the central problem of attracting an adequate share of the best brains of medicine into public health. It also begged the question of how to attract the best brains from other professions such as engineering, nursing, and the social, behavioral, and natural sciences to confront the problems of population health.

With the adoption of the Welch-Rose Report by the Rockefeller Foundation, Abraham Flexner's influence again became dominant. The task now was to establish the first Institute of Hygiene or School of Public Health. The principal matter requiring resolution was the extent to which it was to be a part of or allied with a medical school. Relations with a school of engineering was a secondary matter, and need for involvement of the social sciences, including attention to the economic and political aspects of public health problems, was given lip service at best.

Elizabeth Fee observed that Rose did not share Flexner's strong commitment to the "medical model" of public health; this is a crucial issue. What exactly was the "medical model" that was emerging in medicine, as America gradually assumed world leadership in medicine and related fields toward the end of World War I? Was it to be a reductionist model, based on the germ theory of disease augmented by the burgeoning, and highly successful, field of bacteriology with its proliferation of research laboratories, increasing specialization, and the fragmentation of the patient as James Mackenzie recounted? Or was the medical model to be an ever-expanding paradigm that continued to embrace a broad spectrum of environmental, occupational, cultural, social, psychological, economic, and political influences on health and disease at the micro and macro levels, in addition to a broadened biological base? Who was to decide or, in more practical terms, whose views were to prevail? On what evidence was the "model" to be constructed for organizing society's efforts to cope with ill health at the individual and population levels?

Although Osler embraced the germ theory and was a supporter of laboratory medicine, he was also a humanist with a zest for new knowledge and fresh ideas. Among other things he believed that undue reliance on the full-time faculty system would deprive students of exposure to practicing clinicians who were closer to the natural habitats of their suffering patients—the primary care physicians of the day. Other leaders of clinical medicine such as Richard Cabot and Sir Henry Acland, as well as the latter's colleagues in The London Epidemiological Society, saw poverty, deprivation, and environmental pollution as major determinants of the public's health status; such matters should be important concerns for the medical profession. The narrow paradigm espoused in the Flexnerian medical model was now to be further aided and abetted by the removal of the population perspective from medical schools to the new schools of public health. Henceforth, this essential perspective was to be isolated from the mainstream of "scientific" medicine.

Flexner, Rose, and Welch overlooked other lessons from European experience. The numerical method embedded in the enormously influential French school founded by Louis went by the board with one exception. A Boston surgeon, E. A. Codman, attempted to introduce a system for assessing the outcomes of clinical care at the Massachusetts General Hospital. For his pains he was roundly attacked and had to move to a more modest institution.[69] His ideas and methods were forgotten for five decades. Vital statistics were not forgotten in the Welch-Rose Report, and Welch even suggested that "there are other important applications of statistical science to hygiene."[70] There was no thought, however, of developing in schools of public health methods to assess the impact either of micro interventions at the clinical level or of macro interventions at the institutional or population levels.

Epidemiology was mentioned from time to time, but usually as an ancillary and technical subject related to the study of infectious disease epidemics. There was no awareness of the widespread applications envisioned by The London Epidemiological Society. No consideration seems to have been given to epidemiology as the fundamental "basic science" of public health, nor was there any recognition of the applications James Mackenzie had in mind when he spoke of "the new epidemiology." The basic sciences of public health were bacteriology (and in some settings, parasitology), physics, and chemistry. The essential technology was to be engineering.

True, better sewerage, pure water, and clean food had a measurable impact on the community's health, but what about better housing, productive employment, fair wages, adequate nutrition, care, support, and hope? Opportunities were lost to influence the nature and scope of the model that was to guide the overall health enterprise. Instead of working within the heart of the academic medical enterprise, the new schools of public health chose to go it alone.

Surely the eminent scholars who were the architects of this split would have benefited from a review of the attempts by many clinicians over the previous two centuries or more to improve the public's health? A different strategy might also have evolved had the Foundation's officers had the benefit of wider and more frequent consultations. Closer examination of underlying assumptions, more critical analysis of the general problems they sought to tackle, and much greater attention to the central matter of attracting an adequate proportion of the best possible medical minds to the field of population health might have minimized or avoided the impact of the schism they institutionalized.

Whether this separation between medical and public health education and research was the result of Welch's disaffection with the attitudes of his medical faculty toward the latter, or whether it was his own wish to establish this endeavour apart from the narrowing confines of the emerging medical model is unclear. His slowness in providing the Rockefeller Board with his plan for the new school and the latter's insistence in the terms of the grant to Hopkins that Welch be the Director of the new Institute certainly suggests that the Foundation more than Welch was the prime mover in institutionalizing the schism.[71]

The Johns Hopkins School of Hygiene and Public Health opened in 1918 with William Welch as its first Director. He selected a first-rate faculty and from the start sought to maintain high standards of instruction and, given his perspective, a broad approach to the field of public health. The School and others that were modeled after it did their best according to their lights. The second School of Public Health was established at Harvard in 1921; it combined the earlier School for Health Officers, Richard P. Strong's School of Tropical Medicine, and elements of William Sedgwick's Y-Plan.

The Rockefeller Foundation then proceeded to launch a worldwide program of support for schools of public health and institutes of hygiene. The University of Toronto came next in 1924; it had had a chair of Hygiene and Sanitary Science in the Faculty of Medicine since 1912. Again the medical school department, patterned after the European departments, was to be hived off into a new and separate School of Hygiene. The University of Michigan was the fourth school of public health in North America supported by the Foundation, although not until 1940. All four of these universities, like most that followed, received substantial funds for new buildings; there was to be no doubt that each school of public health had to be, and be seen to be, an institution separate and distinct from the school of medicine—Rose had made that clear in his original draft of the Report. As late as 1945 the Foundation made it a condition of further support for the Harvard School of Public Health that it remain separated from the Harvard Medical School.[72]

Establishment of the London School of Hygiene and Tropical Medicine was another major element in the Foundation's global strategy. Sir Patrick Manson, introduced earlier in this chapter as the father of tropical medicine, was a veteran with 24 years experience of research and service in China and the Far East. As part of Britain's imperialistic expansion, Manson urged that all physicians working in what became the British Colonial Medical Service have formal training in tropical medicine. Based on his admiration for British achievements in the control of hookworm in the colonies, Rose brought together a group of competing interests and advanced the possibility of merging the London School of Tropical Medicine with the Department of Hygiene in University College's Medical School. Manson opposed the scheme and just before his death pleaded with Rose not to "swallow up" his School of Tropical Medicine (personal communication, Professor Roy M. Acheson, Cambridge University, March 12, 1990). According to Rose's plan the new institution was to emphasize the preparation of Medical Officers of Health for both "state medicine" in the United Kingdom and for the Colonial Medical Service. In 1922, following prolonged negotiations with officials of the University of London and the government, including the Cabinet, the Foundation offered a substantial grant in support of the merger. In 1924 the London School of Hygiene and Tropical Medicine was founded, and University College Medical School's department disappeared for some decades. The new school opened the doors of its building in 1929; again the bulk of the Foundation's money was for buildings.[73]

From Britain the Foundation moved on to establish similar institutions in Prague, Warsaw, Copenhagen, Budapest, Oslo, Belgrade, Zagreb, Madrid, Cluj, Ankara, Sofia, Rome, Tokyo, Athens, Bucharest, Stockholm, Calcutta, Manila, and São Paulo. Of these, the experiences of the University of Zagreb are among the most instructive. The lessons provided, as in the case of other institutions, stem from the individuals who built them.

One of those individuals, a giant of international public health in the twentieth century, was Andrija Štampar (1892-1958). No account of efforts to improve the public's health would be complete without a brief review of this remarkable man's influence. Born in a rural village of Croatia, he attended medical school at the University of Vienna. There he was greatly influenced by one of the founders of social medicine, Professor Julius Tandler (1869-1936), both a theoretician and a practical innovator, who pioneered the integration of medical and social services. In Vienna, Tandler first articulated his observations about the influence of social and environmental factors on health and disease. To test his theories he later developed a model network of kindergartens, welfare clinics, dental clinics, hospitals, and "relieving institutions" (i.e., what we would now call "respite care").[74]

Štampar was so impressed by Tandler's discourses on the interrelationships among education, health, and the population's social and physical environments that he embarked on an administrative and academic career with few equals. As a latter-day Johann Peter Frank, Štampar made major contributions not only in his native Yugoslavia (and its predecessor state "The Kingdom of the Serbs, Croats, and Slovenes") but also internationally through his later work with the World Health Organization. Although undoubtedly "progressive" in his social views, Štampar did not belong to any political party. His ideas, nevertheless, distressed many in the medical profession and he was "retired" at the age of 42 from his position as Head of the Department of Hygiene and Social Medicine of his country's Ministry of Health. The University of Zagreb appointed him first as a lecturer and later as a full professor to teach these subjects in the Faculty of

Medicine. Throughout his career Štampar persisted in his views: first, that the preventive and curative aspects of medicine had to be linked, and second, that the social, occupational, and physical environments and, above all, the education of the population, were as important as clinical interventions to the health status of individuals and populations. His third point was that strong and effective leadership, including administration and management, were critical to the success of efforts to improve the public's health.[75]

To this end he played a major role in the development of the School of Public Health at the University of Zagreb. Štampar's initial academic efforts in the Faculty of Medicine at Zagreb had resulted in the establishment of an Institute of Social Medicine, supported intellectually by his two-volume text on *Social Medicine*. Matters were proceeding constructively when, as a result of Štampar's widespread international activities, he came to the attention of the Rockefeller Foundation's officers in Europe. About 1925 they offered to support construction of a building (more buildings!) and the founding of a new School of Public Health at Zagreb. Today, the School retains its original address on the street named "Rockefellerova." What is of much greater interest is the shifting back and forth of the School's administrative locus within the university hierarchy. At times it was a separate entity; at others it was an integral part of the Faculty of Medicine, and at still others a semiautonomous body within the Medical School. Votes were taken, and the faculty was frequently ambivalent and divided about the School's most effective administrative location. In many ways Zagreb provides perhaps the best case study of the impact of attempts at institutionalizing the schism. Given Štampar's views and the School's checkered organizational history, one wonders whether the Foundation's largesse did more harm than good.

A trip sponsored by the Rockefeller Foundation in 1938-1939 to North American universities, including a sojourn at the University of California, provided Štampar with broad insights into public health education in diverse settings. Like his friend Professor C. C. Chen during the sentimental odyssey a half century later, discussed in Chapter 1, Štampar was less than enchanted with the collective impact of the medical and public health establishments on the provision of adequate health services, especially to the underprivileged in the United States. On returning to his own country he was appointed Dean of the Faculty of Medicine for a brief period from 1940 to 1941. He set to work reforming medical education, but the 1941 invasion by the German army put an end to this initiative; Štampar was interned in a concentration camp for 4 years.

In 1945 he resumed his academic endeavors both as Professor of Hygiene and Social Medicine in the Medical School and as Director of the School of Public Health. He published another book entitled *The Physician, His Past and Future*. Štampar's biographer observes that "all those who accused Štampar of being against the medical profession could have seen from this book how mistaken they were. He made in the book a point of the greatness of the medical calling but rightly added that just because of this exceptionally important social role of the physician it was imperative that he be no business man but a social worker."[76]

Štampar, consistent with his belief that improvement in the health of populations depended not only on physicians but on the work of nurses, engineers, chemists, veterinarians, agronomists, and others, set about fostering further integration. The Nursing School was already an integral part of the Faculty of Medicine with full voting status on the Faculty Council.

> He wanted to give a practical example of [further] collaboration by the work of the Zagreb School of Public Health, his pet institution, which in 1947, as a result of his endeavors, became an integral part of the Medical School, accredited with the task of providing training for undergraduate medical students and for physicians and for other workers dealing with health matters. The School organized postgraduate courses on public health, environmental sanitation, occupational health, social pediatrics, nursing, anesthesiology, etc. At first the School was concerned only with the organization of postgraduate training of physicians, engineers, and nurses in preventive-medical work, but according to Štampar's intentions it was meant to take over the organization of all postgraduate training.[77]

Štampar was Rector of the University of Zagreb in 1945-1946, and in 1952 he was again elected Dean of the Medical School and subsequently, contrary to the usual practice, he was elected to a second 5-year term. Contributing to this legacy of administrative and intellectual leadership was a strong, and internationally renowned, Department of Epidemiology in the School of Public Health and, therefore, also in its Medical School. In addition, Štampar's successor as Professor of Preventive and Social Medicine and Head of the Department of Public Health Administration was Ante Vuletic, an eminent clinician. Vuletic (and later his son) played major roles in the rejuvenation of primary care in Europe, with particular emphasis on imbedding the population and preventive perspectives as integral components of clinical practice. Under the senior Vuletic's leadership the faculty conducted an extensive evaluation of the competencies required for this level of medical practice and defined the related educational requirements.[78]

Štampar's final assessment of his own accomplishments found much that remains to be done. He was not happy with the medical profession's leadership, and in 1957 at the end of his term as Dean of the Medical Faculty of the University of Zagreb he wrote:

> In no country—and in this country in particular—can Medical Faculties exist as institutions isolated from the happenings in the field of public health administration. Of course, the willingness to collaborate should exist on either side. Our health service, it is sad to say, is still very far from integrating the main medical branches into one whole, while in the field there is poor coordination and an unsettled situation in institutions themselves, even among physicians who should be the stronghold of advanced ideas in medicine.... It is beyond any doubt that the Medical Faculty should play an important role in the evaluation of the candidates designed for leading public health administrators, lest the large, important institutions should be headed by physicians who have only just obtained their degree, as is the case now. It can be said without much hesitation that without reforms in the health service based on the principles of technical qualifications the Faculty's endeavors will be bound to come to grief....

One of the extremely important duties of the Faculty is also the provision of health institutions with experts specially trained for individual positions in the health service, such as general practitioners and specialists in different branches of preventive, curative, and social medicine.[79]

These observations by one who spent a lifetime trying to *heal the schism* only serve to emphasize the widening gulf between clinicians and the populations they serve. The social contract between the medical profession and the public was unraveling. More than $25 million had been spent by the Rockefeller Foundation in establishing separate schools of public health.[80] By 1985 there were some 101 separate schools in 37 countries worldwide; there is an even greater number (115) of medical schools with departments of public or community health, social, community, or preventive medicine offering postgraduate degrees in public health or a related field, involving an additional 17 countries.[81]

Twenty-six of the schools of public health are in the United States where the population-to-school ratio is the highest in the world. Some countries, however, such as Australia, Canada, and New Zealand, with high levels of health status as measured by the usual indices, now have no schools of public health. Others such as France have only 1, as do the combined Nordic countries; the United Kingdom now has 3. The numbers in Third World countries tend to be low also. Brazil and India each have 2; Chile, Colombia, Cuba, Egypt, Indonesia, Mexico, Peru, Philippines, Thailand, Venezuela, and Vietnam all have 1 each. China, on the other hand, following the Soviet model, has 14 schools of public health; the Soviet Union itself has 15.[82]

The schism was well in place throughout the world by the last half of the twentieth century. What would Petty, Frank, Pettenkofer, Louis, Chadwick, Shattuck, Virchow, and Farr, to say nothing of Sydenham, Bright, George Paget, Acland, Mackenzie, Osler, and Štampar, think of it all? There are no right or wrong answers, only choices. Undoubtedly the choices were made from the best of motives, but that is different from saying that they are the best for all time. In the next chapter we examine other choices designed to soften the impact of the *schism* on the public's health.

References

1. Grundy F, Mackintosh JM. *The Teaching of Hygiene and Public Health in Europe.* Geneva: World Health Organization, 1957:27.
2. Ibid, p. 2.
3. Sand R. *The Advance of Social Medicine.* London: Staples Press, 1952:181.
4. Garrison FH. *An Introduction to the History of Medicine.* 4th Ed. Philadelphia: Saunders, 1929:717.
5. Osler W. *The Principles and Practice of Medicine.* 4th Ed. New York: Appleton, 1901.
6. Cushing H. *The Life of Sir William Osler.* New York: Oxford University Press, 1940:183-184.
7. Ibid, p. 346.

8. Ibid, p. 379.
9. Ibid, p. 791.
10. Ibid, pp. 878-879.
11. Ibid, pp. 1291-1292.
12. Wilson RM. *The Beloved Physician: Sir James Mackenzie.* London: John Murray, 1926.
13. Mair A. *Sir James Mackenzie: 1853-1925, General Practitioner.* Edinburgh: Churchill Livingstone, 1973.
14. Wilson RM. *The Beloved Physician: Sir James Mackenzie.* London: John Murray, 1926:300,301, 304.
15. Mair A. *Sir James Mackenzie: 1853-1925, General Practitioner.* Edinburgh: Churchill Livingstone, 1973:323-335.
16. Ibid, pp. 272-273.
17. Flexner A. *Medical Education in the United States and Canada.* Bull. No. 4. New York: Carnegie Foundation for the Advancement of Teaching, 1910.
18. Ibid, p. 326.
19. Ibid, p. 326-327.
20. Ibid, p. 330.
21. Fosdick RB. *The Story of the Rockefeller Foundation.* New York: Harper, 1952.
22. Brown ER. *Rockefeller Medicine Men: Medicine and Capitalism in America.* Berkeley: University of California Press, 1979.
23. Berliner HS. *A System of Scientific Medicine: Philanthropic Foundations in the Flexner Era.* New York and London: Tavistock Publications, 1985; and Berliner HS. *Philanthropic Foundations and Scientific Medicine.* D.Sc. thesis, School of Hygiene and Public Health, The Johns Hopkins University, Baltimore, Maryland.
24. Bowers JZ. *The Health of Mankind: The Contributions of the Rockefeller Foundation, 1913-1980.* (Unpublished manuscript containing quotations and references from the Rockefeller Archive Center, Pocantico Hills, New York; given to KLW by JZB in 1982.)
25. Jonas G. *The Circuit Riders: Rockefeller Money and the Rise of Modern Science.* New York: Norton, 1989.
26. Fosdick RB. *The Story of the Rockefeller Foundation.* New York: Harper, 1952:22.
27. Stifel LD, Davidson RK, Coleman JS, eds. *Social Sciences & Public Policy in the Developing World.* Lexington, Mass: Lexington Books, 1982:57.
28. Brown ER. *Rockefeller Medicine Men: Medicine and Capitalism in America.* Berkeley: University of California Press, 1979:120.
29. Cushing H. *The Life of Sir William Osler.* New York: Oxford University Press, 1940:455.
30. Osler W. *The Principles and Practice of Medicine.* 4th Ed. New York: Appleton, 1901.
31. Fosdick RB. *The Story of the Rockefeller Foundation.* New York: Harper, 1952:24.
32. Williams G. Schools of public health—Their doing and undoing. Milbank Memorial Fund Quarterly: Health and Society 54 1976:489-527, 504. and a more extensive draft manuscript on which this article was based given to KLW by GW in 1966.
33. Fye WB, and Witte CL, MH. William Osler's Departure from North America, Correspondence. New Engl J Med 1989:321:1199.
34. Williams G. Schools of public health—Their doing and undoing. Milbank Memorial Fund Quarterly: Health and Society, 1976:506.
35. Acheson, RM. The epidemiology of Charles-Edward Amory Winslow. Amer J Epidiol, 91 1979:1-18.

36. Williams G. Schools of public health—Their doing and undoing. Milbank Memorial Fund Quarterly: Health and Society, 1976:506.
37. Jordan EO, Whipple GC, Winslow C-EA. *A Pioneer of Public Health: William Thompson Sedgwick*. New Haven: Yale University Press, 1924:78.
38. Williams G. Schools of public health—Their doing and undoing. Milbank Memorial Fund Quarterly: Health and Society, 1976:509.
39. Ibid, p. 501.
40. Ibid, p. 509.
41. Ibid.
42. Ibid.
43. Ibid, p. 507.
44. Acheson RM. Three Regius professors, sanitary science, and state medicine: the birth of an academic discipline. Br Med J 1986; 293:1602-1606.
45. Ibid, p. 1603.
46. Ibid, pp. 1602-1606.
47. Fee E. *Disease and Discovery: A History of the Johns Hopkins School of Hygiene and Public Health, 1916-1939*. Baltimore: Johns Hopkins, 1987:36.
48. Rose W. School of public health (Mimeographed memorandum), May 15, 1915, R.G. 1.1, Ser. 200, Rockefeller Foundation Archive and Institute of Hygiene, *Annual Report*, 1916. New York: Rockefeller Foundation, 1916.
49. Williams G. Schools of public health—Their doing and undoing. Milbank Memorial Fund Quarterly: Health and Society, 1976:513.
50. Ibid.
51. Ibid.
52. Fosdick RB. *The Story of the Rockefeller Foundation*. New York: Harper, 1952.
53. Brown ER. *Rockefeller Medicine Men: Medicine and Capitalism in America*. Berkeley: University of California Pres, 1979.
54. Williiams G. Schools of public health—Their doing and undoing. Milbank Memorial Fund Quarterly: Health and Society, 1976.
55. Fee E. *Disease and Discovery: A History of the Johns Hopkins School of Hygiene and Public Health, 1916-1939*. Baltimore: Johns Hopkins, 1987.
56. Ibid, p. 39.
57. Rose W. School of public health (Mimeographed memorandum), May 15, 1915, R.G. 1.1, Ser 200, Rockefeller Foundation Archive and Institute of Hygiene. 1915:10.
58. Ibid, pp. 10-11.
59. Ibid, pp. 11-12.
60. Ibid, p. 12.
61. *Annual Report, 1916*. New York: Rockefeller Foundation, 1916.
62. Ibid, p. 417.
63. Fleming D. *William Welch and the Rise of Modern Medicine*. Baltimore: Johns Hopkins, 1954.
64. Ibid, p. 181.
65. Rose W. School of public health (Mimeographed memorandum), May 15, 1915, R.G. 1.1, Ser. 200, Rockefeller Foundation Archive and Institute of Hygiene. 1915:4.
66. Ibid, p. 17.
67. *Annual Report, 1916*. New York: Rockefeller Foundation, 1916:416.
68. Ibid.
69. Codman EA. The product of a hospital. Surg Gynecol Obstet, 1914; April:491-496.
70. *Annual Report, 1916*. New York: Rockefeller Foundation, 1916:425.

71. Fleming D. *William Welch and the Rise of Modern Medicine*. Baltimore: Johns Hopkins, 1954:182.
72. Freymann JG. Medicine's great schism: prevention vs cure: an historical interpretation. Med Care 1975;13:535.
73. Bowers JZ. *The Health of Mankind: The Contributions of the Rockefeller Foundation, 1913-1980*. (Unpublished manuscript containing quotations and references from the Rockefeller Archive Center, Pocantico Hills, New York: given to KLW by JZB in 1982.) 1982:III-25.
74. Sand R. *The Advance of Social Medicine*. London: Staples Press, 1952:224.
75. Grmek MD, ed. *Serving the Cause of Public Health: Selected Papers of Andrija Štampar* (Halar M, Waring LF, trans.) Zagreb: Andrija Štampar School of Public Health, Medical Faculty, University of Zagreb, 1966.
76. Ibid, p. 43.
77. Ibid.
78. Vuletic A. *Evaluation of Medical Education for General Practitioners* and Annex, (Mimeographed). Zagreb: Andrija Štampar School of Public Health, Medical Faculty, University of Zagreb, 1971.
79. Štampar A. After five years: problems of the medical faculty at Zagreb (1957). In: Grmek MD, ed. *Serving the Cause of Public Health*. Zagreb: Andrija Štampar School of Public Health, Medical Faculty, University of Zagreb, 1966:254.
80. Fosdick RB. *The Story of the Rockefeller Foundation*. New York: Harper, 1952:42.
81. World Health Organization. *Directory of Schools of Public Health and Programmes in Public Health*, 3d Ed. Geneva: World Health Organization, 1985.
82. Association of Schools of Public Health. *Reach*. Washington, D.C.: ASPH, 1988.

5
Miscellaneous Medicine

The Rockefeller Foundation's initiative in supporting schools of public health unquestionably has had a beneficial impact on the health of populations in both developed and developing countries. By the last quarter of the twentieth century there were growing numbers of these schools' graduates, who could document, publicize, and initiate the process of redefining the unacceptable. Official agencies—including international ones such as the World Health Organization and UNICEF—national Ministries of Health, and state, provincial, and local health departments throughout the world have been strengthened. To varying degrees they were staffed, but as discussed in Chapter 1, not always led by physicians who were graduates of these schools. Professional societies were formed, national and international meetings organized, journals launched, diplomas and certificates awarded, and accreditation teams established to approve one another's institutions. During the second quarter of the twentieth century, public health became something of a growth industry among society's service enterprises.

As a group, public health workers eagerly sought to stake out preventive medicine as their territory. They distinguished it from an increasingly laboratory-oriented, hospital-dominated, reductionist, and treatment-based medicine. But for all this there were long-term costs.

Aided and abetted by the *Flexner Report*, medical school faculties and students had little exposure to the population perspective. Physicians were trained to study and cure disease based on laboratory diagnosis, and the site for all this was the hospital's wards. The lines were drawn ever more sharply between curative and preventive medicine. The population with its health problems was no longer the concern of the medical school faculty or of its graduates. Out of sight, out of mind! Resources, or lack of them, to help and support both those at risk and those who had succumbed to illness were the responsibility of some other institution, agency or—as the public health workers argued—some other profession.

Nevertheless, the new sciences of bacteriology and immunology reinvigorated the concept of prevention. Medical faculties, especially those in universities without a school of public health, came to recognize that it was incumbent on them to provide some instruction on subjects initially labeled hygiene, sanitary science, preventive medicine, and sometimes public health. Not all the original departments of hygiene had been converted to schools of public health. Many, especially in Germany and the United States, sensing the need to have a scientific base, opted to merge with bacteriology units, laboratories, or departments. Alternatively, the latter expanded to embrace hygiene or preventive medicine, especially as it applied to the infectious diseases. The concept of prevention, in particular, had considerable appeal, especially from a political point of view. Medical school faculty members with a bent for social reform and a vision of prevention that extended beyond immunization, clean water, safe food, and effective sanitation often found their most hospitable reception within these departments.

Later, other topics thought to merit some attention but said to be beyond the responsibilities of clinicians were added to the portfolios of the new departments. Following the discovery of vitamins, nutrition received some attention. Then came a spate of more specific industrial concerns with noxious substances inhaled, ingested, or absorbed cutaneously, with chemical toxins, ionizing radiation, smoking, traffic accidents, occupational "stress," food additives, and medicaments of dubious quality, safety, or efficacy. The list goes on to genetic abnormalities, to screening for developmental abnormalities and then for specific diseases. Tuberculosis, venereal diseases, alcoholism, mental illness, and malnutrition were soon matters for which these evolving departments were either assigned or assumed responsibility. Next was added a series of related skills, disciplines, or topics. These included operations research, planning and evaluation, medical sociology, and sometimes anthropology and psychology. Together with the schools of public health, departments of social and preventive medicine made their contributions to redefining the unacceptable.

Soon patients lacking access to medical care for specific diseases such as tuberculosis, venereal diseases, and other targeted conditions were identified as concerns of "public health clinics." Following the introduction of categorical services in Britain and the early establishment of outpatient departments for the indigent in the United States, problem- or disease-specific clinics for each unacceptable state were established. Then dedicated clinics were created for immunization, for the care of pregnant women and their children, for provision of school health services, and for family planning. Later came specialized clinics under the aegis of health departments for the care of patients with chronic diseases such as hypertension, mental illness, cancer, and the screening of newborns. These categorical, vertical programs required discussion with medical students. Each new health problem that did not attract the interest of one of the major clinical departments was added to the portfolios of what have been referred to as Departments of Miscellaneous Medicine.[1] Anything that the traditional clinical departments did not want to embrace for whatever reason was hived off to these often willing, but understaffed and underresourced departments.

In all of this, where was *numeracy*? Vital statistics were usually taught by these departments as cold abstractions that dealt with aggregated national causes of death. Little attention was paid to the problems of labeling patients' illnesses, the changing fashions in nosography, the structures of nomenclatures and classification schemes, or the role of clinicians in providing the original data from which vital events and other medical attributes are transformed into statistics. Nor was the importance of observer error and variation in labelling and coding taught. Methods of statistical standardization were often expounded without relating the precision of the mathematical maneuver to the quality of the underlying clinical data. John Graunt, William Petty, William Farr, and even Major Greenwood would have been bitterly disappointed to observe the sterile fashion in which their seminal thinking was too often obscured by stodgy recitals of disembodied statistics.

From the teaching of vital statistics there were few extensions to matters of health statistics. The former were largely concerned with counting the dead (and recording births); the latter were concerned with the problems of the living. The faculty in expanded statistical units in these medical school departments, as well as in schools of public health, focused increasingly on what came to be called biostatistics. This meant primarily the application of statistical methods to biological problems studied in bench laboratories and less and less frequently in clinical settings. Undoubtedly the quality of research design in basic science departments and a few clinical departments was enhanced. On the other hand, major improvements in methods for monitoring the public's health came largely from those developing social survey methods.

Epidemiology, the origins and uses of which are among the principal themes throughout this discourse, was taught largely as a descriptive method for understanding the sources, courses, and sometimes control of infectious disease epidemics. The links of the Departments of Miscellaneous Medicine to Departments of Bacteriology served only to emphasize this perspective. The teaching stressed descriptive and shoe leather epidemiology, certainly worthwhile topics, but scarcely the totality of this central scientific discipline or the applications that James Mackenzie had in mind when he spoke of the "new epidemiology." "The big bug hunt" that preoccupied the clinical departments of medical schools was reinforced by adoption of the same theme by most Departments of Miscellaneous Medicine. Prevention tended to focus on finding, eliminating, or controlling the cause of each disease. The monoetiological view of disease and the "magic bullet" theory of treatment became the dominant motifs of Western medicine during the middle two quarters of the twentieth century.

John R. Paul (1893-1971), Professor of both Internal Medicine and Preventive Medicine at Yale, was among those most concerned with the direction being taken by American academic medicine. In his presidential address to the American Society for Clinical Investigation in 1938 Paul introduced the term "clinical epidemiology."[2] This was an effort to broaden the application of the scientific method to the study of clinical problems and their origins in the community. The term is of much less importance than either the concept or the occasion on which he delivered his message. Paul's seminal address started with the observation that:

> In an attempt to predict some of the trends along which Clinical Investigation may proceed in the next few decades, the subject of Preventive Medicine naturally arises as a field for these activities. The term, Clinical Investigation in Preventive Medicine, is cumbersome...and even the term Preventive Medicine has never seemed ideal. It

implies a little too much in the way of propaganda. It presupposes the existence of a sister science, Curative Medicine, and both sciences are committed perhaps too definitely to a therapeutic program. Clinical Investigation in Epidemiology is better for the purposes at hand; Clinical Epidemiology is best, and really what I mean. In fact this is the name I would like to propose for a new science; a new discipline in which this Society might take an important part. It is a science concerned with circumstances, whether they are "functional" or "organic," under which human disease is prone to develop.[3]

Paul went on to relate his concepts and methods to the clinical situation of the contemporary medical academician. He continued:

[N]ow that the emphasis, for this Society at least, has shifted from the home and into the Hospital and Dispensary, clinical epidemiology will be practiced only if we take thought about it. It is a foreign concept for most intramural clinical investigators whose contact with the actual circumstances under which their patients became ill may be limited to a page in the hospital history, or a supplementary talk with a social worker.[4]

After reciting several clinical advances based on combined epidemiological and clinical studies and making certain distinctions between the epidemiology that clinicians might embrace and that which the "orthodox science" of epidemiology uses; his remarks have a strong contemporary ring:

...[W]e may now have to dispel a smoke screen that the folklore of both Preventive Medicine and Curative Medicine has thrown out which consists in a sort of censorship about the meaning of disease, in which there are at least two assumptions. These are: (A) that all disease is bad and hence all attempts to prevent it, or cure it, are good, regardless of its cause or the conditions under which it arises; and (B) that disease is something which an unkind fate has put upon us; in other words disease is not of our own making but it comes from elsewhere....To turn the spotlight of investigation upon these assumptions is the first duty of the clinical epidemiologist.

And further:

If these fields are eventually to be investigated, it is the man (*sic*) with clinical judgment who can best blaze the trail, for it is the prime responsibility of the clinician to do the work. It is his responsibility far more than that of the public health man, or the bacteriologist, or the chemist. To do this the clinician will, however, have to adopt a new technique, and a new uniform. Gone is the glamorous role of the microbe hunter for this type of investigation, and in his place all we can see is something like a rank sociologist.[5]

Paul was echoing the thoughts of Petty, Frank, and certainly of Rudolf Virchow. But his message fell on deaf ears. The institutionalized schism was already both wide and deep; clinical curiosity about causes and interventions had been replaced by a deterministic search for certainty in the wet laboratory and an aggressive view toward diagnosis and therapy that would have shaken to the core the likes of Louis.

Another prominent clinician who sought to stem the tide was John A. Ryle (1889-1950). Following a distinguished career in clinical medicine at Guy's

Hospital Medical School he was appointed Regius Professor of Physic at Cambridge, heading up its new Department of Medicine. In 1943, after 8 years in this prestigious position, he moved to Oxford as first Professor and Director of that university's new Institute of Social Medicine. Ryle's keen social consciousness, his intense clinical interest in the personal lives and circumstances of his patients, and his recognition that medicine was in danger of developing an excessively narrow perspective encouraged him to take up this new appointment. He was much ahead of his time as evidenced by the views set forth in a remarkable little volume, *Changing Disciplines*; it should be of interest to all who aspire to merge the micro and macro levels of the medical endeavor.[6] The book is based largely on lectures given by Ryle in 1947 during a visit to Canada and the United States sponsored by the Rockefeller Foundation. In the Introduction to this classic, Ryle wrote, more than 40 years ago:

> Looking back, it has seemed to me that, while Medicine—through scientific and technical advances—has greatly gained in potentiality during the past quarter of a century, it has, in the process, become less surely attuned to some fundamental human needs—to the deeper personal needs of the individual and to the broader social needs of the group or community. Reforms which should be a particular concern of medicine are still overdue or have found their chief support elsewhere....We are still as a profession, thinking more about curing than preventing, more about medical care and its huge costs than about the economies which could be effected by attacking the basic causes of disease.[7]

Ryle claimed that he was "ever bad at sums" but nevertheless he was a great admirer of William Farr. Whereas it was the postmortem examination that provided retrospective insights into the individual patient's disease, Ryle observed that it was what he termed Farr's social postmortem that was equally important for the health of populations. "Such analyses provided a mathematical refinement of the broad and historic social surveys of Edwin Chadwick. The two great branches of human pathology thus had their beginnings almost simultaneously. The social postmortem examination employs statistical methods and techniques to reveal death rates and their trends in the population, whether from all causes or specific causes, and these rates and trends can be correlated with specific social factors and social change."[8]

Ryle had much to say about nearly all aspects of medical education, practice, and research, but here we are concerned primarily with the *schism*. Sir Charles Symonds in his obituary of Ryle wrote that "he was convinced that the orientation of medicine was wrong, that health and its causes should be actively studied, that normal health should be defined by scientific methods, and departures from the normal related, on the one hand, to the range of individual variation and, on the other, to all the operative factors in the social system."[9] Ryle's own views on the separation of medicine and public health are worth quoting:

> Outside a few great research institutes...such as the London School of Hygiene and Tropical Medicine—which has served broad national and imperial needs but has had only a slender association with the life and work of the hospitals and the medical

schools or with other scientific departments of the university—social pathology has, until lately, been accorded no position of its own. Its students, whether they work in the fields of public health bacteriology, of epidemiology and vital statistics, or other subjects, have tended to do so in various places and in detachment and without the advantages of a presiding and coordinating discipline....Its outstanding importance notwithstanding, social pathology has not notably influenced clinical teachers and the regular instruction of the medical student.

....Lacking the necessary time and associations for expansion, the medicine of the hospital ward and the research unit has been contracting its field and becoming by degrees an exercise in bedside pathology, pharmacology and therapeutic detail. The broader natural history of disease in man has been too little considered....

....It is curious that aetiology, in its wider sense, should have so far lost the interest which it had for the older physicians. While specific agents are still assiduously sought for, the contemporary neglect of more comprehensive inquiry—taking into account the influence not only of specific factors and of age and sex and race and heredity, but also economic circumstance, domestic environment, occupation, nutrition, and education—would I believe, have attracted the adverse comment of [many of the] great physicians.[10]

Research methods and the need to broaden the application of epidemiological concepts and methods to the noninfectious diseases and to a host of other social and community disorders and problems were of deep concern to Ryle. He distinguished between the study of *man* and study of the *environment*, between the study of *individuals* and the study of *groups*. There was a need for all and there was an equal need to link them together within a broader view of health and disease than seemed to prevail within either of what had become the two camps of medicine and public health.

"Thirty years of my life," Ryle wrote, "have been spent as a student and teacher of clinical medicine. In these thirty years I have watched disease in the ward being studied more and more thoroughly—if not more thoughtfully—through the high power of the microscope; disease in man being investigated by more and more elaborate techniques and, on the whole, more and more mechanically. Man, as a person and a member of a family and of much larger social groups, with his health and sickness intimately bound up with the conditions of his life and work—in the home, the mine, the factory, the shop, at sea, or on the land—and with his economic opportunity, has been inadequately considered in this period by the clinical teacher and hospital research worker."[11] John Ryle was an intellectual descendant of Petty, Frank, Louis, von Pettenkofer, Virchow, Farr, and closely related to Osler and Mackenzie; steeped in the clinical medicine of the day he said that in embracing social medicine he was "merely taking the necessary steps to enlarge my field of vision."[12] In 1949 Ryle resigned his Chair at Oxford because of ill health; he died a year later—some said of a broken heart.[13]

There were others in Britain who saw the need for change. In 1953, Thomas McKeown of the University of Birmingham, whom we met in Chapter 3, was another early Professor of Social Medicine. He summarized the state of affairs at that time in an address to the First World Conference on Medical Education.[14]

Based on study of the contemporary reports of the Goodenough Committee on medical education in Britain and the interim report of the Social and Preventive Medicine Committee of the Royal College of Physicians, McKeown concluded that:

- Medical education was in some danger of losing sight of the continuing importance of prevention of disease. It was recognized that an account of the public health services was usually provided in formal lectures; but this instruction was divorced from clinical teaching and was thought to make too little impression on the student.

- Insufficient attention was given to the relation of the social environment to health and to the social complications of illness. Much emphasis was placed on the work of social workers in the teaching hospital, the point of view being very similar to that expressed in the American Books, *The Patient as a Person*[*] and *Patients Have Families.*[+]

- The responsibilities of the community for the provision of medical services deserved more attention.[15]

McKeown noted that the situation was similar in Britain and the United States, except that by 1948 Britain had already established the National Health Service, while the United States continued (and continues) to debate the matter of national health insurance. Otherwise, McKeown regarded his analysis as applying to both countries, and I would add, also to Europe and the developing world. His main point was that the departments referred to as "social medicine" in Britain and as "preventive medicine" in the United States were established primarily for teaching. Both of the British reports he referred to, as well as the two American books published by the Commonwealth Fund, emphasized the teaching mission of these departments. Urging them to stress the need for expanding medical students' horizons beyond the walls of the hospital and for considering their patients' natural habitats and social environments served only to remove the clinical departments and clinicians generally from responsibility for these matters. Nonclinicians were told to discuss the responsibilities of clinicians—hardly a recipe for enlisting the hearts and minds of medical students.

But there were other charges. Neither of the two British reports nor the two American books said much about the need for research, the coin of the realm in universities. McKeown wrote that

....the Goodenough Report, which devotes more than a page to the participation of social workers in the teaching of social medicine [dismisses research by observing]: 'To be a stimulating teacher...[the professor of social medicine] ought to have taken part in investigations aimed at furthering knowledge in some province of social medicine'....The report of the Royal College of Physicians is equally vague and brief: 'Interest and training in research are highly desirable, *if only in order that* the

---

[*]Robinson, G.C. *The Patient as a Person.* New York: Commonwealth Fund, 1946.
[+]Richardson, H.B. *Patients Have Families.* New York: Commonwealth Fund, 1945.

department of social and preventive medicine shall attain an equal status with other departments.'....But the nature of the research was thought a matter of secondary importance: 'It is considered immaterial whether this training be in epidemiology, bacteriology, nutrition, child health, social science, statistics or in a field like tropical medicine.'....The reports..did not ask on what terms a new department without routine laboratory or bedside commitments was to make its place within the present competitive framework of university scientific life.[16]

McKeown pointed out that the early links of these departments to bacteriology was largely fortuitous but, insofar as prevention was concerned, most of the measures invoked under the aegis of the sanitary idea were employed years before the discovery of bacteria. He questioned whether attempts to establish the prevention of disease as a new and separate "discipline" or department was sensible. All would agree that "an ounce is worth a pound," but before prevention came the need to understand the genesis of the disease. McKeown concluded his analysis by arguing that the central research focus of the rapidly multiplying departments of social and preventive medicine was the study of the phenomena of health and disease using data gathered from large numbers of people, that is, populations; "[e]pidemiological methods which were successfully used in the investigation of infectious diseases can be applied to a wide range of problems. Thus one of the most neglected methods of medical research could become one of the most fruitful."[17]

In the United States, the term preventive medicine was preferred to social medicine. The latter term was eschewed to avoid inflaming those members of the medical profession who could not distinguish between the words "social" and "socialized." Uncertainties about its own academic status prompted the holding of three major postwar conferences on preventive medicine. The first of these, sponsored by the Association of American Medical Colleges, was held in Ann Arbor, Michigan, in 1946. It called for the establishment of separate departments of preventive medicine in all medical schools. They were to be funded by 5 to 8% of the total school budget, and 160 hours of teaching time was to be allocated to the department.[18] None of this came to pass.

A second conference, sponsored by both the Association of American Medical Colleges and the Conference of Professors of Preventive Medicine, the precursor of the Association of Teachers of Preventive Medicine, was held in Colorado Springs, Colorado, in 1952.[19] Although the published report sets forth aspirations and visions of the future not unlike those espoused by Ryle and McKeown, the whole exercise seemed to lack focus and a sense of direction, according to Alan Gregg, by then Vice President of the Rockefeller Foundation and one of the conference participants. In his concluding summary of the Conference, a classic from which all students of these matters could profit, Gregg observed that he was "fascinated by the procedure simply as a study of confusion." Not only that but he was reminded, he said, "of a sign that used to be outside the railroad station in Tokyo before the war. The sign read: *S. Makamuri & Company, Transfer Forwarding Agents. Your baggage sent in all directions!*"[20]

The Conference was long on theory and broad in content. Like McKeown, however, its report did stress epidemiology first, followed by biostatistics, as the two central disciplines bearing on prevention. Even the definition of epidemiology used by the Conferees is worth noting since it is broader than many:

> ...[E]pidemiology is the study of all factors and their interrelationships which affect the occurrence and course of health and disease in a population. These factors include the characteristics of the host population; the causative agencies—predisposing, precipitating and perpetuating; and the biological, physical and social environment. The objective is to discover the causes of the disease process and to determine the points in its natural history where interruptions may be accomplished in man's favor.[21]

The participants can only be applauded for laying out a creative approach to medical education and a vision of the future physician that would have gladdened the hearts, and even expanded the minds, of the great clinicians and proponents of the population perspective. There was much talk about joint teaching ventures and about the need to inculcate attitudes that favored better understanding of the origins and natural history of disease and greater attention to opportunities for prevention at the individual and collective levels. Where the Conference failed, in my view, was by perpetuating and deepening the separation of clinical medicine and epidemiology.

The critical issue was not so much what should be done as who should be seen to be doing it. Epidemiology was to be taught by nonclinician epidemiologists as a separate subject. "The principles of epidemiology may be taught by reading, lecture and seminar" the Conference Report affirmed.[22] Epidemiology was not seen as a set of essential concepts and skills that all medical students, residents, and clinicians should acquire, together with skills in communication, physical examination, and evaluating laboratory data. Paul and Ryle argued that all clinicians should embrace the population perspective, as well as the clinical and cellular. McKeown argued that epidemiology, together with biostatistics, should be the major scientific disciplines in all departments of social or preventive medicine. The Colorado Conference argued that epidemiology and biostatistics should be major disciplines of these departments but they also diluted this emphasis by including a wide array of other disciplines, topics, areas of concern, interest, and endeavor. Once again, the conferees reinforced the perception that these are indeed Departments of Miscellaneous Medicine. Departments of social and preventive medicine were joining schools of public health in separating themselves ever further from an increasingly narrow view of the task of medicine generally and of clinical medicine in particular.

In 1963, the Association of Teachers of Preventive Medicine held its third Conference, at Saratoga Springs, New York. George A. Wolf, Jr., M.D., Vice-President for Medical and Dental Affairs, Tufts University, delivered a classic paper entitled "The Specialty of ?." His opening gambit left no doubt about his biases: "I have purposely made my title vague because I cannot find a satisfactory definition of what you people are trying to do. You apparently aspire to a single specialty or discipline. The Oxford Dictionary defines a specialty as a body of knowledge that has been made narrow and more intense."[23] Wolf, acknowledging that he was a friend of many of the participants and interested in what they were trying to do, then launched into a blistering critique of their entire operation. Here are excerpts:

> The specialty of ? has no dominant or unifying technology such as the physical examination, the surgical manipulation, the Warburg apparatus, the scintillation counter, the cardiac catheter, or the analyst's couch. It has not attracted our best men (*sic*), lacks something of a status symbol, and has some of the attributes of a minority group. Too often you want to be integrated without being willing to compete on the basis of quality....Withal I detect the feeling of self-pity and defensiveness which characterizes minority groups. The subject indeed suffers more from being ignored than from being discriminated against.

> ....First, assemble your individual—and I stress individual—assets. Stop defending the specialty of ? because you really can't define it. Develop to its fullest extent what each of you has in terms of individual ability and interest....It is possible in the future that you will be in five departments in the medical school instead of one, or that you will individually disappear as you are individually sought to play important roles in the classical departments, so to speak, of medical schools. Of course it is true we all need the feeling of togetherness but why not make quality of performance the unifying principle.

> ....Instead of using your statistical know-how to prove how right you are, use it to disqualify some of the questionable results written in so-called scientific papers produced by other departments. Instead of giving lectures to students on continuing medical care, make the clinicians answer the specific questions relevant to what happens to the *interesting patients* on discharge from the hospital. Use the language of the clinicians and the basic physical scientist....Avoid gimmicks and evangelism. Medical scientists and clinicians, as you know, are trained to doubt but not necessarily in a scientific way. The successful authoritarian professor in the clinical fields...,however unscientific in his approach, is able to cast doubt upon his opponent's viewpoint and thus prevail.

> You and your critics have frequently said that students are not attracted to the specialty of ?. I believe there is evidence to support this in terms, for example, of the number of medical graduates going into the specialty of ?. May I suggest that in developing any program of graduate education you resolve to conduct only high-quality programs or none at all and that you resolve to select only qualified students.[24]

Wolf concluded his remarks with a cogent comment implying the need for medical schools to embrace the population perspective:

> I feel strongly that it is the responsibility of the medical schools and their departments at this point to define community needs in more precise terms and that organizational methods for meeting these needs will become obvious when the data is assembled and interpreted in a scientific fashion. It is not difficult to sit in an office and dream up systems for keeping everybody healthy. It is difficult to define the needs of the community and most difficult to prove that their needs can be met by a given system. In my opinion, there has been too much focus on the system and not enough on the needs and very little concerning the proof that the needs are met or will be met by a

given system. Although the research called for may be considered applied, the approach is basic.[25]

The balance of the Saratoga Springs Conference Report was a gloomy account of the state of research and research training in preventive medicine departments. Great emphasis, it was observed, was placed on teaching a wide spectrum of topics in an equally dispersed array of settings by varied mixes of faculty. There was a paucity of first-rate research that in turn was linked to the relatively few faculty members interested in systematic enquiry. Lack of adequate funding for research, especially by the U.S. National Institutes of Health, was seen as a major impediment. Research training was limited, indeed. The year 1962 found only 42 trainees in the country's medical schools pursuing research careers—and not all were working for advanced degrees. Of the 42, only a quarter were physicians. In the same year, for the collective student bodies of American schools of public health the ratio of physicians to total graduate students pursuing research training was even lower; 97 of the 463 students were physicians, or 21%.[26]

There was much discussion at the Conference about the relative merits of providing graduate training in departments of preventive medicine instead of in schools of public health. Consensus was reached that research training cannot be provided in the absence of faculty who are themselves pursuing important and creative research questions. There was wide divergence of views about other subjects to be taught, but the Conference did agree with McKeown:

> Obviously the first step in gaining acceptance as equal partners in the health sciences within a medical school is the demonstration to the medical faculty and, perhaps even more important, to the students, that public health and preventive medicine are established on as firm scientific bases as the other clinical and preclinical disciplines. The main scientific bases for both preventive medicine and public health are epidemiology and biometry.[27]

One innovation of interest to our present discussion was recorded. Two departments in the Yale University Medical School recently had been merged. John Paul's Section of Preventive Medicine within the Department of Internal Medicine, created by him in 1940, was consolidated with the Department of Public Health, an accredited "School" of Public Health, founded in 1915 by Professor C.-E. A. Winslow and presided over since 1945 by Professor Ira Hiscock. With the retirement of Professors Paul and Hiscock, a new Department of Epidemiology and Public Health was established within the School of Medicine. The merger was justified on the grounds that there was much overlap of interests in the two antecedent departments; closer association should strengthen all components. To date that department continues to function as an accredited school of public health although its links with clinical medicine are tenuous at best.[28]

In 1951 Alexander D. Langmuir initiated a novel approach to strengthening the teaching of epidemiology and providing recent medical graduates with an appreciation of epidemiological principles and methods.[29] As Chief of the Epidemiology Branch and its Epidemic Intelligence Service (EIS) in what was then the Communicable Disease Center of the U.S. Public Health Service, he started a 2-year training program for an entering cohort of about 25 young physicians, most of them headed for clinical careers. After introductory lectures, tutorials, and practical exercises lasting several months, the trainees were assigned to supervised field work, usually in state Health Departments. These assignments were involved with actual epidemics, more often than not associated with communicable diseases as a result of breaches in water, food, or sanitation standards.

Although aided by the fact that the 2-year EIS program was accepted by the Draft Board in lieu of military service, the program had the effect of exposing hundreds of young physicians to both the principles of epidemiology and one practical application—known colloquially as "shoe-leather" epidemiology, in the great traditions of John Snow, William Budd, and others who pioneered the field. This program exists to the present, but now the enrollees are volunteers; from about 200 applicants annually, some 65 are selected of whom 50 or more are physicians. An increasing number of them have had some prior formal training in epidemiology at a school of public health (personal communication, M. B. Gregg, M.D., Centers for Disease Control, April 1989).

Other important contributions to bridging the growing gulf between clinical medicine and public health have been provided by summer short courses in epidemiology and biostatistics. First offered at the University of Minnesota, the numbers and content of these courses have expanded considerably. Among the universities now sponsoring similar courses are Michigan and Tufts, the Johns Hopkins, and McGill. McMaster University has held well-attended courses in "Design, Measurement, and Evaluation" for a dozen or more years. In England, the London School of Hygiene and Tropical Medicine has for many decades provided courses of several months' duration in epidemiology and statistics for both domestic and foreign students; more recently the University of Southampton has been offering a short course in epidemiology sponsored by the British Council for students from Third World countries, and since 1988 a "European Educational Programme in Epidemiology," sponsored by components of the World Health Organization and the Regional Government of Tuscany, has been available at Florence. At a more specialized level the 10-day workshops on cardiovascular epidemiology established in the 1960s by Professor Ancel Keys, Jeremiah Stamler, and Geoffrey Rose had a major influence on research in this field, attracting both clinicians and epidemiologists who worked together. These are examples of attempts to "spread the gospel" from the enclaves of epidemiology, primarily in schools of public health, to the larger health establishment.

Meanwhile in the 1950s the Rockefeller Foundation began to broaden the base of medical education to encompass community concerns. It merged its own programs in public health and medical education. Elsewhere an interest also developed in fostering communication among faculty members in the various departments of social and preventive medicine on both sides of the Atlantic. For just this purpose, in 1954 John Pemberton, Professor of Social and Preventive Medicine, Queen's College, Belfast; Harold N. Willard, M.D., then of Cornell Medical College; and Robert Cruikshank, Professor of Bacteriology, University of Edinburgh, formed the International Corresponding Club. A mimeographed

Bulletin was circulated to a membership that by 1956 had reached 49 individuals from 18 countries. This group rapidly identified epidemiology as the key discipline that united the founding members in spite of their often disparate views on other medical matters.

The Rockefeller Foundation began its long association with epidemiology by funding the initial meeting of the International Corresponding Club at Noordwijk, The Netherlands, in 1957. This close involvement with what soon became the International Epidemiological Association (IEA) has continued to the present. The IEA's membership has grown to almost 2000 members in more than 100 countries. Some two dozen books have been published or sponsored, including the first-ever *Dictionary of Epidemiology*.[30] In 1972 the original mimeographed *Bulletin* was transformed into the International Journal of Epidemiology, now a major scientific journal in the field.

Of particular interest in connection with the present volume has been the IEA's early commitment to stimulating epidemiological research. Initially the bulk of this embyronic organization's efforts was directed at clinicians. Toward this end the Association during the 1960s organized more than a dozen seminars in the developing world designed to assist clinicians in understanding the uses of epidemiology for investigating their indigenous medical problems. For two decades, in addition to 12 triennial international scientific meetings, there have been numerous regional scientific meetings held throughout the Third World. The best evaluation of this entire enterprise has been less the steady growth of the Association's membership and the circulation of the *International Journal of Epidemiology* than the vigorous participation of younger investigators in presenting their research at the regional and international scientific meetings.

Two points deserve mention. First is the emphasis the IEA has always placed on developing epidemiology as an international science directed at fostering improved understanding and amelioration of local problems of health and disease, including improved evaluation and management of health services. Second has been its continuing educational mission of encouraging both the training of more epidemiologists and the diffusion of epidemiological thinking throughout the medical and public health establishments, especially in the developing world. Indeed, if Chadwick and Shattuck can be thought of as zealous proponents of the sanitary idea, the IEA should be thought of as the zealous proponent of population-based research. For this dedication, the Association owes much to its first President, the late Robert Cruikshank, who constantly urged the membership to "spread the gospel" of epidemiology.

But there were resistances to broadening the application of the discipline even within the organization. As late as 1960, at a meeting in Prague, a number of epidemiologists from Eastern European countries were not persuaded that epidemiological methods could or should be applied to noncommunicable disorders— including the "dancing mania" of the middle ages! And in the 1970s there was similar resistance to extending epidemiological methods to the evaluation of health services, in addition to the conduct of randomized clinical trials.[31] Even epidemiologists can be found wearing intellectual "blinders"!

In 1960 William R. Willard, M.D., was appointed founding dean of a new medical school at the University of Kentucky. With a Master of Public Health degree from Yale, Willard was determined that this new school would have a community-oriented and population-based approach to medical education. Accordingly he and Professor Kurt Deuschle, now of the Mount Sinai School of Medicine, New York, selected the name for the first Department of Community Medicine in the United States. Deuschle had participated in important population-based studies while at Cornell University's Medical School. This strong new department staffed by clinicians, epidemiologists, and biostatisticians working side by side played a major role in the early development of the school. Unfortunately, a decade or so later, with the departure of many of the initial leaders, the early promise of the school as a new model and pacesetter for medical education waned. A trend was established, however, and in 1962 the University of Vermont converted its Department of Preventive Medicine to a Department of Epidemiology and Community Medicine. Again, the initial strong population-based approach, combined with substantial clinical involvement, has not been maintained.

In the 1960s there were other changes afoot on both sides of the Atlantic. Community medicine, the term introduced in Kentucky, was gradually becoming the favored label for many former Departments of Preventive and Social Medicine. At least the new title had the advantage of shifting the focus from prevention, which the Colorado and Saratoga Springs Conferences had argued was really everybody's business, to the study of group phenomena and of extra hospital influences on health and disease. Numeracy and the use of statistical methods was fostered by the addition of epidemiology to the titles of the departments at Yale and Vermont, and later several others, all of which, incidentally, had senior faculty deeply involved in the International Epidemiological Association.

In Britain the term "community medicine" was first defined in 1968 by the Royal Commission on Medical Education (Todd Commission).[32] Observing that the term is currently used with different connotations, the Commission declared that:

> Community Medicine is the specialty practiced by epidemiologists and by administrators of medical services—e.g., medical officers of local authorities, central or other government departments, hospital boards or industry—and by the staffs of the corresponding academic departments.[33]

The Commission clearly identified epidemiology as the central scientific underpinning of this new discipline, at the same time linking it closely with administration, the central activity for organizing and managing the provision of health services. The Royal Commission went on, however, to state that Community Medicine was not concerned with the treatment of individual patients but with the broad questions of health and disease in, for example, particular geographical and occupational sections of the community and in the community at large. At one stroke the Commission, while attempting to bridge the gulf between clinical medicine and "public health" and "social and preventive medicine," succeeded in widening it by excluding the treatment of individual patients from the province of the community physician.

The Commission did recognize the critical importance of recruitment to the entire enterprise, by stating that although relatively few medical graduates would be required each year for further training in Community Medicine—a serious underestimate, as discussed in Chapter 1—the candidates must be of high quality. They emphasized that the "interest of young doctors must be aroused [and] a proper system of training must be introduced and trainees should see in community medicine prospects clearly as good as those in other specialties."[34]

Perhaps the ambiguities and paradoxes reflected in the Royal Commission's Report were in part a reflection of the halting evolution of Britain's health services. From 1948, with the inauguration of the National Health Service, the tripartite arrangement placed in one camp the general practitioners, administered by Executive Councils; in a second, the hospitals and the consultant specialists, under the control of Hospital Boards, run by coalitions of physician consultants, nurses, social workers, and lay members who engaged in "consensus management"; and in a third, the health officers, under Local Authority Health Departments. The latter were merged later with the Hospital Boards and administrators, as part of the second component of the National Health Service (NHS). In 1974 these arrangements were replaced by the creation of Regional, Area (abolished in 1982), and District Health Authorities with the hope that the provision of geographic responsibility and control of all personal health services would bring the hospital and community services closer together, and that both acute and chronic illness would be managed in more coordinated fashion. At the same time the position of Medical Officer of Health was abolished.

The reader will recall that there had been local Health Officers in Britain since 1872, and for 20 years after 1929 they were also responsible for administering the old Poor Law Hospitals. With the advent of the NHS these institutions were removed from their jurisdiction. At the same time, the Medical Officers of Health were left with responsibility for managing the clinical functions of domiciliary midwifery, health visiting, vaccination and immunization, and environmental hygiene.[35]

In 1972 as a consequence of the Todd Commission's Report, the Faculty of Community Medicine was established as an integral component of the Royal College of Physicians (U.K.). A precarious alliance of three groups was forged—public health, medical administration, and academic social medicine—each with different traditions, training, and agendas. The hope was that this new professional stew would somehow come to play a major role in rationalizing the provision of personal health services, on the one hand, and in improving the environmental health services that were perceived to be weakening, on the other. To accomplish this the new Community Physicians were assigned to the Health Authority management teams to advise both their clinical colleagues and lay administrators on policy matters. This new breed of physician also advised, but had no authority within, local governments that retained primary responsibility for most environmental control measures. More recently, the Community Physician's role has become even more obscure with the abolition of consensus management and the introduction of professional managers (many from industrial backgrounds) at all levels of the NHS.

Could there be little wonder that the specialty of Community Medicine in Britain had both a shaky start and a confusing history?

There is more. The Faculty of Community Medicine, although administratively embedded in the Royal College of Physicians, took a strong stance against any involvement of Community Physicians in clinical practice. They did encourage candidates for postgraduate training in the field to obtain prior clinical experience in hospitals and general practice but then told them to abandon it when entering this new field. A 1979 Working Party on the State of Community Medicine, acknowledging that it had received a number of submissions supporting the desirability of allowing Community Physicians to undertake clinical practice, stated that it:

> ...strongly disagreed with this point of view on the grounds that the specialist practice of community medicine was concerned with the health of communities, the satisfaction of their needs for services, and the actual standard of those services; the discharge of those responsibilities was incompatible with commitment to clinical practice.[36]

In his analysis of the Working Party's report, Professor Roy M. Acheson takes powerful exception to its position on clinical practice. He argues that many will find themselves, for example, making decisions about the fitness of patients to remain in the community, providing care to mothers and children, undertaking clinical research in academic departments, and discharging responsibilities for infectious disease control.[37]

About the same time, Sir Donald Acheson, currently Chief Medical Officer, Department of Health, but at that time Founding Dean, Professor of Community Medicine, and an epidemiologist at the University of Southampton, conducted a survey of trainees preparing for qualification as Members of the Faculty of Community Medicine, to ascertain their views about clinical practice by Community Physicians. He concluded:

> Most respondents thought that an option to practice part time should be encouraged, and that it would help the specialty to achieve its objectives, encourage recruitment, and improve working relationships with colleagues. An overwhelming majority said they would have no objection to colleagues practicing part-time clinical medicine, and a majority of the trainees said that they would welcome an opportunity to continue to practice when appointed to specialist grades.[38]

Two anecdotes quoted by Donald Acheson illustrate the polar views expressed by respondents in comments to his survey of trainees. From the majority position of those favoring continued clinical practice this opinion is cited:

> Without clinical involvement I do not feel community physicians can be fully effective in their role of measuring need, planning health services, or evaluating the efficiency or effectiveness of services. Neither will they gain the respect of clinical colleagues and be effective in providing the essential link between clinical doctors and other National Health Service workers, especially administrators in the planning machinery. Furthermore, I feel liaison with the public will be greatly enhanced by clinical involvement of community physicians.

And from the minority view there is this opinion:

> The practice of community medicine requires a full-time professional approach and involvement with personal clinical medicine has the danger of narrowing one's focus subtly towards particular subjects and ideas. I would prefer that specialization into community medicine would come after a broad background in clinical medical fields when some application of the problems of various areas of medicine has been obtained, rather than risking the development of an amateur part-time attitude to community medicine.[39]

Another sortie that attempted to improve matters was taken by the Presidents of several of the Royal Colleges and of the Faculty of Community Medicine in a 1983 letter to the *Lancet*. After reviewing the mounting problems they recommended, among other things:

> That [departments of community medicine] should collaborate with suitable qualified and experienced clinicians, on the basis that sessions be assigned to epidemiology in the case of hospital consultants, and suitable arrangements be made for remunerating general practitioners who contract to give such services.

> That training posts in the clinical disciplines should be established in which epidemiological training practice is included in the post description, and that liaisons are created with academic departments of epidemiology or community medicine or epidemiology research units.[40]

The staff of the London-based King's Fund Institute, in their extensive review of the situation in 1988, concluded that "there remains considerable uncertainty as to the role and status of the community physician. Organizational restructurings have contributed to this uncertainty, but it is also due to the failure of community medicine to focus its activities and consolidate its identity. The breadth of skills and interests encompassed within community medicine may be viewed as a strength or a weakness...."[41]

In many ways the machinations of the Faculty of Community Medicine seem to have exacerbated the *schism* between clinical medicine and population-based perspectives as expressed in the changing structure of the National Health Service and related environmental and other health concerns. Strong opinions were expressed and firm stands taken; careers in Community Medicine did not seem attractive in the face of the academic, accreditation, and bureaucratic barriers erected. The most recent shift has been to rename the field so that it is now the Faculty of Public Health Medicine and its members are to be known as Public Health Physicians. *Plus ca change!*

So much, then, for "miscellaneous medicine" in Britain; to the present it remains a confused field with limited influence on medical education and the provision of personal and environmental health services. The greatest contribution comes from the academic side, where British epidemiologists have been in the forefront of developing new methods and a wide array of applications to contemporary problems of health, disease, and health services. Their skills in developing and conducting randomized clinical trials have, in the view of many, fully justified their existence.

Following the Rockefeller Foundation's merging of its public health and medical education interests, especially in the developing world, efforts were centered on community demonstrations of improved ways for providing what was initially described as family and community medicine in rural health centers. In some settings, for example, at Makerere University, Kampala, Uganda, these activities were the responsibility of the Department of Social and/or Preventive Medicine. Given the primitive state of the health services in these countries and the embryonic nature of their medical faculties, this approach was understandable. Most of the faculty members of such medical schools were expatriates from Britain and, to a more limited extent, the United States. Because the prior education and academic careers of the volunteers had provided only limited exposure to the population perspective, epidemiology, and public health, it should not have been unexpected that the departments of social and preventive medicine seem to have had little long-term influence on medical education or practice.

At Kasangati, for example, the health center developed by Makerere University, the staff complement consisted of a Resident Medical Officer with a Master of Public Health degree (obtained in the United States while on a Rockefeller Foundation Fellowship), a Resident Health Educator, an Assistant Health Educator, three Nurses, a part-time Midwife, and a Secretary. Initially, it had been proposed that the London School of Hygiene and Tropical Medicine provide an epidemiologist for the Department; this did not materialize and a member of an American department of preventive medicine was placed in charge of the field training at the Kasangati Center. The latter provided health services and health education for the local populace, but as an exercise for shifting values, skills, and interests of medical students it seems to have had little impact. The responsible Rockefeller officer reported that although the schedule called for the students to spend 2.5 hours at the Center, they were only present about 45 minutes, "wandering about in something of a daze, and returning to the medical faculty in time for tea." They seemed to be so engrossed in the forthcoming examinations and hospital inpatient services that they were unprepared for field work in community medicine.[42]

In 1963 Robert F. Loeb, Professor Emeritus of Medicine, Columbia University, one of America's leading medical statesmen and at the time a member of the Rockefeller Foundation's Board of Trustees, was asked to survey its health programs in East Africa. John Bowers's account of his opinions confirms earlier discussions I had had with Loeb:

Loeb's reaction to the Rockefeller sponsored community medicine program at Makerere was mixed, reflecting in part the well-established system of medical education with emphasis on bedside teaching and disdain for innovations in community and preventive medicine. However, he was impressed with [the staff's] reception at Kasantagi. 'The obvious satisfaction on the part of the villagers with the unit is everywhere apparent and the villagers seem devoted to [the staff].' ...Loeb

expressed his reservations about the [Director's] ability to put together research programs.[43]

Loeb shared the opinion of many other leaders of American medicine that the social
and environmental setting of a patient belonged at the heart of internal medicine and
should not be fragmented, 'I think the separation of a *cult* of Social Medicine will in
the long run do medicine a disservice as did the Departments of Therapeutics.'[44,45]

Looking back almost twenty years after the program in community medicine was
launched, one can see that the opposition of strong professors of medicine such as
Robert Loeb raised a major barrier to the effectiveness of the community medicine
program. Furthermore, this attitude by senior faculty permeated to the bright young
men and women and made their recruitment another problem.[46]

Following these early initiatives, the Foundation in 1963 embarked on a major
international program directed at the problems of overall development in the Third
World. Known initially as University Development, it was renamed Education for
Development in 1974.[47] This two-decade-long venture involved the Foundation's
three divisions of Agriculture, Health, and Social Sciences. Their combined efforts
were designed:

- To strengthen indigenous faculties;
- To develop curricula appropriate to indigenous needs;
- To encourage research relevant to national needs;
- To help structure outreach programs that address themselves to fundamental
  national deficiencies, particularly in rural life.

The health component of this large-scale enterprise was directed at strengthening the basic sciences and expanding the current concept of community medicine
in what were regarded as potentially major universities in Southeast Asia, Africa,
and Latin America. They were, with the dates the programs started: Universities
in East Africa—Makerere, Nairobi, and Dar es Salaam (1961); University of
Ibadan, Nigeria (1961); University of the Philippines (1962); Universidad del
Valle, Cali, Colombia (1963); Universities in Bangkok, Thailand—Kasetart,
Thammasat, and Mahidol (Ramathibodi and Siraraj) (1963); Gadjah Mada University, Yogyakarta, Indonesia (1971); National University of Zaire 1972); and the
Federal University of Bahia, Brazil (1973). In addition to the universities listed
here, there was a separate community medicine demonstration mounted by the
All-India Institute of Medical Sciences.[48]

Not all these universities had community medicine programs but all attempted
to graft on demonstration rural health centers to what were rapidly becoming
Western-type medical schools with their teaching hospitals. Most of the members
of these faculties had received postgraduate training in British and, increasingly,
American medical centers where the top priority was biomedical laboratory research and the development of applied medical technology in clinical settings. The
Foundation's rural demonstrations were attempts to reverse that course. They
served populations ranging in size from about 15,000 to 85,000 persons, scarcely
enough to experience the realities of analyzing the full range of health problems

within a province or state, let alone a nation, or of providing services for them. It was a matter of too little, too late.

Over the years, I have visited most of these community medicine endeavors, some several times, including Ibadan, the Philippines, Ramathibodi, Cali, and Gadjah Mada, therefore gaining first-hand knowledge of them. Two volumes have also been published reviewing the problems, strategies, frustrations, and accomplishments of these important initiatives.[49,50] Some have been more successful than others but none seems to have had an enduring impact on medical education or on the way curative or preventive medicine is organized and provided to the population.

The Universidad del Valle program was centered in the town of Candelaria and its surrounding villages (population about 20,000) near Cali, Colombia. Probably the most successful of the programs, it was terminated in 1974 after the State Secretary of Health declared that "it had accomplished its objectives."[51] A first-rate exposition of the problems and issues surrounding the relationship of governments and universities in the organization and evaluation of health services is provided by Professor Oscar Echeverri, one-time Head of the Department of Community Medicine at Universidad del Valle, responsible for the Candelaria project, and currently a senior official with the World Bank.[52] He reports that one of the program's positive accomplishments was the recruitment and training of medical residents, many of whom (25% of the graduates, by one account) entered careers in government hospitals or in rural communities.[53] The conduct of demographic and epidemiological surveys and the demonstration through well-designed clinical trials of improved ways of providing, for example, mental health and ambulatory surgery services, added to the credibility of the program. But after more than two decades, there was no overarching commitment by either the university or the government to a population-based perspective, and what is more disappointing, there did not seem to be any general understanding of the principles involved. Ideas espoused by some of the faculty may have prompted political unrest in the university; their efforts to change priorities may also have demonstrated to students and others, once again, the truth of Virchow's oft-repeated aphorism (see Chapter 2). Some of Colombia's traditional medical establishment might argue that community medicine had too much influence on the values and priorities that guided the medical enterprise at the Universidad del Valle.

At Ramathibodi in Bangkok, the community medicine program also met with stiff resistance. Here is a Rockefeller Foundation staff member assigned to Rhamathibodi writing back to the New York office in 1971:

> [There is] widespread resistance and even antagonism to the [Community Medicine] program on the part of the clinical staff. I have been aware of apathy and skepticism all along but there was frank hostility from several quarters this time.

> ...[T]hings have become downright discouraging. The reasons, I believe, are quite straightforward. We have not as yet, really developed a close working relationship with the Ministry [of Health], despite numerous overtures from both sides; we have made few definite steps toward developing an adequate operational health care

program for Bang Pa-in (the site of the demonstration Health Center); and there seems to be an erosion of commitment and direction on the part of the [Community Health Program] at Rama.[54]

In 1976 Willoughby Lathem, at that time on the Rockefeller Foundation's staff in Bangkok, observed that medical schools and their universities were rediscovering "a population of people [that] actually existed outside the confines of the traditional university teaching institutions, particularly the teaching hospital..."[55] He wrote of the community medicine programs slowly emerging in the United States in the new departments of that name, discussed earlier, as "transfused or refurbished departments of preventive medicine." He noted their limited accomplishments in improving the way either personal or environmental health services are provided. In the latter respect he coupled them with what he saw as the failure of schools of public health. Moving on to the developing world Lathem recognized the creative attempts in many of the demonstration health centers under the auspices of departments of community medicine to improve the provision of health services. "The emphasis," he wrote, "is on service and not on study, reflection, and evaluation." He continued:

> ...[E]xtraordinarily few, if any, have [achieved their fundamental objectives.] The reasons for this failure are varied. The tradition of Western academic medicine remains strong, and few faculty members have subscribed to or participated in the new endeavors. The students often have not achieved the skills required, because the teaching is based on transplanted urban-hospital outpatient practices, rather than the less familiar epidemiologic concepts of community medicine. Finally it has been rare to find a student motivated by his experience in such a way as to devote himself to a career of community service, particularly a rural one, for the rewards and prestige are to be found elsewhere.[56]

In 1979 a former dean of the Thai medical school under whom the community medicine program was initiated, hardly an unbiased observer, declared that in some quarters, including our own faculty, for ten years community medicine "were dirty words. Now the program is very active."[57] But who is one to believe? During a visit in 1979, the daughter of yet another of this school's deans, a young faculty member trained in Britain in both clinical and social medicine, took a contrary view in an all-male group. She asserted that the community medicine program was anything but a success and was regarded poorly by students and most clinical faculty alike—a brave pronouncement from a young Thai woman in such a setting.

These important pioneering programs were given mixed reviews at best during the 1978 Bellagio Conference that assessed their status.[58] Two major themes ran through most of the papers discussed. First was the idea that community medicine should help faculty and students to focus on the social, cultural, economic, political, and ethical milieu—the societal values—in which both the health professions and the populations they serve, live, work, suffer, and die. Because the Conference dealt primarily with problems in the developing world there were many references to the poor and the intertwining of poverty and disease, especially among those living in periurban slums and rural areas. The views expressed were contemporary manifestations of those enunciated in prior centuries by Chadwick, Shattuck, and even by Frank and Virchow.

Many engaged in community medicine seem motivated by indignation and outrage at the deplorable conditions giving rise to disease. One may also ask whether this motivation is lacking in other physicians and health care personnel; perhaps it is expressed in different ways. If "outrage" manifested by "redefining the unacceptable" is a necessary condition for change, it is rarely sufficient nowadays. Legislators and administrators need to know the dimensions of the problems they are to tackle and they need markers to measure the rate and extent of change. Numbers, therefore, are also a necessary ingredient for effective change.

The second major theme of the Bellagio Conference was the definition of "community" as a necessary precursor to defining community medicine. There were many and varied views offered, but the notion was slow to emerge that a community involves a population defined by geography, political jurisdiction, and occasionally by enrollment. These in turn constitute denominators, to use an epidemiological term; subsets of patients or of the population define the numerators. This central idea of the population perspective and its scientific analysis by epidemiologists was discussed but not emphasized at this Conference. The idea that redefining the unacceptable might be more persuasive to academic colleagues and politicians if done with numbers did not come through. The ideas of Petty, Louis, Farr, Paul, and Ryle were little in evidence.

The Conference report included long lists of problems and issues to be addressed. Prescriptions were provided for bettering the role of community medicine in medical services. One is left with a clear impression that community medicine is a long way from fulfilling the aspirations of its most ardent proponents. John Knowles, then President of the Rockefeller Foundation, included among his reasons for the program's limited impact on the health enterprises of the developing world:

> ...[F]ailure of those most experienced in public health or community medicine activities to rise above anecdotal, rhetorical, or emotional pleas based on "My successful experience in the field" to influence substantially university faculties, ministries of health and planning heads of national and international funding agencies...and political leaders.[59]

To confuse matters further, the term community medicine has been replaced by community health in many places. Is there any difference between community health and public health? And whatever happened to hygiene? As more and more medical care is paid for through government or public agencies, and as more and more diseases include a behavioral and hence a personal component in their genesis, would it not be more logical to speak of public medicine and private health? And where does the environment fit in?

In 1980, in her Presidential Address to the Annual Meeting of the Association of Teachers of Preventive Medicine, Professor Marion Bishop had this to say:

> I believe that we must once and for all come to an agreement about a department name and then regardless of individual and local idiosyncrasies encourage its adoption in

the 125 [U.S.] medical schools....A review of the 1979-1980 Directory of American Medical Education reveals 91 of the 125 medical schools have departments which can be recognized as relating to preventive and community medicine and public health....[In the titles of these departments] there are 40 with 'Community Medicine' alone or in some combination, 29 with 'Preventive Medicine' alone or in some combination, and 9 utilizing 'Community Health' alone or in some combination.

I don't doubt that all of the 39 variations in departmental identification fit into the broad parameters of our discipline and mean something locally. But we have created a jungle of confusion which I believe directly contributes to some of our identity problems. This plethora of names confuses funding agencies, confuses deans, confuses other disciplines and confuses us.

And there is more:

Attempts to determine the number of courses and the number of contact hours required in preventive medicine with some degree of confidence and accuracy are clouded by the amount of creativity and diversity exhibited in developing course titles. No other specialty involved in medical education exhibits such a proclivity for uniqueness in labelling courses.[60]

With this background, is there any wonder that these departments have failed to achieve their noble aspirations?

A case history illustrates the twists, turns, and shifting fortunes of population-based medicine over the past century. The University of Pennsylvania, one of the most distinguished medical schools in the United States, has negotiated the academic thickets that surrounded efforts to embrace the population perspective. An aftermath of the Civil War (1861-1865) had been the establishment of the United States Sanitary Commission. Among other recommendations it urged the American medical profession to pay much more attention to social and industrial conditions affecting health and disease. Accordingly, the University of Pennsylvania, starting in the early 1870s, had appointed part-time auxiliary professors of hygiene who gave lectures to the medical students. Following the European tradition started at the University of Munich by Max von Pettenkoffer, a Laboratory of Hygiene was created at Penn in 1889. The two major courses taught were hygiene and bacteriology. Ten members of the first class were physicians. As interest in bacteriology grew, that in hygiene waned. The former topic became the predominant interest of successive professors, and in 1915 the name was changed to Department of Hygiene and Bacteriology. At that time the University had hoped that it would be selected to become the first School of Hygiene and Public Health, but that designation went to the Johns Hopkins. Following retirement of the incumbent chairman in 1928, the two topics were separated into two departments. Bacteriology flourished and eventually was transformed into the Department of Microbiology.

The chair in hygiene was left vacant for a decade. In 1939 the department's name was again changed to Public Health and Preventive Medicine. The appointment of an "up-to-date" professor with that title also heralded the introduction of two new postgraduate courses leading to the degrees of Master of Public Health (the principal degree traditionally given by schools of public health), and the Doctor of Preventive Medicine. Within 5 years the chairman left to become Health Commissioner of Wilmington, Delaware. For another 5 years the chair was again left vacant; further testimony to the ambivalence of the faculty towards the population perspective.

The next chairman appointed in 1950 strengthened the department in many ways, especially by appointing a Professor of Epidemiology and Medical Statistics. But when this chairman retired in 1963, the position once more was unfilled for 5 years. The Professor of Epidemiology departed and little happened until 1968 when the department again was reorganized and renamed; this time it was to be Community Medicine. The new chairman developed alliances with the University's Wharton School of Business Administration. A Master of Business Administration in Health Care Systems was offered, a far cry from hygiene and bacteriology. Following the illnesses of the chairman and later of an acting chairman, the department underwent another formal review in 1975. The result was a recommendation that epidemiology and biostatistics be strengthened and several additional areas be added including: health management, medical sociology, environmental and industrial medicine, and health information systems. These recommendations were not adopted and 5 more years went by. Extensive deliberations by Task Forces and the School of Medicine's Long-Range Planning Committee were inconclusive. Meantime there had been some strengthening of epidemiology in connection with cancer research and also in the Department of Research Medicine to which Paul D. Stolley, an epidemiologist, had been appointed. Arguments were advanced to create a Department of Epidemiology and Biostatistics, but these provoked further discord among the faculty.

To give them their due, the faculty seems to have been groping throughout a century of deliberations to define the central or core discipline with which these several activities were associated. Epidemiology was gradually recognized as that discipline—more than a century after the London Epidemiological Society was formed. Further, the faculty bodies seem to have realized that epidemiological concepts and methods needed to permeate the entire faculty and student body; they should not be loculated off in a separate department, certainly not one that was isolated from the rest of the school's activities. In 1979 a Clinical Epidemiology Unit was established within the Department of Internal Medicine (see Chapter 7). From there its influence has spread widely.

Through recurrent periods of uncertainty, ambiguity, marginality, even hostility, and a century of academic backing and filling, the population perspective has emerged into a meaningful place within the medical school. The many incumbents who guided this venture sought to win the hearts and minds of faculty colleagues and students. As long as bacteriology (important as it has been) dominated the scene and was thought to encompass all of epidemiology, there was little progress. Once the faculty understood the potential of epidemiology as a fundamental discipline with broad capacities for improving clinical practice, research, and medical education, they embraced it enthusiastically. The University of Pennsylvania has no separate Department of Preventive, Social, or Community Medicine; it has no

School of Public Health. Within the Department of Medicine there is an enlarging group of epidemiologists, biostatisticians, health economists, and social scientists with growing local influence, with undergraduate and postgraduate educational responsibilities, and a strong research program. As a consequence of the faculty's substantial national and international reputations, their expertise as consultants has been in great demand.[61,62]

Skepticism may be understandable on the part of laboratory-based biomedical investigators who have given the world so much since World War II. If specific interventions stemming from the molecular revolution (i.e., "magic bullets") were to obliterate disease, why waste time and effort on vague promises from the advocates of improved public health measures? At the same time deterioration of the environment, ubiquitous exposure to an endless array of toxic substances, the onslaught of the acquired immunodeficiency syndrome (AIDS) epidemic, unlimited need for "behavioral modification" of "lifestyles," and health education generally reinforce the need for improved measures to protect and improve the public's health and to prevent disease.

A major document heralding the need for a new paradigm to accomplish these objectives was the Canadian Lalonde Report, published in 1974. In addition to providing a ground-breaking analysis of that country's health problems, this widely acclaimed publication announced that "[t]he Government of Canada now intends to give to human biology, the environment, and lifestyle as much attention as it has to the financing of the health care organization so that all four avenues to improved health are pursued with equal vigour."[63]

By 1975, "the situation which existed [in the United States] throughout the first half of the century ha[d] deteriorated during the past 25 years."[64] Only after the 1978 Alma-Ata International Conference on Primary Care, sponsored by the World Health Organization and the United Nations Children's Fund,[65] did the U.S. Department of Health, Education and Welfare (now the Department of Health and Human Services) make a serious attempt to "jump-start" the country's health professions into greater concern for health promotion and disease prevention.[66] Increasingly vigorous attempts were made to galvanize its health enterprise into recognition of specific objectives directed at improving the public's health status. A combined effort by the U.S. Public Health Service and the National Academy of Science's Institute of Medicine has involved the collaboration of more than 1000 individuals who developed specific objectives for health promotion, protection, and preventive services to be attained by the year 2000. The report stemming from these deliberations is both comprehensive and specific but little is said about how the knowledge, attitudes, and behavior of health professionals, in addition to those of the public, are to be changed so that they will undertake the recommended interventions and assessments.[67] Many of the latter should also involve state and local health departments. In spite of worthy efforts in many quarters, however, the results of a decade's efforts have been substantially less than satisfactory judging by the Institute of Medicine's report on *The Future of Public Health*, discussed in Chapter 1.[68]

In 1983, the World Health Organization's Regional Office for Europe held a landmark Workshop under the auspices of its Advisory Committee for Medical Research to explore the prospects for broadening medicine's overarching paradigm. The aims were to:

- Review and analyze from a multidisciplinary viewpoint various paradigms, approaches, methodologies and organizations in relation to health and health care issues;
- Identify missing interdisciplinary approaches and methodologies if they existed;
- Consider the possibility of developing integrated approaches;
- Recommend the investigations needed to fill gaps in knowledge and research.[69]

The Workshop included no representatives from schools of public health or departments of "miscellaneous medicine" but the excellent papers attest to the knowledge and vision that is gradually impinging on medicine and its paradigms. With the exception of the Lalonde Report, I have been able to find only one government-sponsored document dealing with the need for an expanded paradigm for understanding the genesis of health problems and developing practical strategies for coping with them: *Issues in Preventive Health Care*. This seminal report was published in 1986 by the Science Council of Canada. In a short but tightly argued and extensively documented treatise, it summarizes some of the policy problems confronting the health establishment:

- The difficulty of making certain health recommendations when the knowledge base is still evolving;
- The problem of acting on incomplete knowledge;
- The problem of generating specific conclusions and recommendations from the advice of expert panels when the panels may well disagree among themselves;
- The way in which present medical diagnosis and treatment may well be distorted by mistaken assumptions and paradigms, built-in or carried over from the way in which commercial and other vested interests may warp interpretations;
- The need to question research priorities;
  and later:
- The rapid advance of knowledge on widely diverse frontiers;
- The entanglement of physical and humanistic sciences—perhaps no other field of applied science is so involved with the emotional, mental, and even spiritual nature of the human being;
- Medical practice, as we are constantly reminded, is an *art* as well as a science (whatever that may be).[70]

Judicious evaluation of the evidence, an eclectic perspective, and above all effective exchange of ideas and knowledge characterize these last two documents. Their perspectives are at odds with the unbounded enthusiasm exhibited all too frequently by both the proponents of curative and of preventive medicine and their colleagues in public health. Much more than the checkered efforts made on behalf of "miscellaneous medicine" since World War II are required if the health establishment generally, and medical schools in particular, are to embrace the population perspective. Doubts about the relative efficacy and benefits of interventions at the individual and collective levels seem all too rare. In the next chapter, evidence is examined that suggests the need for accompanying even efficacious interventions with a measure of humility.

References

1. Grufferman S. The role of foundations in the development of clinical epidemiology programs. In: *Report of the Health Program*. New York: Rockefeller Foundation, October 18, 1982:3.
2. Paul JR. Clinical epidemiology. J Clin Invest 1938;17:539-541.
3. Ibid, p. 539.
4. Ibid, p. 539.
5. Ibid, pp. 540-541.
6. Ryle JA. *Changing Disciplines*. London: Oxford University Press, 1948.
7. Ibid, p. vi.
8. Ibid, p. 2.
9. Symonds C. John Alfred Ryle. Guys Hosp Reports 1950;99:217.
10. Ryle JA. *Changing Disciplines*. London: Oxford University Press, 1948:8-9.
11. Ibid, pp. 19-20.
12. Ibid, p. 19.
13. This was told to me by either one of his colleagues or one of his sons.
14. McKeown T. Social medicine as an academic discipline. In: *Proceedings of the First World Conference on Medical Education*, London, 1953:603-610.
15. Ibid, p. 603.
16. Ibid, p. 604.
17. Ibid, p. 609.
18. Bakst HJ, ed. Research, Graduate Education, and Postdoctoral Training in Departments of Preventive Medicine: Report of the Conference of the Association of Teachers of Preventive Medicine, Saratoga Springs, N.Y., June 10-14, 1963. J Med Educ, 1965;40(2):115.
19. Clark KG. Preventive Medicine in Medical Schools: Conference of Professors of Preventive Medicine. J Med Educ 1953;28(2).
20. Ibid, p. 102.
21. Ibid, p. 16.
22. Ibid, p. 47.
23. Bakst HJ, ed. Research, Graduate Education, and Postdoctoral Training in Departments of Preventive Medicine: Report of the Conference of the Association of Teachers of Preventive Medicine, Saratoga Springs, N.Y., June 10-14, 1963. J Med Educ, 1965:13.
24. Ibid, pp. 14-15.
25. Ibid, p. 19.
26. Ibid, p. 48.

27. Ibid, p. 81.
28. Ibid, p. 81.
29. Langmuir AD. Significance of epidemiology in medical schools. J Med Educ 1964; 39:39-48.
30. Last JM, ed. *Dictionary of Epidemiology*, 2d Ed. New York: Oxford University Press, 1988.
31. IEA. History of the International Epidemiological Association, 1954-1977. Int J Epidemiol 1977;6:309-324. History of the IEA brought up to date. Int J Epidemiol 1984;13:139-141.
32. *Report of the Royal Commission on Medical Education, 1965-68*, Cmnd.3569. London, Her Majesty's Stationery Office, 1968.
33. Ibid, p. 66.
34. Ibid, p. 67.
35. Harvey S, Judge K. *Community Physicians and Community Medicine*. Research Report 1. London: King's Fund Institute, 1988:3.
36. Acheson RM. Community medicine: Discipline or topic? Profession or endeavour? Community Med 1980;2:2-6.
37. Ibid, pp. 3-4.
38. Acheson ED. Clinical practice and community medicine. Br Med J 1979;2:880-881.
39. Ibid.
40. Smith A, Black D, Thomson TJ, Girdwood RH, Taylor PJ, and Rawnsley K. Importance of epidemiology (Letter to the editor). Lancet 1983;i:928.
41. Harvey S, and Judge K. *Community Physicians and Community Medicine*. Research Report 1. London: King's Fund Institute, 1988:4.
42. Bowers JZ. *The Health of Mankind: The Contributions of the Rockefeller Foundation, 1913-1980*. Unpublished manuscript containing quotations and references from the Rockefeller Archive Center, Pocantico Hills, New York, 1982; given to KLW by JZB in 1982, Volume III, Chapter 11, pp.10-13.
43. Ibid, Volume III, Chapter 11, pp. 16-17.
44. Ibid, Volume III, Chapter 11, pp. 17-18.
45. Stifel LD, Davidson RK, Coleman JS, eds. *Social Sciences & Public Policy in the Developing World*. Lexington, Mass: Lexington Books, 1982.
46. Bowers JZ. *The Health of Mankind: The Contributions of the Rockefeller Foundation, 1913-1980*. Unpublished manuscript containing quotations and references from the Rockefeller Archive Center, Pocantico Hills, New York, 1982; given to KLW by JZB in 1982, Volume III, Chapter 11, p.18.
47. *Annual Report, 1977*. New York: Rockefeller Foundation, 1977.
48. Bowers JZ. *The Health of Mankind: The Contributions of the Rockefeller Foundation, 1913-1980*. Unpublished manuscript containing quotations and references from the Rockefeller Archive Center, Pocantico Hills, New York, 1982; given to KLW by JZB in 1982, 1982:1-204.
49. Lathem W, Newbery A, eds. *Community Medicine: Teaching, Research and Health Care*. New York: Appleton-Century Crofts, 1970.
50. Lathem W, ed. *The Future of Academic Community Medicine in Developing Countries*. New York: Rockefeller Foundation, 1979.
51. Lathem W, Newbery A, eds. *Community Medicine in Developing Countries*. New York: Appleton-Century Crofts, 1979:69.
52. Echeverri O. Community medicine as a health system: rationale and patterns. In: Lathem W, ed. *The Future of Academic Community Medicine in Developing Countries*. New York: Rockefeller Foundation, 1979:69-86.

53. Lathem W, Newbery A, eds. *Community Medicine: Teaching, Research and Health Care*. New York: Appleton-Century Crofts, 1970:64.
54. Bowers JZ. *The Health of Mankind: The Contributions of the Rockefeller Foundation, 1913-1980*. Unpublished manuscript containing quotations and references from the Rockefeller Archive Center, Pocantico Hills, New York, 1982; given to KLW by JZB in 1982, 1982:III-119.
55. Lathem W. Community medicine: success or failure? New Eng J Med 1975;295:18-23.
56. Ibid, p. 22.
57. Ibid, p. III-123.
58. Lathem W, ed. *The Future of Academic Community Medicine in Developing Countries*. New York: Rockefeller Foundation, 1979.
59. Knowles JH. Community medicine an overview. In: Lathem W, ed. *Community Medicine in Developing Countries*. 1979:26.
60. Bishop FM. Prevention: wave of the future. J Community Health 1980;5:221-227, 223-224.
61. Corner GW. *Two Centuries of Medicine: A History of the School of Medicine. University of Pennsylvania*. Philadelphia: Lippincott, 1965.
62. University of Pennsylvania, School of Medicine. Department of Community Medicine: present structure and possible alternatives (Mimeographed). Philadelphia: University of Pennsylvania, November 25, 1975; Report of the epidemiology task force (Mimeographed), Philadelphia, University of Pennsylvania, January 29, 1980.
63. Lalonde M. *A New Perspective on the Health of Canadians*. Ottawa: Ministry of National Health and Welfare, 1974.
64. Rosen G. *Preventive Medicine in the United States, 1900-1975: Trends and Interpretations*. New York: Science History Publications, 1975:69.
65. Director-General of the World Health Organization and the Executive Director of the United Nations Children's Fund. *Primary Health Care*. Geneva: WHO and UNICEF, 1978.
66. Anon. *Healthy People: The Surgeon General's Report on Health Promotion and Disease Prevention*. DHEW (PHS) Publication No. 79-55071. Washington, D.C.: U.S. Department of Health, Education, and Welfare, 1979.
67. Stoto MA, Behrens R, Rosemont C, eds. Institute of Medicine. *Healthy People: Citizens Chart the Course*. Washington, D.C.: National Academy Press, 1990.
68. Institute of Medicine. *The Future of Public Health*. Washington, D.C.: National Academy Press, 1988.
69. Nizetic BZ, Pauli HG, Svensson P-G. *Scientific Approaches to Health and Health Care: Proceedings of a WHO Meeting, Ulm, 1-4 November, 1983*. Copenhagen: WHO Regional Office for Europe, 1986.
70. Jackson R. *Issues in Preventive Health Care. Discussion Paper*. Ottawa: Science Council of Canada, 1986.

6
Factor "X"

The preceding chapters have presented the case for expanding the application of epidemiological concepts and methods to restore the population perspective within medicine. For three centuries preceding the twentieth, this discipline played an increasingly important role within the spectrum of approaches used by medicine to understand the multifaceted aspects of health and disease. The goals of prevention and health promotion since the days of Johan Peter Frank, and of value for money (most recently "cost containment" in contemporary jargon) since the days of Sir William Petty (see Chapter 2) have all been advanced by epidemiological measures that helped in "redefining the unacceptable." Efforts to improve the public's individual and collective health, however, require not only clinical and molecular perspectives but also an understanding of how behavioral, social, environmental, institutional, and professional factors impinge on health status. Epidemiology and other population-based disciplines also provide the means for expanding applications of the scientific method to understand better the diverse linkages between medicine and the population served.

In science, measurement and counting offer the most practical bases for communicating and establishing consensual agreement. The essence of the method is "comparison" among sets of observations. But as one well-worn aphorism puts it: Not everything that matters can be measured and not everything that can be measured matters! Mapping and pattern recognition are other equally valid ways to similar ends.[1] Both individual and collective responses to institutional and professional maneuvers designed to improve health can be measured with varying degrees of precision; epidemiology provides one of the most powerful sets of ideas and methods for accomplishing this objective. A specific application of an idea stemming from the days of James Lind (see Chapter 3) was the introduction by the late Professor Sir Austin Bradford Hill (1897-1991), Professor of Medical Statistics in the London School of Hygiene and Tropical Medicine in 1948, of the Randomized Controlled Clinical Trial (RCT). Since then the method has gradually been refined, largely by faculty working in schools of public health.[2,3] When an RCT is employed to compare the relative efficacy of one or more interventions, one of them is usually designed to be innocuous—a "placebo." But in most such trials *all* participating groups show some improvement. This baseline improvement by all those subjects knowingly involved in the ministrations of health professionals working in and through their institutions and agencies deserves much more attention than it has received heretofore both by clinicians and public health workers. There is every reason to believe that what has been called *Factor "X"* has several components that to varying degrees are revealed by epidemiological methods but exert their influences throughout the health care enterprise. I now explore their potential for *healing the schism.*

Consider William Osler's observation in the British Medical Journal of 1910: "Faith in *St. Johns Hopkins,* as we used to call him, an atmosphere of optimism, and cheerful nurses, worked just the same sort of cures as *Æscupalius* at Epidaurus."[4] "Caring is part of the cure!" read the message on buttons worn by the staff of the Johns Hopkins Hospital 60 years later. An institution-wide campaign to make both professional and support personnel recognize their own therapeutic powers was perhaps unknowingly based on scientific knowledge. Awareness that caring was a beneficial force derived originally from the classic experiments conducted jointly by investigators at Harvard University and the Western Electric Company's Hawthorne plant near Chicago during the decade 1927 to 1937.[5]

This wide-ranging series of landmark studies was designed initially to determine the extent to which variations in the conditions and physical environment of the workplace affected the productivity of employees. The investigations were extensive and complex, involving six women who constituted a discrete social group in a dedicated working environment; they assembled telephone relays, the dependent variable the output of which measured productivity. In brief, the investigators found, to their great surprise, that no matter what changes were introduced by the company in the experimental situation, the number of relays produced went up. When the wattage of light bulbs was increased, production went up; when it was decreased, production went up! This ubiquitous phenomenon has been referred to ever since as the *Hawthorne effect,* a Heisenberg effect in human interactions. In other words, the observer's influence is always present in the clinical, research, and educational environments.

On balance the Hawthorne effect was associated with increases in productivity at the Western Electric plant ranging from 8.3% to 17.5% in one series, and from 5.9% to 24.1% in a second series. The mean increases were 12.6% and 15.6%, respectively. In recent years the studies have been criticized methodologically but it still seems reasonable to attribute to the Hawthorne effect some 10% to 15% of the observed benefits from general and specific interventions at the individual and population levels.[6]

Whatever else they did, the company "cared," and caring became the operative influence in the work environment. The outcome at the Hawthorne plant was expressed only incidentally through increased production, other outcomes are readily envisaged. Similarly, negative perceptions and responses by the recipients of attention or concern from administrators and others in positions of leadership or authority can be expected to affect outcomes negatively. The Hawthorne effect permeates health services at both the micro and macro levels; to ignore its presence in the context of the clinical encounter, in a research study involving human subjects, or even animals, and in the context of a new program designed to improve the health of a population is to omit an essential part of reality.

The vital role it plays in the commercial and industrial worlds was placed in context by the guiding intellect behind the studies, a Rockefeller-supported Australian, Elton Mayo (1880-1949). As Professor of Industrial Research in the Harvard Graduate School of Business Administration he described the research in a classic volume, *The Human Problems of an Industrial Civilization.*[7] Mayo also recognized the link between these industrial studies and clinical medicine in a 1938 address at the Harvard Medical School. This wise "nonphysician" summarized his message by observing that:

> When a patient walks into a consulting room he requires two kinds of aid from the physician. The first is medical attention, the second is assurance: in the ordinary consultation the second is as important as the first. The need for assurance is not adequately met by a hearty manner—nor by dogmatism or breezy self-confidence.[8]

Mayo might have extended his observation to note that even when a patient makes an appointment to see a physician or arrives at a hospital seeking help, more often than not the patient is already "feeling better," sometimes, in the former case, to the point of recovery from a relatively transient illness.

Knowledge of the Hawthorne effect has provided the scientific foundation for management and personnel policies and practices throughout the industrialized countries for six decades.[9-11] Widespread ignorance of it on the part of health professions, agencies, and institutions has resulted in lost opportunities for practitioners, administrators, managers, and policymakers of private and public health services to enhance patient care and improve the population's health. Its importance to the health field specifically was documented in land-mark studies conducted during the 1960s by Professor Reginald W. Revans of the University of Manchester. He showed that, when size and other factors were controlled, hospitals where supervisors employed authoritarian attitudes and behavior, compared to those where permissive and supportive management styles prevailed, had much higher rates of staff turnover (especially for nurses) and longer lengths of stay for six common medical conditions and six common surgical conditions.[12]

The public health field has been slow to recognize the importance of this phenomenon. Appointment of a new health officer, or introduction of a new program, no matter how specific or efficacious one or more components of the overall intervention may be, are accompanied by a new sense of collective confidence and hope on the part of those giving and those receiving services. The literature of efforts to help those in industrialized urban settings as well as those in villages in the developing world or other geopolitical jurisdictions does not reflect awareness of the Hawthorne effect.

Among 15 textbooks on public health and preventive, social, or community medicine from the United Kingdom, the United States, and Australia published during the past three decades, there are only three brief references to this phenomenon. The first textbook reference I have been able to find was in 1968; it is especially apt in the present context since it defines the Hawthorne effect as a "halo of non-specific social and personal influences [that] inevitably surrounds any medical or psychiatric or social treatment and sets subtle traps for the evaluator of the long-term social experiment." Although writing about community care for mental illness, the author continues:

> ...[I]t is necessary to distinguish between the influence of change itself, and of the influence of the enthusiasm and interest that so often accompany experiment....These effects of change and enthusiasm are not to be neglected even with the most precise of material treatments. They take on extra significance when they must be dissociated from less tangible psychological and social treatments.[13]

Presumably the same reasoning applies to other individual and public health interventions. A formal definition for the social sciences, also provided the same year, stated that the Hawthorne effect was "the influence that participation in an experiment may have on the behavior of the subjects."[14] Both of these definitions and the concept arising from the original experiments in the Hawthorne Plant seem too restrictive. Surely the phenomenon applies to all interventions—experimental and operational—where an individual, agency, or institution is perceived to be concerned or caring about the well-being of others, whether clients, patients, or citizens. The converse may also be true.

Only one of the current major textbooks on clinical epidemiology refers to this phenomenon and provides a definition that would be more apt, in my judgment, if the phrase included in brackets were added:

> The *Hawthorne Effect* is the tendency for people to change their behavior because they are the target of special interest and attention in a study [*or any other setting*], regardless of the specific nature of the intervention they might be receiving....[15]

In 1980 a second public health and preventive medicine textbook provided a one-line reference without a definition;[16] the third brief reference was in 1984.[17] If mentioned at all by teachers in schools of medicine and public health, there is little evidence that this widespread phenomenon is accorded much attention in textbooks on public health and preventive medicine, particularly as an important potential contributor to individual and collective well-being. The most extensive definition, and explanation with practical examples of its application, is to be found in *Biomedical Bestiary: An Epidemiologic Guide to Flaws and Fallacies in the Medical Literature*.[18] In addition to these works on public health and clinical epidemiology, a recent text entitled *Epidemiology and Health Policy* mentions the Hawthorne effect as an important element under "Epidemiologic Perspectives".[19]

Two extensive volumes published recently by the World Health Organization (and jointly sponsored by the International Epidemiological Association) consist of contributions by authorities from developed and developing countries. They set forth the conventional wisdom on evaluation of population-based health services. The first is concerned with *Measurement of Levels of Health* (1979)[20] and the second with *Measurement of Health Promotion and Protection* (1987).[21] Neither volume mentions the Hawthorne effect. The term is defined, however, in the IEA's *Dictionary of Epidemiology* and should now become more widely recognized, if not always emphasized, by epidemiological investigators.[22] To the extent that its importance has been recognized by epidemiologists and other investigators in both medicine and public health, progress has been made. That still leaves emphasis on its practical implications for all manner of interventions at the individual, institutional, and collective levels a matter for much greater study and application.

The strands of knowledge that lead to greater understanding and, perhaps, eventually greater wisdom are complex indeed. Lawrence J. Henderson (1878-1942), was a renowned Harvard biochemist, physiologist, and sometime social scientist. Henderson was close to many clinicians and influenced countless more with his broad-based teaching of medical students. He is best known to scholars concerned with medicine as part of larger social systems that influence health and disease for his famous 1941 article in *Science* entitled "The Study of Man."[23]

Henderson is less well known for his close association with Elton Mayo and the team conducting the Hawthorne experiments. Knowledge of both the natural and social sciences and Henderson's "systems approach" to understanding complex human phenomena made him an ideal collaborator. These interests had been prompted initially in Henderson by his early work as head of the Fatigue Laboratory established in the Harvard Graduate School of Business Administration to study physical and mental stress in workers.[24] This interest, in turn, had been stimulated by World War I research at the British Industrial Health Research Board (later a branch of the Medical Research Council). Both initiatives were built on the nineteenth-century legislative reforms associated with redefining the unacceptable factory conditions. In turn, these were inspired by classic observations in Manchester that showed that reducing working hours from 53 to 48 per week resulted in increased productivity, surely an early manifestation of the Hawthorne effect.[25] Who knows? Perhaps the idea derives from the factory studies conducted by Charles Turner Thackrah in Leeds a century earlier, as mentioned in Chapter 3.[26]

Ever the scientist, Henderson moved back and forth among the social and natural sciences, especially as these involved matters of health and medicine. Both his population perspective and his extensive competence in mathematics prompted him to say this of numeracy in medicine:

> ...[T]he practice of medicine slowly eliminates fallacies of misplaced concreteness...One thing is lacking that would greatly contribute to the efficacy of this elimination of the fallac[ies], namely, a thorough understanding of the[ir] logical nature and easy familiarity with the complexity of the usual mathematical interrelations among many interdependent factors. For the interdependence of many variables can only be treated mathematically.[27]

A better known psychosocial or psychophysiological intervention that improves health status is the *Placebo effect*. For centuries a wide assortment of exotic, sometimes innocuous, often unpleasant and costly, and frequently dangerous interventions have been employed by doctors of all persuasions to alleviate pain and suffering. In spite of experiences and of some measure of wisdom accumulated over the centuries, serious scientific attention to the importance of the Placebo effect dates only from the early 1950s following the formal introduction in 1948 of the RCT by Bradford Hill.

Clinical "trials" had, of course, been used over the centuries in virtually every case when a new treatment was introduced. What Bradford Hill did was to substitute formal experimental methods for informal observational methods in studies of clinical medicine and public health. By introducing principles that are the hallmarks of contemporary RCTs, he has had enormous influence on the rational practice of medicine and public health. These require the systematic allocation of interventions or maneuvers (e.g., pills, vaccines, operations, diagnostic tests, counseling, and educational campaigns) and subjects (e.g., individuals, families, institutions, services, and communities) by use of a table of random numbers or similar device, concurrent controls, and "blinding." The latter ensures ignorance of the purportedly active ingredient of the maneuver by the subjects and in a "double-blind" study by the responsible physician, nurse, or administrator, etc..

Throughout early discourses on the use of experimental methods and RCTs, the words chance, disturbing causes, or some other factor were used to explain outcomes or benefits not believed to be associated with the active ingredient of the intervention. To minimize investigator, subject, and design bias and error, methods have evolved for controling many of these so-called distorting factors. A few of the better known are design error, sampling error, observer variation, observer error, selection bias, and so-called confounding variables associated with the nature of the particular analysis or experiment. But when all of these have been accounted for in studies that involve humans (and perhaps animals)—individually, in groups, or populations—there is still a residual improvement or benefit observed in the control or comparison groups unaccounted for by other factors. The tendency has been to attribute this to unknown factors assumed to be of little or no consequence. At best, these improvements are said to be "just the Placebo effect." In the more recent epidemiological literature, when not attributed to the use of a specified placebo these are sometimes referred to as the halo effect.[28]

One of the first investigators to draw the medical profession's attention to the Placebo effect was Henry K. Beecher, Professor of Anaesthesiology at Harvard. His classic paper entitled "The Powerful Placebo" reported that in 15 studies of patients suffering from nine conditions, the mean placebo response rate was 35.2 ± 2.2% or between 31% and 39%; the actual range was from 15% to 58%. We are, therefore, talking about a factor that appears to exercise overall a very substantial influence on health and disease, some 35%.[29]

Psychiatrists have made major contributions to both identifying and explaining this phenomenon, particularly in controlled double-blind studies.[30] One definition of the Placebo effect states that "a placebo may be any object offered with therapeutic intent" and adds "the 'placebo reaction' occurs in psychotherapy even without a pill, in the so-called 'transference' cure."[31]

Professor Howard Brody of Michigan State University has culled from the literature four definitions of the Placebo effect that characterize the "increasing breadth and the increasing range of phenomena that fall under them":

- A therapeutic effect produced by a biomedically inert substance (Pepper, 1945).
- A therapeutic effect or side effect attributable to a treatment, but not to its pharmacologic properties (Wolf, 1950).
- A nonspecific effect of a therapy that may or may not have a specific effect in addition (Shapiro, 1968).
- What all treatments have in common (Modell, 1955).[32]
  He provides his own definition:
  A placebo effect occurs for person "X" if and only if:
- "X" has condition "C";
- "X" believes that he is within a healing context;
- "X" is administered intervention "I" as part of that context, where "I" is either the total active intervention or some component of that intervention;
- "C" is changed; and
- the change in "C" is attributable to "I", but not to any known pharmacologic or physiologic property of "I".[33]

If the words problem or complaints were added to condition, if the words helping, informing, and supporting were added to healing, and if the word efficacious was substituted for pharmacological or physiological, the definition would be more realistic and have much wider applicability. In particular, it could attract increased interest from the public health and community medicine constituencies. Indeed this broader definition of the Placebo effect comes very close to that for the Hawthorne effect, theoretically and practically. Both may operate at the micro (individual) and the macro (population) levels.

The matter is even more complicated. There is wide variation in the way individuals and probably types of individuals or groups respond, just as there is wide variation in the capacity of physicians, other health professionals, and even different institutions to evoke the beneficial responses referred to as the Placebo effect. For starters, in one analysis of six studies, at least four types of individuals who could be called "placebo reactors" were identified:

- Positive placebo reactors, or patients who report decreased symptoms;
- Negative placebo reactors, or those who describe exacerbation of their symptoms;
- Neutral or nonplacebo reactors or patients without change of symptoms; and
- Patients who report new symptoms or side effects, referred to as placebo-induced side effects.
  The authors continued:

Patients who react negatively or positively to a placebo tend to develop placebo-induced side effects more frequently than do neutral placebo reactors. In these studies, which used a standardized 1-hour placebo test at initial evaluation, the range was 40% to 54% for positive placebo reaction, 30% to 41% for neutral placebo reaction, 10% to 21% for negative placebo reaction, and 44% to 71% for placebo-induced side effects. Our studies indicate that it is important that these types of placebo reactions be identified, since each of them may be associated with a different origin, significance, and findings.[34]

Professor Howard M. Spiro of Yale confirmed Beecher's figure of 35% as a reasonable estimate of its overall beneficial influence, but noted that in clinical trials of duodenal ulcer the benefit may amount to 60% with an overall rate of at least 50%. More interesting still are the variations in the Placebo effect among countries and institutions:

> The healing rate on placebo for duodenal ulcer craters in controlled clinical trials runs from 20 percent in London to 70 percent in Switzerland. In the United States it ranges from 50 to 60 percent. A very interesting study was conducted in the United Kingdom a few years ago. An anti-ulcer drug was compared to a placebo in a trial carried out in Dundee and in London. The study was identical at both hospitals, but the healing rates for placebo were quite different: in Dundee 73 percent of ulcers healed on a placebo, in contrast to only 44 percent in London. The reasons for the differences in the healing rates in the two centers were unclear to the observers, who wondered whether there was a difference in the patients, in the doctors taking care of the patients, or in someone's expectations of cure. A study in the United States foreshadowed this observation. In one hospital...antacids relieved pain 79 percent of the time, but in another hospital the same antacids were effective only 17 percent of the time. In one hospital placebos gave relief to 45 percent of the patients, but in another only 25 percent were helped. In both the British and American studies the experimental design, definition of terms, and criteria were the same, but the responses were different, suggesting there are fundamental differences in responses to placebo as well as therapy.[35]

These findings suggest the presence of mixtures of the Hawthorne and Placebo effects. The presence of substantial variations in behavior of groups and institutions has important implications for public health and population-based medicine. These studies also document the differences between the assessment of "efficacy" under rigidly controlled situations and the assessment of "effectiveness" in different clinical, institutional, and community settings. The Hawthorne and Placebo effects must surely accompany all population-based, community, and public health interventions, especially those informative exercises focused on prevention, health education, and health promotion. Few engaged in efforts to improve the public's health can ignore the potentially great influence of "tincture of enthusiasm" or the converse, bureaucratic apathy and administrative indifference, that accompanies many such programs.

Alvan R. Feinstein, Professor of Medicine and Epidemiology, also of Yale, offers a tabular summary of these effects which have modified to reflect the foregoing discussion.[36] If it is assumed that in any endeavor designed to improve the health of individuals or populations there are three factors operating: the allegedly specific *Efficacious Maneuver*, the *Placebo effect*, and the *Hawthorne effect*, then the results of a hypothetical study with four groups, if each had one, and only one, discrete response, might look like this:

Efficacious Maneuver effect:	50% improvement
Placebo effect:	35% improvement
Hawthorne effect:	10% improvement
No intervention and no observation:	0% improvement

In practice, of course, there is a mixture of all three basic responses, as well as of individual and group responses depending on the composition and characteristics of those exposed to the phenomena. The Hawthorne effect would occur with any nonspecific observation or human interaction between "health care personnel" and patients, clients, or populations. Some elements of the Placebo effect would be present to varying degrees even in the individuals comprising both the experimental and control groups given a specific intervention or some form of attention. For example, a hypothetical experimental group might exhibit 25% improvement associated with the efficacy of a specific maneuver, another 35% associated with the Placebo effect, and a further 10% associated with the Hawthorne effect for a total improvement of 75%. The control group might only experience a 45% improvement, of 35% from the Placebo effect and 10% from the Hawthorne effect. If a third observational group (aware that they were participating) were included and assessed at the start and finish of the study, they might exhibit only a 10% improvement from the Hawthorne effect. Even the phenomenon of regression toward the mean may reflect aspects of the Placebo and Hawthorne effects worthy of further study. There is no basis for concluding that analogous responses are not associated with most, if not all, population-based or public health programs and services. Ideally, each type of response should be recognized and where appropriate measured; everything should be called by its right name.

From the available evidence we may conclude that overall the Placebo effect must, on average, account for about 30% to 40% of beneficial outcomes associated with interventions or maneuvers designed to be helpful, healing, educational, or informative. If to this we add the 10%-15% beneficial impact of the Hawthorne effect, we have a total overall influence that must on average approach 50%, not a trivial benefit. At the same time, negative influences, including undesirable or even harmful side effects, may be almost as great, although they have not been studied as extensively as the positive effects.

Just as concerns for individual and population health did not arise in recent decades, so the view of the human condition espoused by Western medicine, especially by a narrowly defined biomedical model, is not the repository of all knowledge, let alone wisdom, about these matters. Nor is the admittedly negative emphasis on redefining the unacceptable, the only approach to achieving man's aspirations for a higher and more tranquil state of well-being or happiness. The numeric method and appropriate applications of numeracy may be important, indeed essential, aids to interpreting many aspects of human behavior and function, but they are certainly not sufficient to afford complete understanding of the mysteries that continue to characterize the diverse states we experience as health and disease.

Physiologic reactions to the *Relaxation Response*, a Western version of Transcendental Meditation and of some forms of yoga, can be measured by contemporary laboratory instruments. The input or active ingredient associated with these states is less easily identified, however, and is difficult but not impossible to quantify.[37] Holistic and so-called alternative medicines may be other expressions of intangible striving toward attitudinal and behavioral changes directed at the attainment of better "health." By the middle of the 1970s, there was growing recognition of the limits of orthodox curative medicine as currently conceived in the West.[38]

John Knowles, as President of the Rockefeller Foundation, understood the significance of these developments and helped organize two major conferences to discuss them; each was attended by several hundred health professionals.[39,40] In the Foreword to the first volume resulting from these deliberations, Knowles and his two colleagues wrote:

> The *Conference on Future Directions in Health Care* was conceived in our conviction that a new perspective of health is essential if we are to achieve substantial improvement in the health status of the population. The examination and discussion reported here have encouraged us to believe that continued challenge to the way health is defined, and continued exploration of new concepts and holistic approaches to health services, offer promising, even exciting opportunities. This conference was a positive start, and we intend to pursue its objectives further.[41]

A decade later we are indebted to Dr. D. B. Bisht, former Director-General of Health Services, Government of India, for adding greater specificity to our deliberations by bringing the concept and the term Factor "X" to the attention of the global health community.[42] In 1984 the World Health Assembly passed a resolution that he introduced recognizing its ubiquitous presence.[43] This landmark official statement provided a quantum leap forward from the health enterprise's ephemeral preoccupations with such mundane matters as costs, nosology, and technology. There are wide differences of opinion about both the existence of Factor "X" and its importance and even wider differences in notions about its manifestations. The consensus among the numerous authorities Bisht brought together to discuss the matter, and certainly among the majority of delegates attending the World Health Assembly that passed the resolution, was that this dimension does exist and that somehow it should be added to WHO's traditional definition of health as "complete physical, mental and social well-being and not just the absence of disease." Bisht summarizes matters well when he writes:

> ...[I]n the East, we often call that aspect of human being which makes one transcend the animal as being 'spiritual.' But this word has been used in many different ways and has acquired various connotations according to perception of this word in relation to one's own socio-religious and traditional backgrounds. There are many people who simply do not believe that there is anything like 'spiritual' which exists in this world. Ignoring the semantics of the word, it can generally be conceded that there is 'something' that makes us human beings, and hence, differentiating us from a pack

of wolves. This 'something' may be called *Factor 'X'* since it is necessary to have word labels.[44]

Whatever the power manifested by the phenomena labeled the Hawthorne and Placebo effects and Factor "X", their collective influence does appear to find tangible expression in behavioral and functional changes in health status. Call their influence the power that heals, or call it faith, hope, or charity (or the converse of all these—negative, destructive attitudes and behavior). For the present, however, I prefer the all-inclusive term Factor "X".

These phenomena are all too real for those who experience them. The contemporary biomedical model is unlikely to admit them as elements of received wisdom, however, until they have been clearly linked to physiological, biochemical, cellular, and molecular changes that in turn produce alterations in functional states or diseases. Perceptions, memories, feelings, values, attitudes, and behavior in turn must be shown to be mediated through the central and autonomic nervous systems, the immune system, and the endocrine and other humoral systems, all with their myriad receptors and transmitters.[45] This is as it should be. In the long run, expansion of medicine's theoretical and practical understanding of health and disease is the surest road to progress in ameliorating suffering and controlling ill health. Investigation of these phenomena as an alternative to the "magic bullet" approach could prove equally rewarding.

To act beneficially, information derived from such fundamental biomedical and behavioral studies, although supportive, is not essential for contemporary practitioners and administrators at the patient and population levels. From Frank through Virchow to Osler, Paul, and Ryle, clinicians and advocates of social reform alike have argued about the importance of associations between social (and by implication, psychological) states and ill-health—however tenuous the evidence about the nature of the linkages at the time. Indeed most of the evidence they used came from population-based, that is, epidemiological, studies. We may paraphrase Osler's famous dictum by stating that: "It is as important to know the characteristics of the population within which the disease arises, as it is to know what kind of a disease the population has."

Lawrence J. Henderson, writing half a century ago, had this to say:

> The medical sciences have suffered and continue to suffer from [the fallacy of misplaced concreteness]. The rise of bacteriology and its influence upon medical thought and practice may be taken as an example. About the time of Pasteur's first discoveries, the thought of Claude Bernard and of other physiologists seemed to indicate a movement toward the study of the interrelations between many things and a recognition of this kind of study, synthetic physiology, as one of the foundations of the medical sciences and as the source of an indispensable point of view in all kinds of medical work. The discovery of specific pathogenic microorganisms seems to have led back to an oversimplification of thought about the origin and nature of disease. For some time at least, the tendency was to think of diseases as entities hardly less definite than atoms of oxygen or molecules of hemoglobin....The disposition was even more marked to think of the specific organism as the cause—the sole cause—of a

specific disease and later to think of the specific antitoxin as the specific cure of that disease.[46]

During the heyday of bacteriology, physiologists such as Walter B. Cannon of Harvard and Curt P. Richter (1894-1988), Director of the Psychobiological Laboratory of the Johns Hopkins Medical School, tried to broaden the horizons of the medical profession. In 1942 the former published his classical article on the history and prevalence of "Voodoo Death," including reports by, among many others, Dr. S. M. Lambert of the Western Pacific Health Service of the Rockefeller Foundation who reported instances of rapid, unexplained death associated with "bone-pointing."[47] Following this report Richter published his famous account of rats who ordinarily swam for an established period of time in a specially constructed water bath, but who swam much longer after being rescued temporarily and then returned to the water bath. This phenomenon, repeated in many different ways, suggested to Richter that rats have some center that responds to what humans call "hope."[48] Professor Hans Selye of the University of Montreal spent his entire career investigating what he called the "adaptation syndrome," but his work was accepted more by the popular press than by the biomedical establishment.[49] Similarly, the impact of careful psychosomatic investigations over several decades by Professors Harold G. Wolff, Stewart Wolf, and their colleagues at Cornell University School of Medicine has been largely ignored by the academic medical and public health communities.[50]

Bacteriology and later the molecular revolution overshadowed the work of these and other pioneers. Even Pasteur's early interest in immunology (as distinguished from bacteriology) seems to have attracted only modest attention compared to the enthusiasm generated among the hygienists and other followers of the sanitary idea and their successors. Most immunologists, until quite recently, were concerned largely with the immune system's responses to exogenous organisms and its "training" over time as a guide to predicting future reactions and behavior. They were much less interested in considering nonorganic influences on the immune system, and hence of assessing individual or group susceptibility to a host of noninfectious experiential and environmental stimuli.

One of the first clues to the mechanism of the Placebo effect (and possibly also to the Hawthorne effect and Factor "X") came from an observation which suggested that, at least as far as pain relief is concerned, the physiological effects may be mediated through the release of endorphins, one of the body's many naturally occurring peptides.[51] Following these and other observations, there emerged the new field of psychoneuroimmunology (PNI; another gerrymandered word, like "biopsychosocial," that lamely tries to label new perspectives on health and disease). PNI is now a flourishing biomedical growth industry. This is not the place for a detailed progress report on this exciting new dimension of research but only to draw attention to its potential importance.[52,53]

Knowledge about Factor "X" has important implications at both the individual (micro) and the population (macro) levels. It should be used to support and reinforce positively, through words, attitudes, and behavior, the application of an intervention of established efficacy (or in the case of the macro level, of established effectiveness). To do otherwise is to run the risk, indeed the probability, that the agent will prove much less effective in both patients and populations living in their natural habitats than the original demonstration of its efficacy or effectiveness suggested. Failure to recognize the negative as well as the positive potential of Factor "X" may well account for wide differences in the outcomes not only of controlled clinical trials but of public health maneuvers in community settings, as the evidence cited above by Spiro and other studies document.[54]

There is also a need to pay much greater attention to the role of cultural, social, economic, and political fluctuations, including wars and revolutions and so-called natural disasters (earthquakes, famines, tornados, floods, etc., and fear of these) as factors, apart from their direct material destruction of human life and function, that influence health, disease, and well-being. Although the links between the determinants of disease and better understanding of some aspects of the web of causality are slowly emerging, there is enough evidence in the epidemiological literature to suggest strong associations between these states and ill-health.

For example, there is a vast literature on the impact of unemployment on health status and the use of health services.[55] Much of this work is hampered by contamination with the "ecological fallacy," which holds that two or more population-based measures moving in predicted directions do not establish positive association, let alone causation, because different individuals may have been observed when each of the measures was made. When social class trends show persistent differences in mortality and use of health services over the decades in Britain, however, the arguments for recognizing the impact of social, political, and economic factors on health are compelling.[56] Many other parts of this literature are anecdotal and clinical in nature, and although they may lack statistical rigor they add poignancy and depth to our appreciation of the raw statistical tables. Once more, combined clinical and the community approaches provide greater understanding of the determinants of health and disease, but the third dimension from the bench laboratory is still needed to complete the circle.

One of the first epidemiologists to study systematically many of the relationships among social factors and health status was the late Professor John C. Cassel (1921-1976).[57] As Founding Chairman of a new Department of Epidemiology in the School of Public Health at the University of North Carolina, Cassel pioneered the creation of what used to be called "social epidemiology." In the best tradition of Virchow, Cassel's theories and his investigations foreshadowed the emerging advances in PNI. Although he was not then in the mainstream of contemporary epidemiology, his views are now widely respected and often emulated. Apart from Cassel's many conceptual papers synthesizing available findings, his most important contribution was in demonstrating the impact of cultural change on morbidity. He predicted and showed that rural citizens who were the first generation to enter factory employment experienced more ill-health than a similar cohort whose fathers had been factory workers before them.[58] A related study did essentially the same for coronary heart disease. Cassel and his colleagues showed that mortality rates from this disease were highest among rural dwellers living in the midst of rapid urbanization and that the risk was probably related to their lack of readiness for a so-called modern lifestyle.[59]

Widowhood, bereavement, and separations of all types, isolation, loneliness, "sensory deprivation," change of abode, and crowding have all been shown to be associated with ill-health. Music, dancing, churches, community social groups, ownership of pets, yes—and ready access to a caring, compassionate, scientifically competent personal physician—have all been associated with improved health status. The extensive literature on this and related influences has been synthesized recently in two important publications. The first, by physician and epidemiologist Leonard A. Sagan, is captured in the following quotation:

> All cultures create their own theories of disease and death. Although there are variants, theories fall into two categories—those that emphasize behavioral factors (health-related theories) and those that emphasize the importance of environmental factors (disease-oriented theories). During the thousand years prior to the modern period, western medicine focused on behavior, illness was seen as evidence of a disordered physiology, which was in turn seen as the result of unhealthy or immoral behavior. Even as recently as the nineteenth century, cholera epidemics which affected the poor almost exclusively, were viewed as divine punishment of those who were considered slothful. Consistent with this person-oriented theory of disease, physicians prescribed diet, medications, or a change in location to restore health.
>
> With the onset of the Enlightenment and the appearance of Newtonian physics, a paradigmatic shift in medical theory appeared. Just as defendants were considered innocent until proven guilty, individuals were assumed to be healthy until proven sick. Medical attention largely moved from the individual to the environment as the source of illness and disease....Because the major causes of death in the premodern period were the infectious diseases, the discovery of bacteria and their insect vectors appeared to substantiate the environmental source of disease. Tuberculosis was "caused" by the tubercle bacillus. In the twentieth century, we continue to place major emphasis on external agents and ignore behavioral factors in health.[60]

Both sets of factors require attention by the entire health establishment as it seeks to help both individuals and populations with their health problems.

The second synthesis is by James S. House and his colleagues at the University of Michigan. Their major conclusions are summarized in the following quotation:

> It is clear that biology and personality must and do affect both people's health and the quantity and quality of their social relationships. Research has established that such factors do not, however, explain away the experimental, cross-sectional, and prospective evidence linking social relationships to health. In none of the prospective studies have controls for biological or health variables been able to explain away the predictive association between social relationship and mortality. Efforts to explain away the association of social relationships and supports with health by controls for personality variables have similarly failed. Social relationships have a predictive, arguably causal, association with health in their own right.[61]

"Caring" is indeed part of the cure, as well as part of prevention, part of health promotion, and part of cost containment. Factor "X" in its many manifestations seems to account for as much as half the benefits experienced by individuals and populations exposed to the health establishments' ministrations. Factor "X" must be much more than the unexplained residual improvement observed in clinical trials. Are we certain that its influence on the health status of neglected villagers in a developing country is less important than the installation of latrines and the immunization of children, important as these are? After all, during a cholera epidemic, not every village succumbs to the plague, not every family in an affected village is taken ill, and not every member of a household develops the disease. Max von Pettenkofer taught us this unlearned lesson more than a century ago.

These matters are at the heart—yes, the heart—of both the medical and public health enterprises. The extent and importance of Factor "X" is being illuminated by contemporary applications of the numeric method and by wider uses of epidemiology. Pervasive social epidemics diminish host and herd resistance to external agents of disease. They too can be measured by epidemiological methods and publicized in the best tradition of William Farr as "health and vital statistics." Now laboratory investigators, as a direct result of the molecular revolution, are discovering the links between the two. For clinicians and public health workers Factor "X" remains what the eminent British epidemiologist Professor Geoffrey Rose calls "the physician's friend." Extensive exposure to all three perspectives—the population, the laboratory, and the clinical—and recognition of their essential interdependence and unity is essential for all students of the health professions. Without this breadth of exposure how will it be possible to attract and prepare professionals who can formulate policies and manage the precariously unbalanced and excessively expensive health care "systems" the developed world has created and the developing world strives to emulate? Coping with the "Principal Problems" and "Root Causes" examined in Chapter 1 requires this broader perspective. We turn now to a discussion of the Rockefeller Foundation's new program in response to them.

References

1. Ziman J. *Reliable Knowledge: An Exploration of the Grounds for Belief in Science.* Cambridge: Cambridge University Press, 1978.
2. Medical Research Council. Streptomycin in tuberculosis trials committee. Br Med J 1948;2:769-782.
3. Hill AB. *Statistical Methods in Clinical and Preventive Medicine.* Edinburgh: Livingstone, 1962.
4. Cushing H. *The Life of Sir William Osler.* London: Oxford University Press, 1940: 909.
5. Roethlisberger FJ, Dickson WJ. *Management and the Worker.* Cambridge: Harvard University Press, 1939.
6. Roethlisberger FJ, Dickson WJ. *Management and the Worker.* Cambridge: Harvard University Press, 1939:56,76,132,148.
7. Mayo E. *The Human Problems of an Industrial Civilization.* New York, Macmillan, 1933.

8. Mayo E. *Frightened people.* Harv Med Alumni Bull, 1939;13:2-7.

9. Roy RH. *The Administrative Process.* Baltimore: Johns Hopkins, 1958:172-175.

10. Ashton D. Elton Mayo and the empirical study of social groups. In: Tellett A, Kempner T, Wills G, eds. *Management Thinkers.* Harmsworth: Penguin Books, 1970:294-311.

11. Peters TJ, Waterman RH Jr., *In Search of Excellence.* New York: Warner Books, 1982:5-6.

12. Revans RW. *The Measurement of Supervisory Attitudes.* Manchester: Manchester Statistical Society, 1961:32.

13. Susser M. *Community Psychiatry: Epidemiologic and Social Themes.* New York: Random, 1968:197-198.

14. *International Encyclopedia of the Social Sciences*, Vol. 13. New York: Macmillan, 1968:88.

15. Fletcher RH, Fletcher SW, Wagner EH. *Clinical Epidemiology—The Essentials.* Baltimore: Williams & Wilkins, 1982:134-135.

16. Last JM, ed. *Maxcy-Rosenau Public Health and Preventive Medicine*, 11th Ed. New York: Appleton-Century-Crofts, 1980:47.

17. Acheson RM, Hagard S. *Health, Society and Medicine: An Introduction to Community Medicine.* Oxford: Blackwell, 1984:213.

18. Michael M III, Boyce WT, Wilcox AJ. *Biomedical Bestiary: An Epidemiologic Guide to Flaws and Fallacies in the Medical Literature.* Boston: Little, Brown, 1984:59-65.

19. Ibrahim MA. *Epidemiology and Health Policy.* Rockville, Maryland: Aspen, 1986: 10.

20. Holland WW, Ipsen J, Kostrzewski J, eds. *Measurement of Levels of Health.* Copenhagen: World Health Organization, Regional Office for Europe, 1979.

21. Abelin T, Brzezinski ZJ, Carstairs VDL, eds. *Measurement of Health Promotion and Protection.* Copenhagen: World Health Organization, Regional Office for Europe, 1987.

22. Last JM, ed. *A Dictionary of Epidemiology*, 2d Ed. New York: Oxford University Press, 1988:56.

23. Henderson LJ. The study of man. Science 1941;94:1-10.

24. Barber B, ed. *L.J. Henderson on the Social System.* Chicago: University of Chicago Press, 1970:102,209.

25. Vernon HM. *The Health and Efficiency of Munition Workers.* London: Oxford University Press, 1940:10-12.

26. Newman G. *The Rise of Preventive Medicine.* London: Oxford University Press, 1932:172-173.

27. Henderson LJ. The study of man. Science 1941;94:1-10 (7).

28. Last JM, ed. *A Dictionary of Epidemiology*, 2d Ed. New York: Oxford University Press, 1988:56.

29. Beecher HK. The powerful placebo. JAMA 1955;159:1602-1606.

30. Shapiro AK. A contribution to the placebo effect. Behav Sci 1960;5:109-135.

31. Ibid, p. 130.

32. Brody H. *Placebos and the Philosophy of Medicine: Clinical, Conceptual and Ethical Issues.* Chicago: University of Chicago Press, 1980:37.

33. Ibid, p. 41.

34. Shapiro AK, Shapiro E. Patient-provider relationships and the placebo effect. In: Matarazzo JD, Weiss SM, Herd JA, Miller NE, Weiss SM, eds. *Behavioral Health: A Handbook of Health Enhancement and Disease Prevention.* New York: Wiley, 1984:376.

35. Spiro HM. *Doctors, Patients and Placebos*. New Haven: Yale University Press, 1986:17-18.
36. Feinstein AR. *Clinical Epidemiology: The Architecture of Clinical Research*. Philadelphia: Saunders, 1985:221.
37. Benson H, Klipper MZ. *The Relaxation Response*. New York: Avon, 1976.
38. McKeown T. *The Role of Medicine: Dream, Mirage or Nemesis*. London: Nuffield Provincial Hospitals Trust, 1976.
39. Knowles JH, Lee PR, McNerney WJ, eds. *Conference on Future Directions in Health Care: The Dimensions of Medicine*. New York: Rockefeller Foundation, 1975.
40. Carlson RJ, Cunningham R, eds. *Future Directions in Health Care: A New Public Policy*. Cambridge, Mass.: Ballinger, 1978.
41. Knowles JH, Lee PR, McNerney WJ, eds. *Conference on Future Directions in Health Care: The Dimensions of Medicine*. New York: Rockefeller Foundation, 1975.
42. Bisht DB. *The Spiritual Dimension of Health*. New Delhi: Directorate General of Health Services, Government of India, 1985.
43. World Health Organization, Geneva: WHA/37/1984/REC/1.6.
44. Ibid, pp. 14-15.
45. Kreiger DT. Brain peptides: what, where, and why? Science 1983;222:975-985.
46. Henderson LJ. The study of man. Science 1941;94:1-10 (6).
47. Cannon WB. Voodoo death. Am Anthropol 1944;44:169-181.
48. Richter CP. On the phenomenon of sudden death in animals and man. Psychosomat Med 1957;19:191-198.
49. Selye H. *The Physiology and Pathology of Exposure to Stress*. Montreal: Acta, 1950.
50. Wolff HG. *Stress and Disease*. Springfield: Charles C. Thomas, 1953.
51. Levine JD, Gordon NC, Fields HL. The mechanism of placebo analgesia. Lancet 1978;ii:645-657.
52. Ader R, Cohen N, eds. *Psychoneuroimmunology*. New York: Academic Press, 1981.
53. Pelletier KR, Herzing DL. Psychoneuroimmunology: Toward a mind body model. Advances 1988;5:27-56 (49).
54. Gracely RH, Dubner R, Deeter WR, Wolskee PJ. Clinicians' expectations influence placebo analgesia (letter to the editor). Lancet 1985;i:43.
55. Westcott G, Svensson P-G, Zöllner HFK. *Health Policy Implications of Unemployment*. Copenhagen: World Health Organization, Regional Office for Europe, 1985.
56. Black DAK, Morris JN, Smith C, Townsend P. *The Black Report*. London: Penguin, 1982.
57. Ibrahim MA, Kaplan B, Patrick RC, Some C, Tyroler HA, Wilson RN. The legacy of John Cassel. Am J Epidemiol 1980;112:1-7.
58. Cassel JC, Tyroler HA. Epidemiological studies of culture change. I. Health status and recency of industrialization. Arch Environ Health 1961;3:25-33.
59. Tyroler HA, Cassel JC. Health consequences of culture change. II. The effect of urbanization on coronary heart mortality in rural residents. J Chronic Dis 1964; 17:167-177.
60. Sagan LA. *The Health of Nations: True Causes of Sickness and Well-Being*. New York: Basic, 1987.
61. House JS, Landis KR, Umberton D. Social relationships and health. Science 1988; 241:540-544.

7
To Heal The Schism

By the last quarter of the twentieth century, the leadership of the Rockefeller Foundation had concluded that past efforts to bridge the gulf between medicine and public health, as well as between curative and preventive medicine, although undoubtedly worthy and constructive left much room for improvement. The task in 1978 was to develop a different and potentially more effective long-term strategy for dealing with the "Principal Problems" and "Root Causes" associated with the decline in medicine's concern for the public's health discussed in Chapter 1.

From 1916 to the early 1950s, the Foundation had played a major role in the development of medical education, biomedical research, and public health both domestically and internationally. In the 1960s its focus shifted to agriculture and population control; health was relegated to the position of an "allied interest," largely as a component of the Education for Development Program discussed in Chapter 5. With the appointment of John Knowles, a physician, as President in 1972, health gradually returned as an interest and starting in 1973 it became part of a reorganized Population and Health Division. But by 1976 health-related programs still were receiving only 2% of the Foundation's annual appropriation.[1] The retirement of several of the Foundation's officers concerned with health affairs provided an opportunity for a fresh start.

In July 1977, Kenneth S. Warren, formerly Professor of Medicine at Case Western Reserve's Medical School, assumed directorship of the Rockefeller Foundation's Division of Health Sciences. Knowles promptly asked him to develop a broad-based program that would rejuvenate the Foundation's traditional concerns with the health sciences. This he did. At the September 14, 1977, Board of Trustees meeting he presented a three-part interrelated program. The first component, to be called *The Great Neglected Diseases of Mankind* (GND), was to focus on improving the quality of fundamental research on the major diseases of the developing world—great in number and long neglected by the Western biomedical research community. The second component was *Population-Based Medicine as an Integral Part of Clinical Medical Education*. The object was to establish divisions of clinical epidemiology within departments of medicine and pediatrics in medical schools in the United States, Europe, and the Third World. Warren's rationale was that population-based medicine, together with its concepts and methods, had not been established within the mainstream clinical departments. In his presentation to the Board he drew attention to the burgeoning interest in clinical epidemiology manifested by the major clinical research societies in the United States (American Federation for Clinical Research, American Society for Clinical Investigation, and the Association of American Physicians). The third component of the program was to be called *Quality-Based Information Systems: Improving Scientific Communication.*[2]

The Foundation's Board accepted this tripartite program, which guided the Division of Health Sciences for the next dozen years. Successes in the biomedical arena, including the burgeoning fruits of the molecular revolution, had been substantial—at least for the developed world. The Foundation's earlier efforts to enlarge the scope of what appeared to be the ever-narrowing "medical" enterprise, however, had at best been only marginally successful. Although impossible to quantify, investments in schools of public health, departments of preventive, social, and community medicine, and their analogues did not seem to be having the same impact as the Foundation's investments in the biomedical sciences, especially in molecular biology. Rising costs, misallocated resources, widespread innumeracy among the medical profession, and the growing tendency to mistake technological fixes for scientific progress were serious enough in the developed world, but they were wreaking havoc in the developing world. An unambiguous commitment was required to new initiatives that would foster coordination of the medical and public health establishments' collective energies.

To help formulate the population-based medicine component, Warren held a small informal meeting in New York on October 12, 1977. Five knowledgeable academicians[*] gathered to discuss the feasibility of initiating a program of support for clinical epidemiology. The group emphasized four goals that, although expanded and refined since, have guided the program throughout its course. In their judgment, the program should strive to:

- Produce practicing physicians better able to interpret population-based data, make better use of such data, and contribute data and knowledge to research problems concerned with evaluating health care.
- Produce faculty members working in clinical departments who would serve as role models for medical students by their teaching and creative investigations in this field.
- Develop medical professionals able to evaluate data and formulate guidelines appropriate to the care of the normal person and the practice of prevention.
- Train medical professionals to participate in the development of public policy.[3]

---

[*] Thomas C. Chalmers (Mount Sinai, New York), Alvan R. Feinstein (Yale), John Hoopis (Vermont), Edward H. Kass (Harvard), and Frank E. Speizer (Harvard).

The individuals present stressed the importance of linking epidemiology with clinical medicine to achieve these goals; they argued that priority should be given to training internists but that other clinical specialties would also be appropriate. The goals themselves reflected society's growing concerns with what came to be labeled quality assurance, resource allocation, equity of access, cost containment, risk assessment, and outcomes research.

Encouraged by this preliminary response, the Foundation held a second larger meeting on December 9, 1977, also in New York. Four members from the original group were joined by 14 other physicians. They spent a day discussing the prospects for such an initiative, largely for medical schools in the United States. Again the response was strongly positive with the suggestion that two or three pilot programs be started initially. These two preliminary gatherings to test the waters included vice presidents of medical centers, medical school deans, professors of medicine and of pediatrics from American medical schools—but no one from institutions in the developing world. There was great enthusiasm for the idea of establishing epidemiology within clinical departments.

The assembled academics were unaware, however, of the internal and external criticisms that would be associated with the proposed component. They were even less aware of the problems of getting it through the hoops and hurdles of the Rockefeller Foundation's bureaucracy and its Board. Warren, as a renowned authority on schistosomiasis and tropical diseases generally, had given top priority in the reinvigorated Division of Health Sciences to establishing the *Great Ne-glected Diseases Network* (GND). Engrossed in launching this major initiative, he had little time to devote to the *Health of Populations* component. In October 1978 Warren and Knowles asked me to join the Division and develop this new venture. I was in complete agreement with the Division's plans, all three components. The opportunity to develop specific ideas that had long intrigued me was especially attractive. John Knowles and I had discussed these frequently over the years and I believe he shared most of the views reflected in the previous chapters of this volume.

My initial task was to review the dimensions of the problems and assess the opportunities for change. From this exercise we concluded that the principal problems and root causes cited in Chapter 1 could really be boiled down to one central question: How can an adequate proportion of the brightest young minds in medicine be attracted to careers in population health? This was not an original finding. It will be recalled, from Chapter 5, that in the 1950s Alexander Langmuir had made a point of seeking out the "brightest young medical graduates" for training in the U.S. Epidemiologic Intelligence Service as the best way to improve the nation's capacity to monitor and control disease.[4] Similarly, when Britain's National Health Service was being reorganized in the 1970s and the new specialty of community physician was launched, a prominent committee urged that "senior respected physicians" be appointed to these new posts to serve as role models for young aspirants.[5]

For the officers of the Health Sciences Division, a not-so-hidden agenda was the need to change priorities in medical education, research, and eventually health services. New sets of priorities should be guided by young clinicians trained in epidemiology and the population perspective. Ultimately they would guide deployment of resources so that services would become more responsive to the public's needs. In this connection, choice of the term Health of Populations deserves comment. The initial name for the component recognized that population-based medicine was gaining currency at the time and it had the advantage of linking the concerns of medicine and medical education directly with populations. The disadvantage was that it emphasized the dominant current concerns of medicine with disease and treatment, rather than with prevention and health. If the term public health were used, there could be confusion with those functions that were seen to be primarily public or governmental responsibilities, in contrast to those which could reasonably be expected to be undertaken by private practitioners, although their services increasingly were financed from public sources. If we now are trending, as I commented earlier, toward public medicine and private health, we still have to deal with the health of populations. This term was also introduced because (as observed at the outset) the phrase "public health," like it or not, still has a powerful and irrational capacity to dissuade far too many clinicians from having much to do with it. They resist attempts to understand the objectives of this essential social activity. The term public health has so muddied the academic and professional waters over the years that new language to describe old concepts was needed.

There is no certainty that the new term will fare any better than prior ones, but there was the hope that it might attract the interest and energies of new recruits from medicine to the greater health enterprise. The future might well take us back to the perspectives of Frank, Louis, Semmelweis, the founders of the London Epidemiological Society, Virchow, Osler, Mackenzie, Ryle, and Paul. By changing from Population-based Medicine to Health of Populations, we hoped to focus on the study of health and disease in groups or populations, in addition to research at the one-to-one clinical and the molecular levels. This new perspective was not to substitute for either of the latter two but was to be an addition.

For the most part, physicians who pioneered attempts to expand medicine's horizons have been distinguished clinicians. The most promising place to start the Health of Populations initiative, therefore, must surely be with clinical departments at the heart of the power structure in the academic medical establishment. There seemed little point in trying to expand medicine's view of its collective mission by tinkering at the periphery or starting new professions or specialties, certainly not new types of schools. Something different was required.

Gunnar Biörck, a cardiologist of international repute, a founding member of the International Epidemiological Association, formerly Professor of Social Medicine at the University of Lund and later Professor of Medicine at the Karolinska Institute, once observed that he taught far more epidemiology and public health to medical students in the latter job than he was ever able to do as a professor of social medicine. My own earlier experiences as a member of a department of internal medicine amply confirm this observation.

The first targets of the new Health of Populations component, as Knowles and Warren envisaged and I concurred, would therefore be clinical departments. Of these, Internal Medicine, or simply Medicine as such departments are labeled outside the United States, seemed the best bet. There is little question that in the last quarter of the twentieth century Departments of Medicine are where the power rests in virtually all medical schools in the developed world and increasingly in the developing world. Surgery may have been the dominant clinical department at the turn of the century, and behavioral medicine may be in the ascendancy in the next century. For the present, Medicine is now in the forefront of intellectual activity and resource deployment in contemporary academic medicine. Pediatrics, surgery, obstetrics and gynecology, psychiatry, and family medicine would certainly not be excluded, but Medicine was to be the primary target.

The first major consideration focused on the concepts and skills to be learned by the students who would participate in the new program and of their relationship to the task of clinical medicine. To interest young academic clinicians in this new field, or more accurately in the renaissance of this old set of ideas and methods, the content had to have a direct bearing on their day-to-day work. They needed to see and believe that epidemiological concepts and methods would help them to practice better medicine. The clear choice was the numeric method or what had come to be labeled clinical epidemiology.

The pioneers of this "re-union" of clinical medicine and epidemiology and the advocates of contemporary applications were John Paul at Yale and his successor there, Alvan R. Feinstein, Professor of Epidemiology and Medicine, in the United States; J. N. Morris, Professor of Social Medicine first at the London Hospital Medical School and later at the London School of Hygiene and Tropical Medicine, a close friend of Paul and a frequent visitor to Yale; Walter W. Holland, Professor of Clinical Epidemiology and Social Medicine (later, Community Medicine, and currently, Public Health Medicine) at St. Thomas's Hospital Medical School, who has trained numerous clinicians and epidemiologists from not only Britain but Australia, Canada, the United States, and elsewhere; Professor Geoffrey Rose, first of St.Mary's Hospital Medical School and more recently of the London School of Hygiene and Tropical Medicine, who also has influenced clinicians from Britain, the United States, and other countries through his research and teaching; and David L. Sackett, Professor of Clinical Epidemiology and Medicine at McMaster University in Hamilton (Ontario), whose seminal ideas and teaching dominated an entire medical school as well as influencing countless colleagues in other institutions.

Once again—a century after Louis and three quarters of a century after the demise of the London Epidemiological Society—these and other physicians had demonstrated the utility of applying epidemiological concepts and methods to the problems of clinical medicine and the wider arena of health problems in the community and population. Clinical epidemiology offered the greatest promise for broadening the minds of contemporary medical faculty and their students. We saw it as a subset of the related concepts of population-based medicine, the population perspective, and the generic term Health of Populations used for the Foundation's new component.

The second decision was not to support training in "public health" as such or to support training of clinicians in epidemiology at schools of public health. That decision did not change the Foundation's commitment to improving the public's health and "the well-being of mankind." Strategies and tactics were changed, not goals or objectives. Practicing clinicians using epidemiological concepts and methods in their research and practice were to be the role models for transmitting the fundamental messages we sought to disseminate. The object was to help aspiring young clinicians internalize the population perspective as a consequence of their propinquity to a critical mass of teachers who would be suitable role models. "Learning" was seen as more important than "teaching."

We hoped that students immersed in suitable settings would develop an awareness that much of clinical value could be learned from studying groups of patients and subsets of populations, in addition to research involving individual patients, organs, cells, and molecules. In studying groups, we expected that students and their faculty mentors would need to investigate populations in the community. In doing so they would be exposed to problems well known to those laboring in the public health vineyard. The contemporary hospital-based perspective would be expanded to embrace that of the entire community; experience with the problems of primary care would balance those of tertiary care. For this the students would need to acquire an understanding of epidemiological, essentially statistical, concepts and methods. Biostatistics, health economics, and health social sciences would be added later.

The third matter to be decided was the point of entry into the system. Was it to be through established senior faculty members, additional faculty, junior faculty, residents (house staff), or directly through medical students? The first group was excluded on the grounds that they might find it difficult to change their spots in midcareer, most being committed to biomedical laboratory research. Earlier clinical research had consisted largely of descriptive case series; this was still true in many Third World medical schools. Now clinicians were finding it increasingly difficult to compete with fundamental scientists who had Ph.D. training in the new research areas spawned by the molecular revolution. Additional new faculty were out of the question because there were few clinicians trained in epidemiology available, and they would have had a hard time gaining acceptance if appointed as newcomers to a traditional department of medicine. House staff do much, if not most, of the teaching of medical students, but heavy clinical loads precluded their devoting time to learning new points of view and additional skills. Broadening the horizons of medical students was the ultimate goal of the program, but crowded curricula and reward systems that favored tertiary care and widespread adherence to a constricted biomedical model made this initially a tough bastion to crack.

Both strategic and tactical considerations required a different initiative. Much as Louis had done, over a century earlier, we opted for targeting young established faculty members. They should be young so that they possessed the energy, enthusiasm, and aspirations to embrace new opportunities and undertake new challenges. They should have completed all their usual postgraduate training and should have been accepted by their superiors and colleagues as full "card-carrying" faculty members—capable of making their way academically no matter what their subspecialty or research interest. Whatever the Foundation was to provide in the way of additional training would be on top of full acceptance by their superiors and colleagues. These young faculty members were to have completed all the rites of passage; they were to be full members of an academic medical fraternity. We did not want those who rightly or wrongly might be perceived by medicine's academicians as marginal or peripheral people, however compatible their ideas, credentials, or aspirations might be with the objectives of the new Health of Populations program.

Next was the matter of institutional support—intellectual, structural, professional, and financial. We determined that each institution selected as a site for developing the program should have unequivocal backing from both the Department Chairman (usually of Medicine), the Dean of the Medical School, and usually from the Rector or Vice-Chancellor of the university. This was to be more than the usual "altar call" put on for visiting philanthropists in which academic czars testify to their undying commitment to the donor's program! The Department Head and Dean had to nominate young faculty members who had firm positions with guaranteed salaries, but they also had to come up with dedicated space for the proposed trainee and his or her colleagues on their return from training. At least some support staff and equipment were also to be guaranteed. In other words, this was to be a cost-sharing, institutional commitment backed by those who controlled the resources and set the priorities. Not every medical school could provide the same resources or constellation of support, but tangible evidence of a definite decision to develop this additional perspective for medicine was a prerequisite for serious consideration by the Foundation.

A solitary faculty member could be readily swamped by demands for this new expertise. Alternatively, he or she might be adumbrated by the traditional academic priorities and reward systems. Training a single faculty member, no matter how bright, how eager, and how well sponsored he or she might be, was viewed as a waste of time. The Rockefeller Foundation's old bugaboo of "scatteration" was a nonstarter. Each institution's commitment, therefore, had to be for the establishment of a critical mass of young faculty members. Certainly two were needed to spell one another and, applying the lore of group dynamics, three was the minimum required for conflict resolution; five seemed the ideal minimum number and eventually six would be deemed "correct." Everyone would know that a division, group, center, or Unit as they were called eventually, had been created. A real presence within the institution would be assured. If one or two of the members were less than fully successful or drifted into other fields there would still be others to carry on. A six-person Unit had some reasonable prospect of enduring; a smaller number had less chance. Six young established faculty members, primarily from departments of medicine but not excluding others, were to form the core of each Unit in those institutions selected for the program.

The next question was whether the several "Units" could or should be linked together. The dozen centers, largely in the developed world, that were selected eventually for the Great Neglected Diseases (GND) program were linked in a collegial network centered around an annual scientific meeting. The network kept people in touch, developed informal ties, and had a multiplier effect that was impossible to quantify but must have been much greater than the sum of the parts. There was now the prospect of developing a second network, a Clinical Epidemiology Network. If the former was to develop new drugs and vaccines, the latter might assist, among other equally important pursuits, in field-testing the efficacy and effectiveness of products anticipated from the laboratories through the conduct of randomized, controlled clinical trials (or their analogues). The synergism might well be expected to augment the capacity of both networks. My own predilections strongly favored the network pattern for the clinical epidemiology component. As chairman from 1964 to 1976 of a 12-unit, seven-country, international network sponsored in part by the World Health Organization (W.H.O.), I had learned first-hand about the benefits for research from frequent interactions with colleagues from different cultures, disciplines, and environments.[6] Commitment to the concept of a network, however, implied additional costs for annual meetings and the inevitable and substantial expenses of communication and travel. To come later was the question of how large and where the network would start and, eventually, extend. From its inception in 1978, however, the Health of Populations component envisaged creation of a network of affiliated units.

In many ways, the most difficult choice was the next one. Certainly the traditions of the Rockefeller Foundation, especially in the health field, had favored international activities. The need was there, and the concept of a Clinical Epidemiology Network as a companion to the GND favored an emphasis on the developing world. Initial discussions, memoranda, and even plans, called for establishing a network of 12 Clinical Epidemiology Centers at the rate of four per year starting in 1979. Strategies discussed varied between placing all 12 Centers in the United States to creation of a broader international approach. The initial configuration chosen included four in North America, one each in Europe and Australasia, and six in the developing world—possibly two each in Asia, Latin America, and Africa. John Knowles supported this approach. In addition to training the young faculty members, funding was envisaged for the core staff and infrastructure of these Centers. A series of international conferences was also planned to launch the program.[7]

This was as far as our thinking and planning had proceeded in 1978 when I had been at the Foundation less than 3 months. John Knowles became ill at the end of December, was hospitalized after the New Year, and died on March 6, 1979. There is no way of knowing what might have evolved had he lived. His interest and enthusiasm for this initiative were long-standing. In the past we had shared thoughts about what might be done to improve relations between medicine and public health and what was needed for *healing the schism*. The prospect of an early start for the Health of Populations program faded; the entire initiative was placed "on hold."

The late Sterling Wortman was appointed Acting President of the Foundation. Wortman had spent most of his professional career with the Foundation's Division of Agricultural Sciences. He knew the developing world well and emphasized its importance for the Foundation's programs. Domestic health problems were of minimal interest to him. Wortman had some familiarity with the Foundation's traditional concerns in public health, but he had no understanding of the strange notion that epidemiology might be a powerful means of changing medical education and priorities for health care.

Warren and I, therefore, had to start anew on several fronts simultaneously. First, there was the need to inform and interest the Acting President and other skeptical officers of the Foundation about the potential value of clinical epidemiology. Second was the need to identify potential sites for training clinicians in epidemiology and sites for establishing the proposed units. Both Sterling Wortman and the Foundation's Board, understandably, were reluctant to embrace new initiatives until the presidential succession was settled.

We were encouraged, however, to continue our explorations of the field. Although responsibility for developing the Health of Populations Program resided with me, Kenneth Warren provided unstinting intellectual leadership and administrative support. His championship of the concepts, strategy, and tactics for the program made an extremely difficult organizational passage possible. We both shared the conviction that the two major thrusts of the Division of Health Sciences were complementary; each had the capacity to enhance the other.

The overall goals of the new component were taking shape. We now had to develop a clear understanding within the Foundation of the need for such a program both domestically and internationally. Although practices differed over the decades and hindsight is easy, the officers in 1978 were determined to do a more thorough job than that which apparently had launched the program for establishing independent schools of public health. We left few stones unturned in our efforts to tackle old problems in what seemed to be unfamiliar ways but which were really not new.

John R. Evans and I had been friends for a decade. We first met in 1969 when I was a visiting professor at McMaster University, Hamilton, Ontario. As Founding Dean in 1965, Evans had established the first truly innovative medical school of the post-Flexnerian era. An internist and cardiologist trained at Toronto, Harvard, and Oxford he had been on the faculty of the University of Toronto. The new school was to become a global pacesetter, internationally recognized, as the faculty pioneered the use of problem-based learning, a science-based approach to patient care, and the use of quantitative methods for critical appraisal of all the faculty's and students' activities; it had the most advanced medical curriculum extant. With the largest group of clinical epidemiologists and biostatisticians to be found in any medical school, epidemiology had a pervasive influence throughout McMaster. It was part and parcel of the everyday practice of clinician epidemiologists, aided and abetted by departmental colleagues who were statisticians, economists, and social scientists.[8] If there was a model that provided a guide for healing the schism and for what our Health of Populations initiative later established—the International Clinical Epidemiology Network (INCLEN)—McMaster was it.

From founding this pioneering medical school Evans went on to become President of the University of Toronto. There, in 1974, among his many accomplishments, he successfully merged its Faculty of Medicine and its School of Hygiene and Public Health. In so doing, Canada phased out its last separate School of Public Health but by no means its widespread national commitment to improving the public's health. The School, as noted in Chapter 4, had been founded in 1927 with support from the Rockefeller Foundation. Several departments were transferred to the Division of Basic Medical Sciences within the Faculty of Medicine, others to its Division of Clinical Medicine, and the remainder to a new Division of Community Health. Each of the divisions had an Associate Dean. The budget for the Division of Community Health was segregated from the rest of the Faculty of Medicine's budget so that there would be no temptation to shift resources to bolster competing interests and priorities. Having just completed his tenure as President of the University of Toronto in 1978, John Evans was in an excellent position to help us in establishing the new Health of Populations component at the Foundation. At my suggestion, in the last week of December 1978, just before John Knowles's terminal hospitalization, Evans met with Knowles and me and agreed to be a consultant to the Division of Health Sciences's proposed Health of Populations component. He was asked to assess the present state of affairs globally with respect to teaching, research, and practice in "public health" and related matters. The first Rockefeller grant to launch the new component was awarded in January 1979 to the University of Toronto to permit Evans to conduct a feasibility study for his global survey; this was followed in April 1979 by a larger grant for the full study.

In spring of 1979, Evans embarked on a large-scale travel schedule to learn first-hand about the state of education for physicians whose talents would be directed at improving the public's health in the last quarter of the twentieth century. The scope of the enquiry is best described by Evans's own Preface to his final review, initially published as *Measurement and Management in Medicine: Training Needs and Opportunities*:

> The observations in this paper are based on interviews with senior staff in the ministries of health of four industrialized and four developing countries; World Health Organization staff at headquarters and in three Regional Offices; academic leaders in universities, schools of public health, and schools of medicine; senior spokesmen for national and international associations for public health, medical education, and health and hospital administration; and program officers of six foundations in the United States and the United Kingdom active in support of these fields of education and research. Site visits were made to five universities with schools of public health as well as medical schools, and to four medical schools with innovative health programs in the United States and Canada; to the London School of Hygiene and Tropical Medicine and three medical school departments of community medicine in the United Kingdom; to the Andrija Štampar School of Public Health in Yugoslavia; and to public health training centers in four developing countries. Attendance at the annual meetings of the associations of schools of public health in the United States, in Latin America, and in Europe provided a valuable opportunity to review problems in public health education with representatives from a broad section of institutions.[9]

Throughout 1979 and 1980 we had the benefit of Evans's observations and emerging conclusions stemming from his travels and enquiries; his final report was published in 1981. Some 3000 copies of the English version were distributed worldwide, as well as 1000 copies of the Spanish edition and an indeterminate number of a Chinese translation. The report should be of interest to all concerned with the problems addressed in the present volume; they are summarized in less than 60 pages with abundant examples and ample documentation. At this point, however, there is little to be gained by dwelling further on the sad litany of almost universal failure to recruit and prepare adequate numbers of young physicians to assume creative leadership positions in the public health and health care establishments.

Evans confirmed our evolving ideas about the best way to address the root problems we had identified. Somehow the broader population perspective had to be brought back into the mainstream of medicine; the public's health was the business of the entire medical establishment or, as it was starting to be called, the "health sciences", because professions other than medicine are involved. Without physicians, whose steering effect at all points of the system is enormous, little else can be achieved. Evans defined our opportunity succinctly:

> The major problem facing medical schools is the generation of a core of clinical teachers, trained to apply quantitative thinking and the scientific method to populations in the same way they have been applied to physiological problems. They are needed as instructors, role models in clinical training, and as researchers.[10]

A commentator in Australia had this to say about Evans's report:

> The overriding impression of this monograph is that it accurately describes the comprehensive basis of a complex set of problems which collectively lead to poor utilization and application of existing resources in health sciences education, health care delivery, and health management.[11]

The uncertainties and hiatus in leadership at the Rockefeller Foundation that stalled our own development of clinical epidemiology, certainly in the United States, were compensated for by other initiatives from the Charles A. Dana Foundation, the Andrew W. Mellon Foundation, and the Milbank Memorial Fund. The latter, under the leadership of its newly appointed President, Robert H. Ebert, former Professor of Medicine, Dean of the Harvard Medical School, and a one-time member of the Rockefeller Foundation's Board, initiated a program to provide 5 years of financial support for about five young clinical faculty members annually. Most candidates were to be selected from Departments of Internal Medicine and each was to spend an initial year studying epidemiology and biostatistics at the London School of Hygiene and Tropical Medicine under the direction of Geoffrey Rose, Professor of Epidemiology. This was to be followed by a year of combined clinical and epidemiological experience based in one of the Departments of Medicine in Britain. I worked with officers of the Milbank Memorial Fund in formulating the program and was on the Selection Committee for these Fellowships. In search of possible sites for fostering clinical epidemiology I accompanied Ebert on visits to a number of medical schools in the United States, including the Universities of California (Davis), Pennsylvania, Texas (San Antonio), Washington (Seattle), and Yale.

Two points deserve mentioning. First, there was keen competition for the five openings each year, and although it took some time for many departments of internal medicine in the United States to understand fully what the program was intended to accomplish, we did establish the existence of a need for this training, at least as perceived by the candidates and their sponsors. Second, many faculty members in schools of public health in the United States were incensed that none of the latter had been selected as sites for training these young clinicians in epidemiology. The reason was clear. In contrast to most faculty members of American departments of epidemiology, Geoffrey Rose had a strong clinical background from his days at St. Mary's Hospital Medical School, and both his research and teaching were more attuned to the needs of clinicians than was apparent in the United States' schools of public health. A related issue was the ready transfer of Fellows during the second year of training from the London School of Hygiene and Tropical Medicine to the several departments of medicine in Britain hospitable to the application of epidemiological methods of investigation in clinical settings.

The anger of the American schools with these initiatives was not assuaged by the related initiative of the Andrew W. Mellon Foundation. I had several conversations with J. Kellum Smith, Jr., its Vice President. He had formerly been Secretary of the Rockefeller Foundation, and I had known him for some years as a fellow trustee of the Foundation for Child Development. The Mellon Foundation had learned about clinical epidemiology and was interested in supporting its development in medical schools. The resulting program filled the void left by the uncertainty surrounding the Rockefeller Foundation's support of clinical epidemiology within the United States. The Mellon Foundation provided $3.7 million to support clinical epidemiology in six major East Coast private medical schools: Columbia, Duke, Harvard, the Johns Hopkins, Yale, and Pennsylvania. The Charles A. Dana Foundation's program focused more on preventive medicine but it did provide an early 5-year grant to help establish clinical epidemiology at the University of Pennsylvania. These three major programs were largely responsible for putting clinical epidemiology on the academic map in American medical schools. In all of this the Rockefeller Foundation was only an indirect player.

Meanwhile the Robert Wood Johnson's Clinical Scholars program, although not focused primarily on epidemiology, continued apace, and undoubtedly was responsible for sensitizing many young academicians to the potential contributions of epidemiology. Many of the country's leading young clinical epidemiologists were trained with support from this program. All told, more than 600 individuals have been trained so far; six universities (University of California at Los Angeles and at San Francisco; University of North Carolina; University of Pennsylvania; University of Washington; and Yale) currently offer training, two in close affiliation with the INCLEN program.[12] The Clinical Scholars program was the first recent attempt in the developed world to heal the schism, and in many ways it was the forerunner of INCLEN.[13] Unfortunately faculty members in some American schools of public health were said to regard these initiatives negatively, a position difficult to comprehend given the history recounted in earlier chapters and the growing demand for epidemiologists in the United States.

We undertook additional explorations at the Rockefeller Foundation starting early in 1979 as we sought to build the case for the clinical epidemiology component. Our task was to identify potential training sites where there were strong clinical epidemiology groups and departments of medicine or even entire medical faculties committed to developing and applying epidemiological concepts and methods. We were familiar with major developments in the United States and, in addition, once the word was out that the Foundation might be developing a clinical epidemiology component, we received numerous unsolicited informal and formal proposals. In Canada, Kenneth Warren and I visited McMaster University and the University of Western Ontario as potential training sites for clinical epidemiologists.

Given the Foundation's and Sterling Wortman's predominant interests in the developing world, however, we needed to identify possible sites, university rectors, deans, and department heads to lead the development of clinical epidemiology in Third World universities. We decided to approach leading medical schools in these regions with the hope of interesting the administrators and leading clinicians in the new program.

In Southeast Asia John Evans and I visited the Universities of Singapore and Malaya; Gadjah Mada, Airlangga (Surabaya), and Udayana (Denpasar, Bali) Universities in Indonesia; Chulalongkorn University and Mahidol University's two medical schools (Ramathibodi and Siraraj), and Khon Kaen University in Thailand. I also visited the Hindu University at Benares and the University of Srinagar in India, and later the University of the Philippines. In Latin America, I visited the Universidad del Valle in Cali, Colombia; the University of Venezuela; the Universidad Federal do Rio de Janeiro, Escola Paulista, and the University of São Paulo in Brazil; the University of Buenos Aires; and in Central America, the University of Costa Rica. Visits were also made to schools of public health at Mahidol University, and at the Universities of Buenos Aires, São Paulo, and Venezuela. I had visited the University of Ibadan in Nigeria, and other medical schools and schools of public health in Latin America on earlier occasions. Later I visited the University of Southampton in England as a potential training site; it was regarded as the most innovative medical school in that country.

In February and March 1980 Kenneth Warren and I visited the Peoples' Republic of China. Our first stop was Peking Union Medical College (at the time temporarily renamed the Capital Medical College), the country's premier medical school and the earlier recipient of the largest single institutional investment by the Rockefeller Foundation. In spite of a warm welcome and extended discussions we could elicit no interest whatsoever in clinical epidemiology; so imbedded was the schism between clinical medicine and public health that the possibility of developing common interests through the application of epidemiological thinking seemed beyond the faculty's comprehension. A far different reception awaited us at the First Shanghai Medical School (now Shanghai Medical University) where Professor Su Delong, introduced in the Preface, paved the way for establishment of a Clinical Epidemiology Unit. The same was true at Chengdu, Sichuan Province, where Professor C. C. Chen, mentioned in Chapter 1, was instrumental in helping to establish a second unit at Sichuan Medical College (now West China University of Medical Sciences).

Throughout our travels the interviews and experiences varied widely. At some universities, although received graciously, we failed miserably to explain our mission, let alone convince anyone of its merits. At first, practically all the deans and clinical department heads simply could not understand how epidemiology was even remotely related to the work of a clinician. This was "public health" territory and not the function of a medical school, except for transient mentions in a department of social or preventive medicine. So much for awareness of the history of this topic!

One country's leading nephrologist and head of the department of medicine at its leading medical school, trained at McGill and Harvard, simply could not comprehend what I had in mind initially. After two evenings of intense discussion, he revealed that his young son, a pediatrician, was interested in social medicine. At the time his son was training in London with Professor J. N. Morris, my former mentor, who, as I noted earlier, had been a close friend of John Paul's and an early advocate of clinical epidemiology during his tenure at the London Hospital Medical School. When I explained that Morris was an epidemiologist interested in clinical problems, among other matters, this prominent professor of medicine immediately caught on. Ever since he has been one of the staunchest supporters of clinical epidemiology in his own institution and, especially when he was appointed Dean, elsewhere in his own country and globally.

The ready receptivity we encountered at other times is illustrated by an example from a different part of the world—Thailand. Prawase Wasi, Professor of Medicine, was chairman of his department and a biomedical scientist with an international reputation as an authority on thalassemia in one of his country's leading medical schools. He saw the opportunity immediately and expressed great regret about the isolation of his university's school of public health from its two medical schools and about the absence of concern in the latter's faculties for the population's most pressing health problems. When asked what earlier benefactions from the Rockefeller Foundation had done for medicine in his country, this biomedical scientist replied: "It brought our research up to international standards but it took us away from the people!"

On another occasion, we had an enthusiast for clinical epidemiology in the developed world announce that "We'll get those biomedical bastards yet!" This was the last point of view we wished to encourage. Clinical epidemiology and the population perspective were seen as additions to, not substitutes for, the biomedical and clinical approaches; we wanted to expand horizons, not constrict them. From all these visits and interviews we were helped in the later selection of sites for establishing what came to be called *Clinical Epidemiology Training and Research Centers* (CERTCs) and *Clinical Epidemiology Units* (CEUs)—the components of INCLEN.

Early in 1979 I organized two more formal meetings, each based on a set of prepared short statements that described opportunities and constraints in developing epidemiology in clinical departments. These formed the basis for extensive discussions. Both were 2-day meetings held in New York; the first on March 8-9, 1979, was labeled "Primary Care and Balanced Health Care Systems," and the second on May 8-9, 1979, had the title a "Clinical Epidemiology, Priority Setting, and Resource Allocation."[14] The participants in the first conference included seven officers of the Rockefeller Foundation, and John Evans, as well as officers from the Ford Foundation, the W. K. Kellogg Foundation, and the Canadian International Development Research Center (IDRC). Representatives from other international agencies and individuals knowledgeable about the developing world also attended. The object of the first exercise was to consider the health care arrangements of the Third World, and how they might be approached more rationally so that resources would be allocated appropriately to their most pressing indigenous problems.

The second conference focused more directly on the opportunities for expanding clinical epidemiology and especially on identifying potential sites in North America for training young faculty members from the developing world. Again there were six Rockefeller Foundation officers, John Evans, and three officers from the W. K. Kellogg, Josiah H. Macy Jr., and Andrew W. Mellon Foundations present. In addition there were five chairmen and professors of internal medicine and family medicine and five epidemiologists, primarily clinicians. The dean from an innovative medical school in Israel and five professors of medicine from medical schools in Third World countries completed the group. The papers from the two conferences were rearranged for publication in five chapters: Understanding the Health of Populations: Clinical Epidemiology; Balanced Health Systems; The Health of Populations in the Developing World; Strategies for Improving Health in the Developing World; and Summary—Health for Populations.[15] In the latter chapter Paul D. Stolley, at that time, Professor of Research Medicine at the University of Pennsylvania, persuasively stated the case for our proposed program:

> Epidemiology is usually defined as the study of the distribution and determinants of disease in human populations. Morris has summarized the uses of epidemiology to include:
>
> - Studying the history of the health of populations and of the rise and fall of diseases and changes in their character;
> - Diagnosing the health of the community, and the condition of the people, to measure the present dimensions and distributions of ill health in terms of incidence, prevalence and mortality. This investigation helps to define health problems for community action and to determine their relative importance and priority while at the same time identifying vulnerable groups needing special protection.
> - Studying the working of health services with a view to their improvement;
> - Completing the clinical picture of the natural history of disease by investigating disease as it is presented in the community and not just in the hospital; screening; and prevention;
> - Searching for causes of disease utilizing epidemiologic methods to uncover etiology.[16]
>
> Because the amount of investment in the health sector is necessarily limited, more appropriate allocation of manpower, facilities, and services is desirable. If misalloca-

tion of resources and funds occurs, then this wasteful expenditure and activity diverts funds and efforts away from appropriate activities. For example, if a less-developed country places an emphasis on the training of cardiothoracic surgeons rather than primary care practitioners and medical auxiliaries, it is likely that the high priority health needs of the population will be neglected. Similarly, if inefficacious therapies are widely distributed, then this will be at the expense of those that have been proven effective....

The objective of clinical epidemiology is to...[contribute to] analysis and resolution of the following problems:
- Misallocation of manpower, facilities, technology, and services;
- Adoption of unevaluated or inappropriate forms of medical intervention;
- Overemphasis on laboratory and clinical medicine and neglect of population-based medicine;
- Inadequate education and training in population-based medicine, especially in the developing world.[17]

Stolley closed with these observations:

The plight of developing nations is closely connected to the effectiveness and efficiency of the health sector. To the extent that better health care is important in improving the life of the needy people of the Third World, the epidemiologic perspective is an essential requirement to guide health planning efforts. Foundations have a special role in encouraging these efforts by virtue of their unique flexibility and their willingness to experiment with more innovative programs.

The conference participants enthusiastically urged foundations to undertake the support of a consortium of clinical epidemiology units (preferably located in a clinical department of a medical school) in both developed and developing nations. These units would train individuals in clinical epidemiology who would acquire research skills while working on problems peculiar to their own geographic region, even if they studied elsewhere. The units would comprise a network which would meet at regular intervals.

Individuals trained in these units should be uniquely able to integrate the epidemiologic perspective and methods with clinical medicine, and would, it is hoped, have a significant impact on medical education and health planning.[18]

Following our May conference, the first grant was approved by the Executive Committee of the Board to assist in the development and expansion of the Clinical Epidemiology Training Center being created at the University of Pennsylvania; it was for the 3-year period beginning July 1, 1979. This was to be the test case in an American medical school for the program we were launching and marked the birthdate of the International Clinical Epidemiology Network (INCLEN).

Pennsylvania's history of attempts over the decades to develop the population perspective was reviewed in Chapter 5. It is worth recording that this new training center was established by Professor Laurence E. Earley, a distinguished nephrologist, who had recently assumed the chairmanship of the department of medicine. Earley had been a brilliant medical student at the University of North Carolina where I like to think he absorbed some of the ideas being espoused in the 1950s by

John Cassel, T. Franklin Williams, and myself. As chairman of the department of medicine at the University of Texas, San Antonio, he had established the first formal Clinical Epidemiology Unit in the United States under the leadership of Michael Stern. This successful experience surely must have encouraged Earley to replicate the pattern at the University of Pennsylvania and support Paul Stolley in establishing a similar unit.

As noted, the Charles A. Dana Foundation had provided an initial 5-year grant in 1978 to start the clinical epidemiology program at Pennsylvania. The purpose of the Rockefeller Foundation's grant was to strengthen this initiative in the department of medicine, under the direction of Paul Stolley (and later under Stolley and Brian L. Strom, as Co-Directors of the center) and to extend its capacity for training candidates from the Third World. Excerpts from the docket recommending the grant to the Rockefeller Board illustrate the logic behind the entire component—logic required to persuade a skeptical body unaccustomed to looking at the problems in this manner:

> A clear disjunction exists today between the training of most physicians and society's perception of its health care needs. Medical school curricula are directed chiefly toward training future doctors to think only about the problems of the individual patient, with the objective of securing optimal care for that patient regardless of cost and consequences to others—family, community or country. The disciplines of population-based medicine are usually taught in a relatively superficial manner in the first two years of medical school by departments of preventive or social medicine or of community or public health. During the next two years of clinical studies and the three years of hospital experience, however, the student is trained to think solely in terms of individual-based medicine, and especially at the molecular and organ-system levels of disease processes. Virtually all attempts to reorient physicians toward population-based thinking and public health occur after this critical learning period—by which time the great majority are ineluctably embarked upon careers in clinical or laboratory medicine where increased specialization is well rewarded. This medical model had its origins in Europe and flourished in America following the Flexner Report of 1910; since World War II it has evolved with the exponential growth of biomedical research and has been widely copied in the developing world.
>
> But the enormous benefits of biomedical research have been accompanied by substantial imbalances in the allocation of resources for organizing and providing efficient—as well as more effective and less costly—health services based on the application of epidemiological concepts and methods. Many countries are deeply concerned about the geographic maldistribution of physicians and other health workers; the dearth of physicians to provide family and primary care, train other health workers, and organize and manage health care systems; and the rising costs of health care in relation to other costs and to perceived benefits. The less developed countries, in particular, should gain substantially by application of scientific concepts and methods for estimating the burden of illness and evaluating the efficacy of alternative modes of intervention.
>
> In light of these circumstances, the University of Pennsylvania proposes to establish a clinical epidemiology unit within the Section of General Medicine of its Department of Medicine. Space has been provided in the outpatient clinic, and the University has

obtained an endowment for a new chair for Dr. John M. Eisenberg, head of the Section. The new unit will be directed by Dr. Paul D. Stolley, a young clinical epidemiologist with an international reputation...[T]he unit's staff will collaborate with faculty colleagues, medical students, and postgraduate Fellows—including some from the developing world—in applying epidemiological principles and methods to studies of populations drawn from hospital and ambulatory practices as well as the general community...[The faculty all have] patient care responsibilities. Among the activities undertaken will be studies of the relative efficacy, costs, and risks of common treatments for pain and surgical procedures, the preparation of monographs on iatrogenic (physician-related) disease and on epidemiological methods, development of new teaching methods and courses in clinical epidemiology, and population studies of the natural history of common health problems and the influence of social factors on them. All the concepts and methods are applicable to the developing world, although the problems will differ.

The formal development of this unit in the heart of the most powerful department in a major medical school in the developed world will provide a clear example of reoriented priorities in medical education and a climate in which postgraduate Fellows from the developing world can learn attitudes, concepts, methods, and skills that will help them to reorient their own universities and health services.[19]

The initial understanding was that Pennsylvania would start with just one trainee from the developing world in addition to its American Fellows, and that gradually the cohort of Third World Fellows would expand as experience and staff permitted. Progress at Pennsylvania and in other elements of the program will be discussed later, suffice it to say here that all of the expectations from this initial grant and many more have been realized fully. By 1989, not only had 31 Fellows from the developing world been trained in clinical epidemiology at the University of Pennsylvania, but there has been an outpouring of first-rate research and wide-spread requests for consulting services internationally. The University of Pennsylvania has provided increasing amounts of "hard money" support, and Professor Stolley has been established in a named, endowed chair. This is the outcome of the decisions taken by Pennsylvania's School of Medicine described in Chapter 5—a decision that required a century of debate.

Several other related early initiatives should be recorded. The first was a grant in 1979 to Professors Frederick Mosteller and John C. Bailar III, nationally prominent biostatisticians at Harvard. The purpose was to examine the adequacy of the experimental designs and analytical methods employed by clinical investigators as reflected in articles published in the *New England Journal of Medicine* and other leading medical journals, including the *Lancet*, the *British Medical Journal*, and the *Journal of the American Medical Association*. Again, the object of this exercise was to establish the need for more extensive and intensive training in epidemiological and statistical methods. By all accounts the need was great; substantial numbers of articles analyzed were either flawed or required methodological improvement. Arnold S. Relman, editor of the *New England Journal of Medicine* and one of the instigators of this project, described the results as "spectacular"; more than 30 articles based on research supported by this grant were published, in addition to a book.[20]

Another activity was aimed at creating opportunities for establishing clinical epidemiology in medical schools that claimed to emphasize population-based perspectives in their undergraduate education. In 1979 the Network of Community-Oriented Educational Institutions for Health Sciences had been established by the World Health Organization and its regional component, the Pan American Health Organization, at an inaugural meeting in Jamaica. This consortium of medical schools, largely in the developing world, was led by three of the most innovative schools in the developed world: McMaster University (Canada), the University of Newcastle (Australia), and the University of Limburg, Maastricht (The Netherlands).

Two major themes characterized the interests of the entire faculty of each of these schools, not just those of one or two departments. First was the commitment to relating priorities for health sciences education, research, and service to the community's or population's health problems in rational fashion. Second was the commitment to linking medical education to that of other health professionals and to the community's other health facilities and services. Both objectives required active use of the population-based sciences, especially epidemiology. As such they were clearly related to the goals of the Health of Populations program. For 2 years, this network had languished for lack of funding. The possibilities of finding among its members medical schools suitable for developing clinical epidemiology encouraged us to assist the network by organizing an international meeting at the Rockefeller Foundation's Study and Conference Center in Bellagio, Italy. From the papers and deliberations at the meeting a book was published, entitled *New Directions for Medical Education*.[21] This conference (March 30-April 3, 1981) helped to rejuvenate the network that indeed was found to have several universities with strong interests in clinical epidemiology. Not the least of these was represented at the Bellagio Conference by the late David Maddison, Founding Dean of the new medical school at the University of Newcastle, Australia, where clinical epidemiology was embedded as an essential component in the curriculum.

Strategies for encouraging physicians to think about the health of the populations they serve, of necessity, should involve primary care, as well as secondary and tertiary, care. One of the great limitations facing all those concerned with this fundamental level of care—involving responses, as it does, to the bulk of the health problems experienced by any general population—was the totally inadequate set of labels (nomenclatures) and classification systems employed. At the level of primary care, the majority of patients present with symptoms, complaints, conditions, and problems; much less frequently do they arrive with readily diagnosable "diseases," especially at the first encounter. The *International Classification of Diseases* (ICD) has gone through nine revisions with no coherent organizational theme; it is an outmoded mixture of classifications based on organ systems, age and sex groupings, and notions of causation.[22] The ICD is quite useless at the primary care level. If there are no recognized or standardized "labels" for use in primary care, the phenomena encountered can not be counted; if they are not counted, they are thought not to "count". "Catch-22" best describes this absurd state of affairs.

The Foundation, therefore, in collaboration with the World Health Organization, the U.S. National Center for Health Statistics (NCHS), and the World Organization of National Colleges, Academies, and Academic Associations of General Practitioners/Family Physicians (WONCA) helped to finance an international Working Party to develop a classification for primary care. The new array was built on earlier work by the Royal College of General Practitioners, the NCHS, WONCA, and others. After numerous meetings in the course of a decade's work, including field trials in nine countries, the *ICPC-International Classification of Primary Care* was published.[23] Sad to say, the World Health Organization refused to endorse this innovative development and withdrew official support; apparently the guardians of the ICD found the ICPC too threatening. This position was taken in the face of WHO's efforts to advance primary care stemming from the Declaration of Alma Ata in 1978.[24] After all, how can we know how much progress has been made towards the attainment of "Health for All by the Year 2000" if appropriate labels for the people's problems do not exist and we cannot count them? Fundamental lessons about the central importance of nosology taught by Sydenham, Louis, and Virchow, to say nothing of William Farr, seem to have been lost on some officials then at WHO.[25] More recently, the European Economic Commission, and most of its member countries, have embarked on strategies for adopting the *International Classification of Primary Care*.[26]

Because emotional and social problems, as well as the impact of Factor "X," are integral components of virtually all illnesses, we also considered it desirable to develop methods that would encourage clinicians, especially those working at the primary care level, to record their observations along three axes: the biological or physical, the psychological, and the social. The ICPC contains classifications for all three parameters but in the course of its development, further discussion of the desirable attributes of the two latter emerging classifications seemed important. Accordingly, the Foundation provided the World Health Organization with a grant to assist in expanding the social and psychological classifications and to conduct field trials in developed and developing countries for testing and refining them. We also sponsored three meetings to discuss problems and progress: the first at Bellagio, November 6-10, 1979, was a "Workshop on Psychosocial Factors Affecting Health: Assessment, Classification, and Utilization;" the second in New York, February 19-21, 1980, was a "Conference on Recording Health Problems Triaxially: WHO Consultation on an International Collaborative Study;" and the third, again at Bellagio, February 9-13, 1981, was a "Conference on Primary Health Care: Triaxial Recording of Physical, Psychological, and Social Components." From these efforts, in addition to the ICPC, another book emerged: *Psychosocial Factors Affecting Health*.[27]

Because the capacity to estimate population-based rates is essential for comparison across practices or jurisdictions, we gave considerable thought to what has been called "the denominator problem" in primary care. The problem is to devise estimates to serve as a denominator in calculating rates for the population served by a health center, polyclinic, physicians's office, or hospital outpatient facility. To stimulate interest we held a small meeting at Bellagio concurrently with the February 9-13, 1981, Triaxial Recording Conference. The proceedings were published in a volume entitled *Primary Care Research: Encounter Records and the Denominator Problem.*[28]

Epidemiological terms had never been formally codified; usages varied, and definitions were not standardized internationally. Professor John M. Last of the University of Ottawa, a noted epidemiologist and student of the discipline's evolution, was asked by the International Epidemiological Association to undertake creation of *A Dictionary of Epidemiology.* With the help of an international editorial committee, numerous collaborators, and support from the Milbank Fund, the U.S. National Library of Medicine, and the Rockefeller Foundation, the volume was completed in 1983. It has been extremely well received by epidemiologists of all persuasions, and a second edition followed.[29] Among its many contributions was the most widely accepted definition of epidemiology extant:

> The study of the distribution and determinants of health-related states and events in populations, and the application of this study to control of health problems.

Primary care is only one component of a balanced health care system and data from patient encounters at this level are only one source of health statistics, albeit the most neglected. Accordingly from September 8 to 10, 1982, at Le Prieur), Talloires, the Tufts University European Center, in collaboration with the Fondation Mérieux we held an international conference on Health Information Systems. Epidemiologists and statisticians from the developed and developing worlds discussed a series of prepared papers that were subsequently published.[30] One of the papers—"Ecological Fallacies in Epidemiology"—must surely be a classic. Manning Feinleib, a noted epidemiologist and currently Director of the U.S. National Center for Health Statistics, and Paul Leaverton, Professor of Biostatistics in the University of South Florida, examined the underlying assumptions and methodological hazards that face epidemiologists dealing with large population-based data sets, a field of growing importance as the population perspective spreads throughout the health establishment.[31]

The environment was another area that I believed was being neglected as a consequence of current preoccupations with the costs of medical care. Accordingly, also with the collaboration of the Fondation Mérieux, three international conferences on "Environmental Epidemiology" were organized in 1979, 1980, and 1981, also at Talloires. The first considered environmental epidemiology generally. The second focused more specifically on the use of environmental health sentinels or disease "markers" that might herald the existence of an environmental hazard. The final conference discussed the use of sentinel practices as reporting nodes in Ambulatory Sentinel Practice Networks pioneered in Britain and the Netherlands and that at the time, were developing in North America, Australia, and elsewhere; again the papers were published in a book.[32]

Meanwhile, the Health of Populations program, although not yet endorsed formally by the Board, was beginning to take shape. Our first training center at the

University of Pennsylvania, in the absence of a clear decision to focus the program on any particular region or set of countries, had accepted its first Fellow from the developing world (India). The underlying concepts were gaining acceptance within the Foundation, and its Executive Committee, if not the entire Board, was beginning to understand. At best however enthusiasm was muted, and there was precious little help from the overly cautious Acting President. Nevertheless, at the December 1979 meeting of the full Rockefeller Board we were successful in gaining approval of a second grant of $500,000 to train Fellows in clinical epidemiology from the developing world; these funds were to be disbursed by the Foundation's officers over a 2-year period. Although far from a full-fledged Foundation program, the underlying ideas and the proposed strategy were beginning to generate interest. Excerpts from the docket for the second grant state the case we advanced:

> This proposal is aimed at the training of clinical epidemiologists for the developing world who can conduct teaching and research in the more important diseases of the rural and urban poor. There is need to determine the morbidity and mortality caused by these diseases, and the most efficacious means of preventing, treating, and controlling them, through application of the skills of biometry, demography, health statistics, and social survey methods. Such epidemiological tools are essential to the process of estimating the distribution of health problems over time and place, and of measuring and analyzing the projected benefits, risks, and costs of various mixes of health manpower, resources, and available services.

> Moreover, some authorities in the developing world are becoming deeply concerned about the maldistribution, by type as well as geographically, of physicians and the equipment and facilities demanded. They note that the rising costs and questionable benefits of health care in relation to diminishing budgets especially affect the rural poor....

> Under the proposed appropriation, faculty members from interested universities in developing countries would be enabled to obtain training in clinical epidemiology at recognized centers of excellence and to undertake research in their own countries....

> During the training, each participant would be expected to plan an investigation of a health problem important in his or her own country with guidance from an experienced preceptor at the given host institution....On return home, the student would carry out the project under continued supervision by the preceptor, who might make a site visit while the work was in progress....

> Periodic workshops would be held to accelerate the dissemination of knowledge of health problems in the developing world and the methods needed to identify them, and to determine the optimal modes of intervention, the potential for additional research, and the public policy implications of their findings and future work....[33]

Over the years, as discussed in the balance of this chapter and the next, the clinical epidemiology initiative was expanded and modified by experience, but these early docket statements set out the objectives, strategy, and tactics for the Health of Populations program. As in the case of the four goals enunciated at the first advisory group's meeting in 1977, they have not changed fundamentally in the intervening period.

Under the leadership first of David L. Sackett, Professor of Clinical Epidemiology and Medicine, later of Michael Gent, and then of Peter Tugwell, all professors of clinical epidemiology and biostatistics, McMaster University's Faculty of Health Sciences; during its first decade, had built a Department of Clinical Epidemiology and Biostatistics with 24 faculty members and a commensurately large support staff. More than half of its faculty also had appointments in clinical departments. Recently the department's founding chairman, David Sackett, resumed clinical responsibilities for several years as head of medicine at one of McMaster's teaching hospitals. In addition, a substantial number of faculty members from other departments at McMaster, at least equal to the number within the Department of Clinical Epidemiology and Biostatistics, had been trained in clinical epidemiology and had M.Sc. degrees in this field. The presence of more than a dozen biostatisticians is further testimony of the extent to which quantitative methods had permeated the research interests of both the basic and clinical departments.

This was an ideal setting for the second Clinical Epidemiology Research and Training Center (CERTC). Accordingly, in May 1980, our third proposal went before the Executive Committee of the Rockefeller Foundation, and they approved an initial 2-year grant for McMaster University to provide training in clinical epidemiology for candidates from the developing world. Six-month intensive courses were originally envisaged by the McMaster Faculty. Experience rapidly showed that at least a year, and often more, was needed to attain the M.Sc. level; eventually 16 months were found to be optimum. The level of competence required for independent research and the desire of virtually all trainees to return home with a degree guided this decision. The same pattern was adopted at the other training centers as soon as practicable.

We still had before us the task of testing the "market" more thoroughly and of finding out what kinds of medical schools in the Third World might be the most suitable from which to select students for training. We were involved in another "Catch-22" situation; we could not select promising sites if there were no suitable candidates for training and we could not select candidates if there was no hospitable academic environment to which they could return. Our earlier visits had helped, but we still had to identify first-rate medical schools from which to select Fellows for training and we still hoped to develop a global program.

The next move was to plan an International Workshop in Clinical Epidemiology to publicize and test acceptance of the program more widely. We decided to hold the workshop at a prestigious university outside North America and one without a school of public health; these decisions were designed to set the program apart from prior Foundation efforts. Churchill College of Cambridge University was selected as the site, and two of the medical faculty's leaders were approached. Since his earlier days at Guy's Hospital Medical School, Sir John (now Lord) Butterfield had exhibited a keen interest in clinical epidemiology. He was now de facto Dean of the Cambridge Clinical Faculty and Regius Professor of Physic (Medicine)—another in the long line of Regius Professors who have played a role in this saga. Professor Roy M. Acheson, one of Britain's leading epidemiologists, had taught at the London School of Hygiene and Tropical Medicine and at Yale University. He headed an active research department, had had extensive experience in the developing world, especially with the series of Seminars for Clinicians conducted in the 1960s by the International Epidemiological Association, and enjoyed the full support of the Regius. Both agreed to lead the proposed exercise, and accordingly we planned a 12-day Workshop to be held from September 20 to October 2, 1980. Letters of invitation and announcements for posting on bulletin boards were sent to the deans and clinical department heads of all medical schools in the developing world. Advertisements were placed in the leading English language American and British medical journals. More than 150 applications were received, and from these a small selection committee chose 25 participants who were a mixture of deans and clinical department heads from as many medical schools in 16 countries. All travel and expenses for the Workshop were paid by the Foundation.

Our objective was to introduce participants to the concepts and methods of epidemiology and determine their interest and the prospects for establishing a Clinical Epidemiology Unit in their respective institutions. The Workshop Faculty consisted of an international array of epidemiologists, statisticians, and one economist, all with broad teaching experience. In addition to the Cambridge medical group, led by Sir John Butterfield and Roy Acheson, we had faculty members from the Institute of Cancer Research in London, the London School of Hygiene and Tropical Medicine, McMaster University, Shanghai First Medical College, the University of Newcastle, Australia, the University of Western Ontario, and York University, England. Additional guest lecturers included the Director of the Medical Research Council (MRC). Laboratory of Molecular Biology, Cambridge, the Director of the WHO Tropical Diseases Research Programme, Geneva, the Director of the MRC Environmental Epidemiology Unit, University of Southampton, and Professors of Immunology and of Mathematics from Cambridge. The postworkshop evaluations by the participants showed that the overall experience was considered to have been either excellent or good; several did not find it useful.

The whole exercise was of great value to the Foundation in developing the selection process and in identifying prospective sites for establishing Clinical Epidemiology Units. Five extremely successful future directors or sponsors of these units, some of whom we had met previously during our site visits, were identified by the full faculty during the Cambridge Workshop: two in China and one each in Indonesia, Nigeria, and Thailand. Another individual became head of a major funding agency for the health sector in his country and played a leading role in developing clinical epidemiology both domestically and internationally. A professor of medicine from another country translated a clinical epidemiology textbook into his native language and initiated teaching of the subject in his own department.

We also gained insights into the types of medical school deans and department heads who were unlikely to grasp initially the new dimensions we were proposing for medical education. For them, the old dichotomies between the clinician and the public health worker were the ordained way; their capacity to understand, let alone change, was deemed modest at best.

Having been sensitized to the field of clinical epidemiology, the assembled medical leaders were invited to nominate candidates for training at the University of Pennsylvania or McMaster University. Additional announcements of the program were circulated. In 1981, McMaster received more than 100 applications from 27 countries; 8 candidates were selected; the next year another 8 candidates were accepted from 92 applicants. Pennsylvania had fewer applications because at that time it was only prepared to accept 1 or 2 candidates per year.

On August 1, 1980, Richard W. Lyman, President of Stanford University and a trustee of the Rockefeller Foundation since 1976, assumed its presidency. From his service on the Board he was aware of our clinical epidemiology initiatives, but he needed time and opportunities to familiarize himself with the specific plans. Our strategy from the beginning had been to obtain all the advice we could as well as to build a consensus among all the Foundation's officers for what we hoped would become a formally approved Health of Populations component. Accordingly in collaboration with the U.S. National Academy of Sciences' Institute of Medicine and its immediate past and then current presidents, David A. Hamburg and Frederick C. Robbins, we organized a meeting at the Foundation's Study and Conference Center at Bellagio entitled "Health of Populations: Changing Perspectives."

President Lyman was among the 23 participants who met from November 6 to 10, 1980, a month after the Cambridge University Workshop. The others came from the developed and developing worlds and represented ministries of health, medical schools, schools of public health, as well as international health agencies. The papers presented and summaries of the discussions were subsequently published in a 1982 volume: *Population-based Medicine*.[34] One of the principal objectives of this conference was to provide an opportunity for President Lyman to examine the assumptions, strategies, and tactics involved in the Health of Populations component. We hoped that he would ask questions and bring up whatever lingering reservations he had about giving it his unqualified endorsement. In a private talk with Lyman during the Bellagio Conference, I said that we needed a firm decision. I told him that I did not want him to feel under undue pressure and if he wished to abort the initiative, I was prepared to resign from the Foundation. Because I had been hired by John Knowles and Kenneth Warren for the express purpose of developing this program, that seemed the only reasonable alternative; I was neither equipped for nor interested in embarking on some other enterprise at the Foundation.

Most of the arguments and examples set forth earlier in this chapter were advanced once more in the course of the Conference. John Evans's talks with Richard Lyman also helped the latter to understand the nature and potential of the program. And Evans's remarks summarizing the Conference, and by implication the Health of Populations component and its goal of establishing an international network of collaborating institutions, helped to place them in the context of contemporary thinking about health and health services:

How can the population perspective be promoted more vigorously in planning and operations of the health system? The starting point for the process might be in government, health services operations, or a higher educational institution, depending on the circumstances; it will be most successful if it involves all three areas. A logical starting point is the medical school, because of the importance of conditioning the attitudes of the medical profession. The linkage with government and health services operations could be achieved by a joint mechanism for determining priorities for research, cross-appointments of staff, and recognition of the group as a resource for the type of network of institutions in each country that the World Health Organization has designated as a national health development network. The aim would be to establish a resource group with evaluation capabilities in several countries that show evidence of interest in this process.

The functions to be served by the resource group in the medical school are to stimulate the clinical staff to adopt the population-based perspective, to train members of the clinical departments to carry out evaluation research, and to assist in the design and execution of research projects of importance to the clinical departments. The training function should at the outset address the needs of established clinical and administrative personnel at all levels, in order to enhance their skills and critical review of evidence and to orient them to the population perspective. Without the support of these leaders in education and in health service operations, more junior personnel trained in depth will find few opportunities to apply their talents.

The resource group also has an external consultative function to the ministry of health and the ministry of planning, to health agencies, and to the health professions—to sensitize these constituencies to the significance of the population-based perspective in their work, and to stimulate an interest in participating in and using the results of health services research.[35]

And Evans continued:

Where schools of public health exist, they can play a more important role than most have done in the past. To do so, however, they should interact more directly with the operations of the health system, and should also overcome their professional isolation from medicine and their academic isolation from the array of disciplines that have an important bearing on the solution of health problems. Few schools have either the material resources to assemble such diverse disciplinary resources within their own institutions, or the flexibility of administrative structure to permit staff turnover in relation to changing health needs. It is for these reasons that the matrix approach to teaching and research in public health, using the resources of existing schools and agencies rather than creating new and separate institutions, has special appeal.[36]

We followed this conference immediately with a third one at Bellagio (November 13-17, 1980) also designed to build understanding and support for our program by knowledgeable and influential professionals. Attended also by John Evans, Frederick Robbins, and others from the prior Bellagio Conference, this conference had representatives from other international health agencies and several developing countries. Entitled "Resource Allocation and Health Technology," it was organized in collaboration with the Office of Technology Assessment (OTA) of the U.S. Congress, represented by H. David Banta, then the Assistant Director for OTA's

Health Program. Although concentrating largely on experiences from the developed world, the underlying message from the conferees had global implications: both the concepts and methods of medical technology assessment can be readily transferred from one country to another.[37]

Among the other things we asked President Lyman to do in the first year of his tenure was to write a Foreword to John Evans's report of his global investigations. He had this to say:

> The Foundation commissioned this report during the process of reviewing our many efforts over the decades to reduce the burden of illness and improve the organization, appropriateness, and effectiveness of health services. Our support of biomedical and behavioral research directed at major health problems has been coupled with our longstanding interest in the generic problems underlying the transfer of useful knowledge through compassionate and efficient services. From our earliest interest in developing a vaccine for yellow fever and our decision to support separate schools of public health, we have sought to link the products of the laboratory with the pressing needs of society. At a time of escalating health-care costs, gross inequities in the availability of health care within and among countries, and irrational imbalances in the mix of resources and manpower, Dr. Evans's report should serve to stimulate a reconsideration of the diverse approaches to improving those managerial and measurement skills that have maximum potential for enhancing the health of populations everywhere.[38]

His first Bellagio Conference as the Foundation's President apparently helped to persuade Lyman that the Health of Populations program had merit and should continue. He thought we would proceed most constructively, however, if we concentrated initially on one continent rather than attempting to establish units throughout the developing world; he encouraged the choice of Southeast Asia and China as the initial regions. This was a sound decision. It strengthened the embryonic concept of an international network and prevented a number of potential mistakes. We had already accepted young faculty members from Escola Paulista in Brazil and the University of Ibadan, Nigeria in our first cohort of trainees; in a sense, the development of these units was under way. We now shifted our emphasis to developing Clinical Epidemiology Units in the Asian and Pacific region; the majority of the next two or three cohorts of candidates for training at McMaster and Pennsylvania were selected from these countries.

In spite of our progress, a formal Foundation commitment to the development of a full-scale Clinical Epidemiology Network had yet to be made. On September 20, 1981, at its meeting in Puebla, Mexico, I presented the case for the Health of Populations component to the full Board of Trustees. After briefly summarizing the history and arguments to which the reader has been exposed in this volume, I continued:

> ...[O]nly a small proportion (perhaps 20%) of all the specific diagnostic, and therapeutic interventions and maneuvers employed by physicians are supported by objective evidence that they are more useful than useless or even harmful for the purposes for which they are advocated. For example, in at least one Southeast Asian country there are 30,000 drugs sold over-the-counter in spite of a list of 200 essential

drugs recommended by the World Health Organization. The Caesarian section rate in some hospitals in Latin America is 80% of all deliveries. All this proceeds in the face of children dying because available measures for treating infant diarrhea are not readily available and because funds have not been allocated to purchase vaccines of known efficacy.

...[A] strategy is needed to change the information base and attitudes of those who make decisions about priorities and resource allocation in health care. It is our view that this can best be done by reorienting the thinking and priorities of clinical professors to embrace the concepts of epidemiology so that they can develop the essential evidence on which to base clinical, managerial, and political choices. In defining these specific objectives, we also recognize the importance of concurrently modifying the attitudes and behavior of medical students and of practicing physicians to embrace the population-based perspective, in addition to the one-to-one perspective of clinical medicine, and the molecular understanding of disease processes.

In conclusion, I said:

...[I]t may be argued that all of this substitutes a concern for numbers and quantification at the expense of doing worthy things for suffering people. But numbers are the stuff of science and the means by which judgments are made about the credibility of claims both for miracle drugs and for nostrums. As William Petty, the brilliant 17th century economist, mercantilist and physician argued, "we need to weigh the impact of social and health expenditures by comparing them with objective measures of the differences they make to the well-being and health of the populations served." He coined the term "political arithmetic" and that is to a considerable extent what clinical epidemiology is all about. We suggest that traditional expressions of individual compassion by physicians be expanded to include analogous expressions of statistical compassion by all physicians for the populations they serve. As emphasized by Alice in Wonderland, "it is just as well to have all of this done with numbers." If health statistics and epidemiology seem dull to some, one can recall the remark of an early medical statistician that after all health statistics really represent "people with the tears wiped off."[39]

The Board tentatively agreed to further limited development of the Health of Populations program. We could proceed with an Asian and Pacific Clinical Epidemiology Network. There was also the prospect that if this proved feasible we would expand to Latin America and later to Africa, and possibly to the Middle East. Of equal importance, the Board provided a grant for the establishment of a third Clinical Epidemiology Research and Training Center at the University of Newcastle in Australia to be known as the Asian and Pacific Centre for Clinical Epidemiology (subsequently changed to the Centre for Clinical Epidemiology and Biostatistics). We made the initial distinction between Pennsylvania and McMaster as "global" training centers for our clinical epidemiology program and Newcastle as a specifically regional training center; later this distinction was dropped.

Modeled in part after McMaster, Newcastle was a new medical school started in 1975. I referred earlier to my 1981 encounter at Bellagio with David Maddison, the Founding Dean, and his creative approach to problem-based learning, and a community-oriented commitment that related medical education to the needs of the surrounding population. This meeting was followed by a visit to Newcastle later in 1981, where I also met Professor Stephen R. Leeder, a clinician with a Ph.D. in epidemiology and strong commitments to improving the public's health as well as to clinical research. The faculty for this new school were few in number (about 40) and as such afforded an excellent example for the developing world of what could be achieved with an appropriately chosen staff and relatively modest material resources. In accordance with our 1981 mandate from the Board, Newcastle's clinical epidemiology Fellows were to be selected only from institutions in Southeast Asia, the Western Pacific, and China. More specifically they were to come primarily from Shanghai Medical University and West China University of Medical Sciences (as they are now known) where both are among what were then the top five "key" medical schools in that country;* from the University of the Philippines; and from Chulalongkorn University, Khon Kaen University, and Siraraj Hospital Medical School of Mahidol University in Thailand.

Because selection procedures based on our original plans were still in place, and our new ones not fully coordinated among the three training centers, each had selected its own Fellows. As a consequence there were additional single trainees still being appointed from institutions and countries outside those designated in Southeast Asia and China, as well as from the University of Ibadan and from Escola Paulista, São Paulo. For example, one Fellow each had been accepted from the Universidad Federal do Rio de Janeiro in Brazil; the Universidad de la Frontera, Temuco, Chile; the Institute of Child Health, Madras, India; the Institute of Nutrition, Mexico City; and Anhui Medical College and Beijing Heart, Lung, and Blood Vessel Medical Research Center in China. I had diverted two other trainees under an earlier Rockefeller Foundation grant for community medicine at Gadjah Mada University, Yogyakarta, Indonesia to doctoral training programs in epidemiology at the University of Western Ontario, and at the London School of Hygiene and Tropical Medicine.

These arrangements may sound like a haphazard approach but they were occasioned by the wish to select only first-rate students with deeply committed sponsors and institutions and our policy of giving the three training centers maximum discretion in deciding which Fellows to accept. There were those who suggested that Warren and I were ignoring the edicts of the Board by not limiting the selection of Fellows to the Asian and Pacific Region. This was never our intention but we were caught up in the realities of commitments that had been made much earlier both to the CERTCs and to diverse institutions; in many instances the Foundation's credibility was at stake. The on-again-off-again Presidential and

---

* Following liberation, five "key" medical colleges, including the Traditional Medical College at Guangzhou, were recognized in the People's Republic of China. In addition there were six other federally (as distinct from provincially) supported medical colleges in the country. Subsequently, in connection with a World Bank loan to support reforms in medical education, a total of thirteen federally supported colleges were recognized; these now are referred to frequently as the "key" colleges.

Board decisions, although completely understandable, complicated our task immeasurably.

While all this was in train, there were on-going major interpersonal struggles and divisional rivalries within the Foundation that made the work of starting a new program especially difficult. This is not the place to dwell on the ins and outs of "foundation hardball" but suffice it to say that during a 4-year period there were three deaths of senior officers—all associated, at least temporally, with seriously frustrated personal aspirations and perceived loss of status. In addition, there were numerous untimely resignations, onsets of potential fatal diseases, and much personal anguish throughout all ranks of the Foundation. I add these observations lest anyone think that changing course in a Foundation is a straightforward intellectual exercise! What appears in *Annual Reports* reflects only the end results—and not always completely.

In the spring of 1982 the University of Pennsylvania received a second major grant to expand the annual intake of developing country Fellows from one to four. With the three training sites now in place, we introduced more widely terms that had been used previously only by the officers. Henceforth we would refer more openly to Clinical Epidemiology Research and Training Centers or CERTCs; the entities we were establishing in the developing world would be known as Clinical Epidemiology Units or CEUs. We circulated another bulletin board announcement of the availability of fellowships in clinical epidemiology at the three CERTCs to deans and clinical department heads in medical schools throughout the developing world. Our own projections suggested that we would complete the training of Fellows for the Asian Network sooner than the Board of Trustees anticipated. We had to be prepared to move rapidly when approval for expansion was granted if we were to make full use of the established CERTCs.

To foster additional understanding of teaching methods as well as providing an opportunity for the faculty of the three CERTCs and the sponsors of the evolving CEUs to get to know one another, we organized yet another Bellagio Conference. Entitled "Teaching Clinicians Epidemiology: Problems and Prospects," it was held May 3-7, 1982. The papers and discussions focused on both the long-term training envisaged for the Foundation's Health of Populations program and the need for more short-term courses and workshops of the type sponsored by the International Epidemiological Association in the 1960s and described in Chapter 5.[40] The consensus was that both were needed and there was the expectation that the CEUs in the future might undertake short-term workshops in their own countries, perhaps assisted by the IEA. The *Lancet* summarized its reactions to these initiatives in a 1982 editorial:

> A population perspective of medicine is something all clinicians need, because of the effects their decisions have on the distribution of resources. This is especially so in developing countries where massive demand competes for puny supply. The doctors congregate in urban areas, where they aspire to provide first-class medical care; and there is nothing left for the basic needs of the poor who are the majority of the population.

It is too early to judge the likely impact of [the Rockefeller Foundation's] initiatives, but it would be ironic if clinical epidemiology became firmly established in the Third World while in the First World it continued to be balked by the inflexibility of postgraduate training programs.[41]

As 1982 drew to a close it was time for a 5-year review of the overall progress made by the Division of Health Sciences; reviews such as this were carried out regularly for all Divisions of the Foundation. Until that year Health had been grouped with the Population program for budgetary purposes; the two were now separated. The Health of Populations component had been germinating for 5 years, but it had been fully operational for only a little over 3 years. During this period the Foundation's financial status had probably received less attention than it merited; annual grant disbursements had fluctuated from about $39.8 million in 1979 to a high of $42.7 million in 1981 and were $41.6 and $39.5 in 1982 and 1983, respectively. President Lyman's highly constructive efforts, a restructured Finance Committee, and the "bull" stockmarket starting in 1982 improved matters substantially in subsequent years. The Division of Health Sciences started getting larger annual appropriations in 1982. By the end of that year about $3.2 million had been expended on the Health of Populations component. Although much less than John Knowles had originally discussed with me, it was a substantial beginning. There was every reason to be optimistic about the future of clinical epidemiology.

The Health of Populations component had three external reviewers: David A. Hamburg, then President of the Institute of Medicine of the U.S. National Academy of Sciences and now President of the Carnegie Corporation; Carol Buck, Professor of Epidemiology and Biostatistics, University of Western Ontario and at that time President of the International Epidemiology Association, and Seymour Grufferman, Professor of Pediatrics at Duke University. All three were extremely supportive of the program. They also provided a number of constructive criticisms that proved useful in the next phases of the Network's development within the Foundation. Excerpts from their comments follow:

> The program...could benefit from a broader range of coverage. The major issues involved in developing countries are not only those dealing with causation of disease and efficacy of therapy, but also with resource allocation, diagnostic testing, algorithm development for triaging patients, and related matters. The current three centers...emphasize a portion of the spectrum but the coverage is not yet optimal, at least in depth....Implicit...is a focus on certain aspects of the field, e.g., case control studies, randomized clinical trials, and cohort studies. This is certainly an important part of the discipline, but not all of it. In a number of universities in this country (United States) and several abroad, causation and efficacy of therapy are considered less important than resource allocations. The present Rockefeller Foundation units do not put much emphasis on diagnostic testing, cost benefit analysis, cost effectiveness analysis, decision analysis, and algorithm development.

> ...[N]ot...enough emphasis has been placed on the need to develop ties with biostatisticians. For example, it may be useful for biostatisticians in developing countries to come to a training center to be exposed to some medical aspects of clinical epidemiology that they might not otherwise be familiar with. Active involvement of

biostatisticians in randomized clinical trials provides valuable grounding in clinical medicine. This combination of knowledge and skills is badly needed in developing countries. Overall serious attention will be needed in a continuing way to the minimum core size and types of disciplines (e.g., biostatistics, computer sciences) necessary at each...medical school which sends students to technically advanced countries.

Objectives were formulated on a number of occasions during the development of the Program. It is interesting to find that their breadth has varied from one occasion to another. The broadest set of objectives seeks to inculcate in physicians some knowledge of all the population-based disciplines (biometry, demography, health economics, epidemiology, health statistics, and survey methods) so that they will provide better patient care, foster prevention at both the individual and societal levels, and participate knowledgeably in the formulation of health and social policy. The narrowest set of objectives seeks to make physicians aware of epidemiological and statistical principles that would improve their understanding of the natural history of disease and lead them to identify efficacious, effective and efficient techniques for disease screening, diagnosis and therapy....Influential physicians whose style of practice is enriched by epidemiological and biostatistical principles will have an effect on health care economics of their country by diverting expenditures from unprofitable into profitable directions. This is the first link. Another link would be forged if the Clinical Epidemiology Program gave its graduates a sufficient appreciation of demography, health statistics, and environmental epidemiology, so that they could collaborate intelligently with other scientists in the formation of health policies...[T]he Clinical Epidemiology Program might be capable of forging this second link, if its importance were kept in mind.

...[T]he Program would have a wider impact, and one more in keeping with the general goals of the Rockefeller Foundation, if it were associated with efforts to bring together clinicians, politicians, economists, demographers, and behavioral, and environmental scientists in broad discussions of social policy. Improvements in health require more than changes in clinical practice. Population-based medicine is a part of the larger sphere of population-based science.

Each training center should receive students from a variety of developing countries. This would allow students to learn from the experience of colleagues in different settings. Combined with a mechanism for rotation, it would avoid the inbreeding that is bound to arise if all students from one country are trained in the same center. It is also essential that a critical mass be trained in each center of the developing world.

The [Program] should attempt to lure some of the more traditional epidemiologists into clinical epidemiology. It would be quite valuable to enlist the support of the field's strongest critics by getting them involved in the development of more scientifically rigorous methods.

The [Program] should attempt to lure more physicians into the field of epidemiology.... [E]pidemiology is basically a medical subspecialty and requires strong grounding in the biology of medicine and the principles of clinical care. If rational health care delivery systems are to be developed, it is essential to involve persons who understand the basic process of providing medical care.[42]

These comments, as well as others made by the reviewers, were entirely compatible with my own thoughts; the ultimate goal was to improve the public's health and to expand collective efforts from a medical to a health enterprise. The reviewers helped to clarify problems and issues as well as to inform other Foundation officers and the Board about the opportunities and challenges this new approach was generating. The reader should not forget that there was a 60-year tradition in the Foundation, as well as in many universities and governments, that viewed clinical medicine and public health as quite separate enterprises. Most contemporary observers were unfamiliar with the notion that both camps had similar roots and missions.

For the Board's meeting on December 7, 1982, we summarized once again our goals and objectives as follows:

> The goal of the Health of Populations [component] is not to develop another clinical specialty within medicine, but rather to disseminate of epidemiological and biostatistical thinking throughout clinical medicine and health policy making by fostering a focus for epidemiology within the mainstream of scientific medicine in universities. Appreciation by physicians of epidemiology as both a powerful analytic tool and an essential medical perspective should contribute to the intellectual and scientific underpinnings of preventive and clinical medicine and of public health measures. The incorporation of these perspectives and methods within clinical medicine should result in institutional and public policies and health priorities that conform more closely to the real medical needs of the entire population served.[43]

The Health of Populations program continued to garner administrative support within the Foundation, as well as to stimulate curiosity domestically and abroad, but the Board still was not prepared to authorize its full-scale global development. Their reservations were much less about the goals and objectives of the program than about its scale. They believed that we should demonstrate the utility and attractiveness of the training programs and the feasibility of establishing CEUs in medical schools in Third World universities on one continent before we expanded globally—not unreasonable precautions. The Board also wanted further evidence that seemingly isolated academic institutions could influence health policies in their respective countries. According to the repeated testimony of medical school deans and department heads, traditionally there had been little interaction between clinical departments and Ministries of Health or Education. There had been even less interaction among clinicians, health economists, and social scientists; indeed, potential contributions by the latter two groups had been largely ignored. What evidence could be produced that things were now to be different? The minutes for the Board meeting of December 7, 1982, state that the Board "...agreed upon continuation of the Health of Populations component as an experimental effort to establish a number of global or regional Clinical Epidemiology Resource and Training Centers in the developed countries and an Asian Network of Clinical Epidemiology Units, but future expansion into other regions was contingent upon positive evaluation of accomplishments and availability of funding."[44]

As 1983 began, we had at least this limited but now "official" mandate to develop the Asian and Pacific Regional Clinical Epidemiology Network in Southeast Asia. Newcastle took its first six Rockefeller-supported Fellows in 1983. Following discussions I had with officials of the Australian International Development Assistance Board (AIDAB) that year, it began supporting two or more additional trainees annually. Small research grants were given to Khon Kaen and Shanghai First Medical College (as it was known then) to support the first returning trainees. McMaster was for the present still to be regarded as the Global Center, accepting eight Fellows a year from a variety of countries. Pennsylvania was now to be designated, at least for a time, as an unofficial Regional CERTC because it had already accepted two fellows from Latin America and was training as many as four candidates a year. It was anomalous to be training Fellows from Latin America and Africa, albeit in limited numbers, without being able to develop the CEUs in their universities as vigorously as we were doing in the Asian and Pacific Region. On the other hand, the Board was certainly reasonable in requiring evidence that our strategy was successful before embarking on the much larger global operation. This was, after all, a very high risk venture. But is that not what Foundations are all about? All three CERTCs were also training additional domestic Fellows from their own countries. This parallel experience provided a broader exposure for both groups and was seen as a worthwhile by-product.

We now started referring publicly to the International Clinical Epidemiology Network, coined the acronym INCLEN, printed a descriptive brochure, and devised a logo. The growing number of collaborating institutions used the term and the logo and external bodies began to recognize them. From February 27 to March 1, 1983, in Honolulu, Hawaii, we held what was to become the first of a succession of Annual Meetings—this one to be known later as "INCLEN I." Only the faculties of the three CERTCs and the Rockefeller Officers were involved; important collective decisions were taken. The group included senior biostatisticians and health economists who were faculty members of the CERTCs, as well as clinical epidemiologists.[45] More important, the collegial atmosphere and the group's sense that they were embarking on a timely, and perhaps pacesetting, venture enhanced ésprit de corps and commitment. No longer was there any question in our minds that we would, over the next decade, be building an INCLEN.

Written by the collective faculty from the CERTCs, a clear set of goals and objectives for INCLEN was set forth. They have guided the enterprise ever since without substantial modification, except to refine aspects bearing on their practical application. We recognized all too well that the capacity of the program to effect change had yet to be demonstrated and the goals and objectives were introduced, therefore, as "assumptions." All we could say was that other strategies attempted by the Foundation during the previous 60 or 70 years appeared to have been less than adequate. Here is the original set of assumptions on which INCLEN is predicated:

That the establishment of Clinical Epidemiology Units (CEUs) in schools of medicine will have a favorable impact on the provision of effective and efficient systems of

health care which are appropriate for the health status of the population served by
those medical schools, by:

- Educating, within a clinical setting, physicians to use interventions proven to be
  efficacious;
- Educating, within a clinical setting, physicians to establish arrangements for
  providing **effective** care **efficiently**;
- Encouraging (as a result of 1 and 2) a more rational approach to the allocation
  of resources for medical care in relation to the health status of the population.[46]

In addition to these three objectives, I brought up at the meeting the need for
stating a fourth—the importance of recognizing and investigating the Placebo and
Hawthorne effects. As in Chapter 6, I argued that these should no longer be
regarded as merely residual outcomes unassociated with the relative efficacy of a
specific clinical maneuver. They should be regarded as intrinsically powerful
therapeutic modalities. The assembled faculty seemed intrigued by the concept but
thought it premature to include the study of these phenomena in the goals of the
program. My own view is that elucidating the nature and dimensions of Factor "X"
should remain an important goal not only of this program but of medicine and
public health generally. Both individuals and populations can be affected, for better
or for worse, by the attitudes, behavior, and the organization and management of
health personnel, institutions, and agencies.

In addition to the major themes discussed previously the following points were
given further emphasis and greater specificity at INCLEN I:

Selection of each CEU should emphasize: the importance of having an identifiable
leader; adequate space, strong local support and institutional commitment—including
a 'sponsor' high in the academic hierarchy; and administrative location within one or
more clinical departments.

Specific tasks of each CEU should include: the conduct of clinical research and health
care evaluation bearing on local health care needs; development of programs to
integrate epidemiologic and population-based concepts into teaching programs designed for consumers of research results; development of teaching programs, workshops, seminars and short courses for researchers in their respective countries;
obtaining long-term government and other financial support; and development of
clinical role models.

Career development for the trainees would depend on: adequate initial research
funding; appropriate supervision; and 'human support' through CERTC faculty site
visits.

The need for training biostatistical colleagues was reviewed and the Foundation
undertook to fund this, but several problems warranted further exploration: an
established mechanism for ongoing financial support and career development of Unit
statisticians may be lacking in many settings in the developing world; there should
be a thorough investigation of all available biostatistical and computational services
at each CEU site in order to determine the type and level of biostatistical training
required; the training programs for biostatistical personnel should be flexible, based
on the backgrounds and needs of each trainee and Unit; the long-term goal of such

training should be to develop biostatistical personnel who are full colleagues of clinical epidemiologists rather than research associates.

The need for health economists was also explored and the following points made: all three CERTCs' curricula currently included training in health economics although there was debate about the extent desirable or essential; many of the assumptions underlying economic appraisal techniques in health care are not appropriate for developing countries, e.g., techniques such as cost-effectiveness analysis should not be taught as 'value-free technology' since clinical epidemiologists working in developing countries need to be aware that controversial assumptions may restrict the application of health economic analysis; at a minimum clinical epidemiologists should be competent 'consumers' of research using health economic techniques of analysis.

The potential contributions of medical sociology, anthropology and other behavioral scientists to the training of clinical epidemiologists were discussed; selected concepts and methods from these sciences were considered to be useful, and perhaps essential, for the trainees; attitude assessment, scaling, questionnaire design, and interviewing skills were cited as important techniques; in view of the difficulties of transferring social science concepts across cultural boundaries, locally based consultants would probably be preferable to long-term collaboration with CERTC social scientists.

Three other supporting activities were initiated: overall coordination and computerization of CERTC educational resource and teaching bibliographies was to be undertaken by McMaster which had already compiled a Third World Health Resource Bank of cost-effective health care interventions for common health problems in the developing countries; Pennsylvania was to establish computerized lists of ongoing research and teaching programs, and of faculties' and trainees' activities at CERTCs and CEUs, including biographical information on the Fellows as well as abstracts and related information about their research projects; Newcastle was to assemble and distribute information about sources of health statistics and health indicators for Third World countries, especially in the Asian and Pacific region.

To facilitate communication, the sharing of resources, coordination of selection processes and site visits, and needs for a centralized data source and a secretariat were discussed. The Foundation agreed to meet them.

There was also agreement that the CERTCs would each prepare annual reports and that a periodic *INCLEN Newsletter* would be started with McMaster assuming responsibility for the first edition. A brochure would also be prepared describing INCLEN's goals and procedures for distribution to potential trainees, interested institutions, potential funding agencies, and others who might be interested.

The need for critical evaluation of the entire INCLEN program had been raised by Carol Buck in her 1982 review of progress. She provided an extended outline of the criteria that might be used. This was elaborated in considerably more detail as part of INCLEN's formal statement of goals and objectives. Guidelines were also specified for CERTC site visits so that comparable data might be gathered.

The need for a Steering Committee (or eventually of an Executive Committee) for INCLEN was recognized and a small group consisting of the directors of the three

CERTCs and a foundation officer was established; they planned to meet twice each year.[47]

Throughout 1983 the jerky progress of guiding the Health of Populations component through the Rockefeller hierarchy and Board proceeded. Among Foundation officers and the Board there were still pockets of resistance to this strange new venture. Traditional public health, as known to one and all for the past 60 or 70 years, was the way things of this type were to be arranged. Few if any of the other officers were familiar with the long history of efforts by clinicians, statisticians, and social reformers to respond to the public's collective health problems.

In June 1983, yet another full budget review of all the Foundation's programs was conducted in the light of contemporary financial constraints. Once more we documented the need for advance planning, pointing out that from solicitation of applications for Fellowships to the onset of training takes an average of 14 months. We emphasized the potential waste involved in training clinical epidemiologists haphazardly without providing for their institutional base in organized CEUs, adequate follow-up, effective communication, and annual meetings. We pointed out that most of the Asian and Pacific CEUs would be up to strength, at least as far as clinical epidemiologists were concerned, in the next 2 years. In desperation we posed the prospect of cutting back drastically on the whole Health of Populations component and limiting the Foundation's commitment to completing the Asian and Pacific Network if we did not have the prospect of adequate funding that was more in keeping with the original plans developed under the aegis of John Knowles.

We were not alone. External support was growing. On May 20, 1983, Professor D. C. Luo, Head of the Department of Medicine at the West China University of Medical Sciences (then Sichuan Medical College), and a participant in the Cambridge University workshop in 1980, wrote to Professor David Sackett of McMaster University that:

> You will probably be delighted to know that the Ministry of Public Health has decided to set the National Training Centre of Clinical Epidemiology in our medical college; virtually all our department will shoulder the responsibility. Dr. White will also feel very happy because his suggestion to our Ministry of Public Health has been accepted.[48]

In addition, we were now attracting interest not only from the Australian International Development Assistance Board (ADIAB) but also from the International Development Research Center (IDRC) in Canada, the World Bank (WB), the UNDP/WB/World Health Organization Special Programme for Research and Training in Tropical Diseases (WHO/TDR), and the United States Agency for International Development (USAID).

The Health Sciences budget for 1984 was not cut but rather increased modestly (from $4.2 to $4.4 million). Now we could move ahead with our plans for developing INCLEN on a broader scale. Grants to McMaster and Newcastle were renewed, and these CERTCs were given approval to train Fellows from regions other than Asia and the Pacific.

By the end of 1983 we had more than 60 Fellows either trained or being trained. There were three CEUs in Thailand (i.e., almost half that country's medical schools), two in China's original five "key" medical colleges, and one each at the University of the Philippines and Gadjah Mada University (Indonesia). As noted, other solitary Fellows were scattered among a number of other embyronic units.

We were now well on the way to healing the schism! Petty, Frank, Louis, Snow, Virchow, Farr, Osler, Mackenzie, Paul, and Ryle would have been happy. There was still sniping from the side lines but now it came much less from within the Foundation than from without. We continued to hear that faculties of schools of public health were unhappy with the Health of Populations program. This was perceived to be "their territory," and the medical schools were poaching on it. Moreover they were being aided and abetted by the Rockefeller Foundation, which had institutionalized the schism by establishing—perhaps fathering—these schools, in the first place.

Our message was simple. By attracting more young physicians familiar with the concepts and methods of epidemiology and related population-based disciplines to careers in population-based medicine, surely there would be increased demand for further collaboration, if not training, from schools of public health provided their offerings proved attractive and appropriate. In any event, surely there are enough problems to go round to occupy all who can help?

At the end of 1983, I had exceeded my agreed tenure of 5 years to establish the Health of Populations component. It was time to retire and turn matters over to my successor, Scott B. Halstead, formerly Professor and Chairman, Department of Tropical Medicine & Microbiology in the School of Medicine, University of Hawaii. His guardianship of this still fragile initiative has been superb; of greater importance has been his judicious and creative development of INCLEN. This phase of our combined efforts to *heal the schism* is described in the next chapter.

References

1. Report to the Rockefeller Foundation Board of Trustees on the Health Program, and Annexes, December 7, 1982. New York: Division of Health Sciences, Rockefeller Foundation, 1982 (unpublished).
2. Rockefeller Foundation. Working Papers: Meeting of the Board of Trustees, The Rockefeller Foundation, September 14, 1977. New York: Rockefeller Foundation, 1977 (unpublished).
3. Report to Trustees, Annex I (Hamburg, D), December 1982. New York: Rockefeller Foundation, 1987:1.
4. Langmuir AD. *Significance of epidemiology in medical schools*. J Med Educ 1964; 39:39-48.
5. Hunter RB. *Report of the Working Party on Medical Administration*. London: Her Majesty's Stationery Office, 1972.
6. Kohn R, White KL, eds. *Health Care: An International Study*. London: Oxford University Press, 1976.

7. Report to Trustees and Annexes, December 1982. New York: Rockefeller Foundation, 1982 (unpublished) and KLW's notes.
8. Hamilton JD. The McMaster curriculum: A critique. Br Med J 1976;1:1191-1196
9. Evans JR. *Measurement and Management in Medicine: Training Needs and Opportunities.* New York: Rockefeller Foundation, 1981:7. Also published in Lipkin M, Jr., Lybrand WA, eds. *Population-Based Medicine.* New York: Praeger, 1982.
10. Ibid, p. 45.
11. Rigg JRA. *A Review of the Monograph: Measurement and Management in Medicine and Health Services-Training Needs and Opportunities, Rockefeller Foundation, New York, October, 1981 by John R. Evans.* Bentley, Western Australia: Western Australia Institute of Technology, Centre for Advanced Studies, Division of Health Sciences, 1982.
12. Robert Wood Johnson Foundation. Clinical Scholars Program: Roster. Princeton: Robert Wood Johnson Foundation, 1988 (unpublished).
13. White KL. Clinical scholars and health services (Editorial). New Eng J Med 1970; 283:929-930.
14. *Health of Populations: A Proposal for Continued Funding, 1981-1983.* New York: Rockefeller Foundation, 1980 (unpublished).
15. White KL, Bullock PJ, eds. *The Health of Populations: A Report of Two Rockefeller Foundation Conferences, March and May, 1979.* (Mimeographed). New York: Rockefeller Foundation, 1980.
16. Morris JN. *Uses of Epidemiology* (3rd Ed.). Edinburgh: Churchill Livingstone, 1975.
17. Stolley PD. In: White KL, Bullock PJ, eds. *The Health of Populations: A Report of Two Rockefeller Foundation Conferences, March and May, 1979,* (Mimeographed). New York: Rockefeller Foundation, 1980:183-184.
18. Ibid, p. 188.
19. Rockefeller Foundation. Board of Trustees' Executive Committee Docket, Population and Health - 1, May 5, 1979. New York: Rockefeller Foundation, 1979 (unpublished).
20. Bailar JC, III, Mosteller F, eds. *Medical Uses of Statistics.* Waltham, Massachusetts: NEJM Books, 1986.
21. Schmidt HG, Lipkin M., Jr., de Vries MW, Greep JM. *New Directions for Medical Education: Problem-Oriented Learning and Community-Oriented Education.* New York: Springer-Verlag, 1989.
22. World Health Organization. *International Classification of Diseases* (9th rev.). Geneva: World Health Organization, 1977.
23. Lamberts H, Wood M, eds. *ICPC: International Classification of Primary Care.* Oxford: Oxford University Press, 1987.
24. Director-General of the World Health Organization and Executive Director of the United Nations Children's Fund. *Primary Health Care.* Geneva: WHO and UNICEF, 1978.
25. Faber K. *Nosography* (2nd Ed.). New York: Paul B. Hoeber, 1930. Reprinted in 1978 by AMS Press, New York.
26. Report of a Workshop. *The International Classification of Primary Care in the European Community, Noordwijk, 8-11 September, 1988,* (Mimeographed). Amsterdam, November 1, 1988.
27. Lipkin M, Jr., Kupka K, eds. *Psychosocial Factors Affecting Health.* New York: Praeger, 1982.
28. Kilpatrick SJ, Boyle RM, eds. *Primary Care Research: Encounter Forms and the Denominator Problem.* New York: Praeger, 1984.

29. Last JM, ed. *A Dictionary of Epidemiology* (2nd Ed.). New York: Oxford University Press, 1988.
30. Leaverton PE, Massé L, eds. *Health Information Systems*. New York: Praeger Scientific, 1984.
31. Ibid, pp. 33-61.
32. Leaverton PE, ed. *Environmental Epidemiology*. New York: Praeger Scientific, 1982.
33. Rockefeller Foundation. Board of Trustees Docket, Population and Health - 7, December 3-4, 1979. New York: Rockefeller Foundation (unpublished).
34. Lipkin M, Jr., Lybrand WA, eds. *Population-Based Medicine*. New York: Praeger, 1982.
35. Evans JR. In: Lipkin M, Jr., Lybrand WA, eds. *Population-Based Medicine*. New York: Praeger, 1982:164.
36. Ibid, p. 186.
37. Banta HD, ed. *Resources for Health*: *Technology Assessment for Policy Making*. New York: Praeger Scientific, 1982.
38. Lyman RW. Foreword. In: Evans JR. *Measurement and Management in Medicine and Health Services*: *Training Needs and Opportunities*. New York: Rockefeller Foundation, 1981:5.
39. White KL. Remarks to the Rockefeller Foundation Board of Trustees, Pueblo, Mexico, September 20, 1981.
40. *Teaching Clinicians Epidemiology: Problems and Prospects*, (Mimeographed). New York, Rockefeller Foundation, 1982.
41. Anon. Clinical epidemiology in the Third World (Editorial). *Lancet* 1982;2:1448.
42. Report to the Trustees and Annexes, December 1982. New York: Rockefeller Foundation, 1982.
43. Ibid, pp. 25-26.
44. Rockefeller Foundation, Health Sciences Division. Responses for Budget Review, June 27, 1983. New York: Rockefeller Foundation, 1983 (unpublished).
45. *Report of the First Annual Meeting of the International Clinical Epidemiology Network* (INCLEN), Honolulu, Hawaii, February 27-March 1, 1983. (Mimeographed). New York, Rockefeller Foundation, 1983.
46. Ibid.
47. Ibid.
48. Rockefeller Foundation, Health Sciences Division. Responses for Budget Review, June 27, 1983, Exhibit No. 4. New York: Rockefeller Foundation, 1983.

8
The Healing Continues

Epidemiology has roots in six fundamental disciplines—biology, psychology, sociology, demography, economics, and statistics. It joins them in contributing to population-based perspectives that continue the inexorable inroads of science into human affairs. Proprietary views about who is in charge of which ideas makes a mockery of the goals of education, to say nothing of those professions committed to public service. And yet that is precisely what we had in the 1980s. Several examples illustrate the point.

The President's address to the annual meeting of the Association of Teachers of Preventive Medicine in 1980 contained the following passage:

> [An] apparent setback occurred when the Milbank Fund and the Rockefeller Foundation took a stand for prevention, but chose to enter the arena by providing funding to establish epidemiology programs outside departments of preventive medicine. This occurred despite the efforts of several ATPM members. The long term effect is not clear, but in the short term, the demise of and/or the curtailment of at least one department of preventive medicine/community medicine * appears to be related to the perceived support for internal medicine departments as opposed to preventive or community medicine departments.[1]

The Pan American Health Organization (PAHO), the Regional Office for the Americas of the World Health Organization (WHO), held a seminar in Buenos Aires (November 7-10, 1983) on Uses and Perspectives of Epidemiology. In my address I observed that:

> Epidemiology is the one science that can shift the balance in the health care establishment's priorities from a predominant preoccupation with individual transactions between doctors and their patients to a broader collective concern on the part of all health professionals for the care of entire populations. At the very least, epidemiology should help to sensitize medicine to society's health needs and prepare for demands which will inevitably find expression through the political process....[2]

and concluded by saying:

---

* Probably the University of Pennsylvania; see Chapter 5.

Latin America has an unusual obligation, if not an urgent need, to accept the challenge to broaden the base of epidemiological understanding and the range of epidemiological applications in the entire health care enterprise. Several countries have already shown substantial initiatives and PAHO is fostering these. The Rockefeller Foundation offers Fellowships for training young clinical faculty members and additional financial support will undoubtedly be forthcoming from national, bilateral, and international agencies. The opportunity for epidemiology to serve as society's *ombudsman* for health has never been greater. Latin America can show the way.[3]

Judging by the discussion and comments at the meeting, these views seemed well received. And yet a year or so later, two senior epidemiologists expressed quite different views in connection with another PAHO exercise discussing a volume of classical epidemiological papers they edited entitled *The Challenge of Epidemiology: Issues and Selected Readings*. First: Alvaro Llopis, Professor of Epidemiology and Biostatistics at Central University of Venezuela:

At present, we are worried about the future of the schools of public health in Latin America. The Rockefeller Foundation, which has a long history of supporting public health in the region, now says that it is much more concerned with medical schools than with public health schools. So much so that they are funding clinical epidemiology programs through medical schools in several Latin American countries.[4]

Second: Professor Milton Terris, a distinguished epidemiologist, and a Past-President of the American Public Health Association, of the Association of Teachers of Preventive Medicine, and of the Society for Epidemiologic Research commented:

I have yet to meet a teacher of preventive medicine in a medical school who is happy. Once a teacher told me how happy she was teaching epidemiology at her university and how wonderful it was because the students were eating it up. A few months later there was a strike of the students against her teaching program...[5]

My experience has convinced me that we are deluding ourselves if we think we are going to change most medical students. However, I firmly believe that we should have departments of community, preventive, and social medicine in medical schools....

...I really was a big failure, and every time I visited a school that said it had a successful epidemiology training program, I found after I talked with them for a while, that epidemiology was a failure there too.[6]

The Rockefeller Foundation people are selling this [population health] program, with real money to back it up, all over Asia, Africa and Latin America. They are going to divert promising people into doing drug trials. Both the Rockefeller Foundation program and the Robert Wood Johnson Foundation's "clinical scholars" program avoid public health schools like the plague. I think it is an absurdity. Here we have the Third World with all its terrible problems of famine, malnutrition, infant diarrhea, malaria, and all the other infectious and noninfectious diseases, and all this money is being spent to teach clinicians how to do clinical trials. These foundations operate under a false banner. They are misusing the term epidemiology. Why? Because of the great prestige of epidemiology in the world today, because of the fact that schools of public health are the outstanding centers of teaching and research in epidemiology. This is threatening. They want the medical schools to continue to be dominant; they want all clinicians to keep their political power; they want to make sure that health services don't infringe on the narrow professional interests of clinicians.[7]

Information is readily available to counter such assertions. The Annual Reports of the Robert Wood Johnson Foundation, the Andrew W. Mellon Foundation, and the Milbank Memorial Fund provide ample evidence that the first two foundations support training in U.S. schools of public health and that the third used the London School of Hygiene and Tropical Medicine exclusively for its clinical epidemiology program, as observed in Chapter 7. In addition to the Rockefeller Foundation's Annual Reports, the conference proceedings, and books described earlier, the widely distributed brochures describing International Clinical Epidemiology Network (INCLEN), and an ongoing series of *INCLEN Newsletters* are all readily available from the Foundation and any of the Clinical Epidemiology Research Training Center (CERTCs). The schism has created an intellectual and operational gulf that is indeed both wide and deep; much remained to be done before it is healed.

By the end of 1983 all the initiatives agreed upon at the Hawaii meeting were under way: the International Teaching and Methods Resources Program was being developed at McMaster; the Statistical Packages and Programs at Pennsylvania; the Information System for Health Statistics in the Asian and Pacific Region at Newcastle; and the Abstracts of Ongoing and Planned Research Being Conducted by Trainees in the Clinical Epidemiology Units (CEUs) at Pennsylvania. The first issue of its *Newsletter* included a complete recapitulation of the assumptions, objectives, strategies, tactics, and evaluation plans for INCLEN.

As the first step in broadening the horizons of the five INCLEN Fellows who had returned home, particularly in Thailand, provisions were made for them to attend the Regional Scientific Meeting of the International Epidemiological Association, on "Changing Patterns of Health and Disease," held in Singapore, October 3-6, 1983. These Fellows, all established clinical faculty members from the three emerging CEUs in Thailand, met in Singapore and determined to develop their own national forum for exchanging experiences. A Clinical Epidemiology Club (shades of The London Epidemiological Society) emerged and in January 1984 the members ran a 2-week National Epidemiology Workshop before the second Annual INCLEN Meeting. The Workshop was attended by participants from the seven Thai medical schools.[8] All of this was a prelude to formation 4 years later of a national Network to be known as THAICLEN.

"INCLEN II," planned in 1983, was held from January 29 to February 3, 1984 in Pattaya, Thailand. The keynote address was given by the then sponsor of the CEU at Chulalongkorn University, Professor Charas Suwanwela, a neurosurgeon who subsequently became Dean of the School of Medicine and is now President of his University. He highlighted the challenges faced by clinical epidemiology. Likening the flow of medical knowledge from Europe initially and later from America to the flow of water, following what was then Siam's opening to Western ideas in the nineteenth century, he said that filters were needed. At first the intellectual desert in Southeast Asia was in need of water of any kind but now there was a need to examine critically what was and was not useful for Thailand's population. Clinical epidemiology with its emphasis on design, measurement, and evaluation, and its commitment to using these quantitative methods for allocating resources to meet the people's medical needs, was seen as providing the essential "filter." Said Professor Charas:

> The universities have all along served as pipelines without filters for knowledge from Western countries. No attempt was made to be critical or selective. We are presently seeing the consequences which include the lack of critical thinking. Many medical graduates are interested in easy knowledge for immediate consumption and use. Even those who have gone through postgraduate training in clinical specialties abroad have the same mentality. Many are of the opinion that articles published in reputable journals such as the *Lancet*, the *British Medical Journal,* or the *Journal of the American Medical Association* can be accepted as the truth and no critical judgment is required....It is evident that clinicians' and clinical teachers' ability in scientific reasoning seriously needs improvement. This kind of mentality is certainly in conflict with an attempt at critical appraisal of evidence and at research development. This brought us to [a] second...content-oriented mentality in contrast to a methodology-oriented one. Teachers and students alike are more interested in the way to treat a patient than the way to judge the suitability of a treatment....

> The medical doctors who are the most knowledgeable persons on health problems and their solutions in the district have to serve a different function. He or she needs to have a perception of the whole population in the district with its social, cultural, economic, and political set-up. He needs to use science and technology as his tool to assist in the development efforts of the community....
> In order to reach that status a change is needed to swing the pendulum toward a scientific basis of clinical medicine and population-based medicine...[Cl]inical epidemiology would handily serve as a tool toward this goal. Unfortunately the word "epidemiology" carries a certain set of values among clinical teachers which poses the first obstacle to change. Misunderstanding regarding clinical epidemiology prevails in many circles. The term in Thai language is worse than in English. Epidemiology in Thai literally means the science of epidemics.[9]

Professor Charas continued:

> Clinical epidemiology cannot cover everything because it will dilute its effort. In my opinion, traditional epidemiology as a discipline taught in schools of public health still has a big role. It has successfully developed to serve many functions from national health planning to the management of epidemics. Clinical epidemiology should not be expanded too far in this regard. A distinction between clinical epidemiology and epidemiology should be sufficiently [distinct] so that no territorial problem is created. Conflict from this basic psychology of the animal kingdom must be avoided. This is not to say that there is a hard boundary between the two areas. Interchange and mutual contribution must be encouraged. Clinical epidemiology needs to draw resources from [our] epidemiology colleagues....Collaborative research projects are a good means to develop expertise.[10]

The reader will detect in Charas's remarks further fallout from the *schism*. The unhealthy influence on academic territoriality, knowledge, and innovative responses to the people's health problems is all too apparent. At the same time there have been gratifying moves by clinicians at Chulalongkorn who are using epidemiology. Gradually they are venturing into the community by linking these studies to more narrowly hospital-based manifestations of disease. Only gradually can the Fellows and faculty be stimulated to study problems such as malaria, dengue, malnutrition, and "community health" generally. Critics of the Rockefeller Foundation's initiative with clinical epidemiology may not fully appreciate that INCLEN Fellows, their peers and superiors, are the products of long and constricted associations with tertiary care academicians. The latter, in turn, have had little or no exposure to illness at the level of primary care in the community. The top-down view from the teaching hospital traditionally has guided their priorities; the faculty investigate the diseases to which they are exposed in the teaching hospital.

In another connection Professor Charas contrasted the traditional mentality that resists change (left-hand column) compared with a mentality that accepts critical appraisal and analytic thinking (right-hand column) in the following:[11]

Information-oriented	vs.	Critical Appraisal-oriented
Answer-oriented	vs.	Question-oriented
Knowledge- and Content-oriented	vs.	Methods-oriented
Anecdotal and Descriptive	vs.	Analytical and Experimental
Qualitative	vs.	Quantitative
Molecular and Cellular	vs.	Societal and Community Interests
Pursuit of International Standards	vs.	Local Relevance

A major objective of INCLEN is to expand the perspectives of students and faculties so that they achieve a balanced view of society's health problems and a constructively critical stance toward what can be done to ameliorate them.

Comments at a meeting of the CERTC Faculty during the Pattaya Conference, illustrate the realities of the problems INCLEN is attempting to address:

Clinicians in Thailand have a very heavy clinical load which causes the Fellows difficulty and concern in terms of doing research, particularly outside the hospital setting. There is need to approach the issue of population medicine slowly as the Fellows have to maintain their credibility with their peers and population medicine is not as yet given a credible rating by these peers. However, there are changes occurring in the health services and new graduates are much 'turned-on' to working beyond the confines of the hospital.[12]

A major tenet of the INCLEN program is to enlist the returning Fellow in asking questions about the efficacy, risks, benefits, and costs of what he or she is doing and gradually to relate educational and research priorities to the health problems of the entire population, that is, the community.

When applying epidemiological concepts and methods in clinical settings those doing so sooner or later should come into contact, if not merge, with those doing the same in the community. The top-down and bottom-up perspectives inevitably meet, as Professor Charas pointed out. As described further on, successful strategies were developed later for bringing together field and clinical epidemiologists. Both groups should participate in "redefining the unacceptable" through use of the numeric method. How else can scarce resources be allocated more rationally in the interests of improving the public's health? How can any reasonable member of the medical profession openly take an opposing position?

Another example of the importance of making epidemiological principles and skills accessible to clinicians in their day-to-day work is provided by Professor Ernesto Domingo. In 1983, during my first encounter with Domingo, then chairman of the department of medicine, later Dean of the University of the Philippines College of Medicine, and now his University's Chancellor, I failed to help him understand the relationship of epidemiology to clinical medicine. Gradually, he grasped the concept, became the initial sponsor of his own University's CEU, and now is one of INCLEN'S most ardent supporters. This CEU has flourished both within the University and the country. In 1989 President Corazon Aquino presented Mary Ann Lanseng, one of its first Fellows, with the Philippines National Academy of Science and Technology's "Outstanding Young Scientist Award in Medicine."[13] At the 1984 Annual INCLEN meeting in Thailand, Domingo described "the adverse effects on past generations of medical students of boring epidemiology lectures unrelated to clinical problems conducted by people from the school of public health. He outlined an ambitious plan to integrate clinical epidemiology throughout various levels of a new curriculum being adopted by the College of Medicine. The major need he identified was for more people to receive training at the CERTCs and return to carry on this new approach to teaching and research."[14]

At Escola Paulista in São Paulo, Brazil, returned Fellows are provided with tangible incentives to pursue their careers in clinical epidemiology. They are given an increase of 2 years in seniority, and their patient care responsibilities are reduced to provide more time for research. A "problem with territory," however, was recognized in concerns expressed over the "definite division" between preventive medicine and clinical epidemiology.[15] The schism again intruded. Why should departments of preventive medicine be upset that clinicians are now doing what the faculty of these departments have been vigorously advocating for lo these many years? For the long haul, surely success will be measured by the extent to which the population perspective and preventive strategies are integrated into the entire health establishment. For the short haul, it should be gratifying to think that clinicians are not only getting the message about the population perspective but have the skills to conduct independent population-based research.

The Health of Populations component with its emphasis on clinical epidemiology and INCLEN were never seen as "quick fixes." As in the case of the Rockefeller Foundation's 1916 decision to fund schools of public health apart from medical schools, the decision to support the Health of Populations component was taken for the long term. The bright, young, established clinicians selected, in time, should become influential academicians, familiar with the concepts and skills of epidemi-ology. Having internalized the population perspective, the expectation is that the next generation of academic leaders will be advisors to Heads of State, to Ministries of Health, Education, and Finance, and to national and international health agencies. In turn they should argue for more rational deployment of resources to improve the population's health than is currently the case.

INCLEN II was attended by 84 participants from 15 countries. Twenty-four Fellows from nine countries who had completed their training and returned to start CEUs presented scientific papers. Here are the types of studies (with numbers of each on the right) reported at this first Scientific Meeting:[16]

Type	Number of Papers
Case-control study	1
Randomized, double-blind efficacy study	10
Disease prevalence study	5
Disease etiology study	1
Evaluation of epidemiologic methods	1
Evaluation of clinical decision making	1
Evaluation of "health provider system"	2
Evaluation of diagnostic methods	3
Total	24

Scott Halstead, who had just taken over the INCLEN program from me, wrote in a memorandum to President Lyman:

Neither [I] nor others outside INCLEN were prepared for the outstanding quality of the presentations. High intelligence marked the Fellows individually. Careful preparation, command of English, quick and thoughtful answers to questions characterized most presentations. I heard many remarks, such as, 'This is the best scientific meeting I have ever attended in a developing country.' The results attest to high standards of selection by the CERTCs plus an unusually successful tutorial training program. It was notable that several Fellows had immediate offers of research support from funding agencies in attendance. From the standpoint of quality INCLEN could not have gotten off to a better start.[17]

The Abstracts of all submissions were published but the following examples indicate the range of interests:

- Mail follow-up of patients with chronic diseases;
- Prevalence of iron deficiency anemia among female textile workers in Shanghai;
- Promoting rational antimicrobial prescribing of clinicians in primary medical care in Thailand;
- Risk factors for infant mortality and morbidity in the ninth region of Chile;
- Randomized trial of health centre versus hospital laparoscopic sterilization;

- Controlled trial of the village health worker program in Indonesia;
- Effectiveness of chemoprophylaxis against malaria for nonimmune migrant workers in eastern Thailand;
- Randomized controlled trial to assess the efficacy of prenatal nutritional intervention on the outcome of pregnancy;
- Case-control study of risk factors for stroke in Nigerians.

Are these activities components of "public health"? Should these matters be studied only by the faculty or graduates of schools of public health? Is involvement in these kinds of studies likely to sensitize clinicians to the importance of the population perspective? Is it likely to make them more knowledgeable colleagues and better collaborators with more traditional public health workers? What possible harm can come from a contemporary initiative that merely restores the status quo ante, that is, before the schism? Scott Halstead emphasized the challenges and opportunities:

> An important goal of clinical epidemiology is to influence health policy. To this end, better communication is needed between Health Ministries and medical schools. The joint World Health Organization-[U.S.] Centers for Disease Control (CDC) epidemi-ology training program in Thailand offers one such opportunity. The competence acquired in priority epidemiological research by medical school faculty should increase areas of shared interests between the public health and tertiary care sectors. Increased collaboration and consultation may be the ultimate outcome.[18]

At the Pattaya Meeting the decision taken at Hawaii to have the INCLEN candidates for training obtain data on the most important health problems in their own bailiwicks was reaffirmed. One of the requirements of a newly appointed Fellow is that, before departure for training at the CERTC, he or she obtains or develops statistics, expressed as rates, for the diseases and health problems in the municipality, district, region, or nation (i.e., catchment area) from which his or her medical school and teaching hospital(s) receive patients or for which these institu-tions assume responsibility. Arrangements for formal follow-up to ensure that each Fellow arrived with the necessary data were agreed on. Annette Dobson, Professor of Biostatistics at the University of Newcastle, reported on the Role of Health and Vital Statistics in clinical epidemiology as follows:

- Training programmes in clinical epidemiology should include experience in using health statistics to determine priorities for research and health care delivery and to assess economic implications.
- Clinical epidemiologists need to know how and where to obtain the data they require and to be able to assess the quality and analyze and interpret the information.
- Collection of documents relating health and vital statistics is probably best done within the countries concerned since people in these countries are in the best position to judge the accuracy of the data. Therefore, the CEUs should have the primary responsibility for identifying sources and collecting such information.

- Assistance with methodological aspects such as standard data collection instruments, quality control, and statistical analysis should be provided by CERTCs.

- There is a need to find out about work on health statistics being done by governments and other organizations. The Information System for Health Statistics in the Asian and Pacific Region in Newcastle will be responsible for this task.[19]

A second Hawaii initiative also was followed up with the formal appointment of a Health Economics Subcommittee consisting of Jane Hall (Newcastle), Greg Stoddart (McMaster) and John Eisenberg (Pennsylvania), Chairman. The subcommittee was charged with making recommendations for selecting and training individuals to develop this aspect of the program.[20]

Beyond the Rockefeller Foundation other international agencies were taking an active interest in INCLEN. Of special importance was the World Bank's initiative in China where a loan for upgrading medical education provided core support for five specific components. These included a program in Design, Measurement, and Evaluation at each of the 12 participating federally sponsored medical colleges. In addition the Bank agreed to support the CEUs at the Sichuan Medical College (now the West China University of Medical Sciences) and the First Shanghai Medical College (now the Shanghai Medical University) and their expansion into two National Training Centers for Clinical Epidemiology. The Guanzhou College of Traditional Medicine, although not an integral part of INCLEN, also was supported by this loan to provide 4-month courses in clinical epidemiology for other medical colleges supported directly by the Ministry of Public Health.

The Bank's initiative got off to a running start in 1984 at Chengdu where a "Workshop on Design, Measurement, and Evaluation" was conducted by a faculty drawn largely from INCLEN staff for the Presidents or Senior Vice Presidents of the 12 participating medical colleges. The ideas and methods introduced marked a new beginning in Chinese medical education. As in the case of INCLEN itself, however, assessment of the long-term impact must await future developments.

Administratively, one of the most important conclusions stemming from the Pattaya Meeting was the realization that the Asian and Pacific Regional Network was developing very rapidly. Given the several Fellows who had already been trained from Latin America and, although fewer in number, from Africa, there was no longer any logical reason why progress had to proceed sequentially. Parallel developments in all three major regions of the Third World now seemed feasible.

In his memorandum to President Lyman summarizing INCLEN's progress to date, Scott Halstead concluded by stating:

> Because of the virtual completion of the training goals for Asia, it is recommended that the Rockefeller Foundation proceed with the orderly selection of four CEU-designates in Latin America. The funded training is such that ten Fellowships beyond Asian requirements will be available in 1985. By 1987, the four Latin American CEUs will have been staffed and training for African/Middle Eastern Units can begin to complete the global Network by 1990. It is likely that the process will be accelerated by the

addition of training funds from other donors. A plan for the establishment of CEUs at a reasonable and constant rate, including the subsequent maintenance of INCLEN is envisaged.[21]

At its meeting on June 15, 1984, the Executive Board of the Foundation approved an allocation to the officers for further development of INCLEN. More specifically, the grant provided funding for a commission composed of representatives of the CERTCs and the Rockefeller Foundation to visit medical schools in Latin America. The purpose of this exercise was to select suitable sites for developing CEUs in addition to Escola Paulista, which had already been selected informally in 1981, and to interview prospective Fellows for training. From this allocation it was now also possible to fulfill the earlier promise of modest research support for each returning Fellow. This was to be a one-time grant of $5,000, for each Fellow, apart from any other competitive research funds received from the Rockefeller Foundation or other agencies.

In July 1984 the Commission visited 14 of the leading medical schools in six Latin and Central American countries: Mexico, Costa Rica, Colombia, Chile, Argentina, and Brazil. An Executive Committee for INCLEN had by now been established and, based on the report of the Commission, they approved formal Network affiliation for Escola Paulista, São Paulo; Pontificia Universidad Javeriana, Bogota, Colombia; and the University of Chile, Santiago. It was also agreed to accept, on a "space-available" basis, additional Fellows from the Faculty of Medicine of the Universidad Federal do Rio de Janeiro, Brazil, the Faculty of Medicine of the Universidad de la Frontera, Temuco, Chile, and the National Institute of Nutrition, Mexico City, each of which had already sent one Fellow for training.

"INCLEN III," held at Cavite, The Philippines, January 27-February 1, 1985, was attended by 91 persons including 40 Fellows, 14 CEU sponsors, and 18 CERTC faculty. The papers presented were again said to be of high quality. Some 27 (64%) of them were directed at community problems in open (nonhospitalized) populations; the other 36% were hospital based. Again all the abstracts were published; examples of the range of papers presented are:

- A study of occupational pesticide exposure among Filipino farmers;
- A cross-sectional study of the risk factors and predictive score for the development of protein energy malnutrition in pre-school children of Bangkok slums;
- Research methodology in Thai medical journals;
- A prevalence investigation of chronic leukopenia in Chengdu;
- A survey of antibiotic use in medical wards of a university hospital;
- Clinical epidemiological study of nosocomial infection in Hua Shan Hospital.[22]

By this time 44 Fellows had completed their training and five CEUs each had 5 or more trained Fellows: Siriraj, Chulalongkorn, and Khon Kaen (Thailand), Sichuan, and First Shanghai (China). In Thailand a second national meeting, opened by the Minister of Health, was designed to explain clinical epidemiology to department chairmen of the country's medical schools. Both of the CEUs (now National Training Centers) in China were running 2-month workshops attended by faculty from 12 other medical colleges in their country. The Ibadan CEU also had organized national workshops in clinical epidemiology.

All three CERTCs were now awarding M.Sc. or M.S. degrees on completion of training; these required submission of a satisfactory thesis based on a research project. The last to obtain approval from their Board of Trustees was Pennsylvania. Here the medical school, bucking tradition, became the first in the United States to offer the M.S. degree in clinical epidemiology, a clinically based graduate academic program, in addition to the M.D. degree. Previously all graduate degrees had been awarded by the University's Faculty of Arts and Science. Two of the Thai CEUs were planning to develop formal graduate programs in clinical epidemiology and to award an M.Sc. degree.

On April 2, 1985, the Rockefeller Board allocated further support for development of INCLEN. This included research grants to CEUs, distribution of a 15-journal microfiche library collection including 3 years of back issues, a microfilm reader, and several textbooks of epidemiology, including a recently published volume entitled *Clinical Epidemiology: A Basic Science for Clinical Medicine* by Professors Sackett, Haynes and Tugwell of McMaster.[23] Distribution of the McMaster computerized catalogue of teaching materials in clinical epidemiology and production of the *INCLEN Newsletter* were also supported. At the same Board meeting the University of Pennsylvania's CERTC had its major support grant renewed for a third 3-year period.

In October 1984 the Health Economics Subcommittee had its first meeting and, in 1985 at "INCLEN III," put forward specific recommendations. In contrast to programs of other foundations that exposed clinicians to economic thinking, the Subcommittee argued for the attainment by selected INCLEN Fellows of specific competencies in health economics, rather than acquiring a smattering of knowledge about the subject. Petty and Frank would have been delighted! I question whether as much attention has ever been given to determining the most appropriate level of understanding of economic concepts and methods desirable for clinicians. The Subcommittee's analysis was based on extended travel and consultation by Ms. Jane Hall, a health economist at the University of Sydney, who worked with the Newcastle CEU. The material available to the Subcommittee included interviews with Fellows and faculty in both the CERTCs and the CEUs, as well as with health economists in university economics departments; experiences in both the developed and developing worlds were canvassed.

A knowledge of economic principles is essential for clear thinking about priority setting and resource allocation within the health care sector, as well as among the many other sectors (education, food policy and nutrition, employment, housing, the environment, and "safety nets") that materially affect individual and collective health status. Without this knowledge the medical profession is unlikely to be able to make material contributions to coping with contemporary problems revolving around the provision of personal health services. The importance of helping Fellows examine all the underlying assumptions (often highly controversial) in any economic analysis was stressed. To ensure that the subject was not considered to be a "value-free technology," the Subcommittee originally distinguished four levels of competence in health economics training; these were later collapsed into three levels. Because of their importance for both undergraduate and postgraduate medical education generally, they are worth recording is some detail:

Level One. Individuals trained at Level One will be able to:
- Use the principles of economic evaluation in medical education, medical practice, and research, specifically to:
  - collaborate in their research projects with investigators who have more advanced skills;
  - appreciate the economic implications of their clinical decisions (identifying the resources that are consumed and the related expenditures), understand the rationale for reforms to engender more efficient health care within their own economic and social system, and help to create a climate of understanding of the economic constraints on medical practice among clinicians;
  - be intelligent users of the results of economic evaluations of clinical practice;

Level Two. Individuals trained at Level Two in addition to the objectives above will be able to:
- Carry on economic evaluations of clinical services, assessing the resources that are consumed by clinical interventions, the resources that may be saved, and the outcomes that are obtained for the expenditure;
- Identify the relationship between their own and others' medical practice, teaching, and research, and the characteristics in which the health care delivery system is set;
- Encourage other faculty to incorporate economic considerations into their clinical research, clinical practice, and teaching.
- Serve as consultants to their colleagues who would like to incorporate economic evaluation into their clinical research;
- Teach other researchers economic evaluation methods for inclusion in their clinical research.

Candidates for these two levels of training would normally, but not necessarily, be clinicians with an identified interest in conducting economic evaluations. The Level Two Fellows would earn an M.Sc. degree.

Level Three. Beyond these first two levels of training, a third level might be considered—doctoral level training in health economics. The Subcommittee suggests that individuals trained at Levels One and Two eventually will need access to doctoral level economists or health services researchers once they return to their home institutions. These individuals will be important as consultants for the Fellows, particularly with regard to new developments in health economics methods as well as in providing the informal collegial relationship that will be important for these individuals to maintain their interest, enthusiasm, and expertise.[24]

The Health Economics Subcommittee was under no illusions that all this could be accomplished easily, and they set out a number of constraints and problems. Among these was another example of the schism they sought to anticipate and bridge:

> Some of the Fellows interviewed felt that a potential problem exists with regard to the administrators of the hospitals and health care system in the developing countries. These individuals may be threatened by Fellows who return with special skills in economic analysis. If these individuals are clinicians, they may challenge the authority and reputation of administrators who had previously been the most expert individuals in assessing economic implications of medical care. Such administrators may need to be educated in the use of research results. This concern probably parallels a concern about possible conflict between individuals who emphasize clinical epidemiology and experts in public health at their home institutions, who might be threatened by clinicians returning with expertise in epidemiologic methods.[25]

One approach to such matters is more education for all concerned with the peoples' health. The following were among the Subcommittee's recommendations:

* Identification of health economics resources at the CEU sites and the strengthening of resources outside the INCLEN program;
* Programs at Levels One and Two, should be termed *Clinical Economics*, and consist primarily of principles of economics as applied to economic evaluation (e.g., cost-effectiveness, cost benefit, and cost utility), and selected broader topics in health economics;
* Economics should be integrated into clinical epidemiology education materials;
* The Clinical Economics component should be evaluated against the criteria of the clinical economic skills that the Fellows demonstrate and incorporate in their research projects;
* The development of the Clinical Economics program should proceed in 1985 and a detailed review of the requirements of Level Three programs be prepared for the Annual INCLEN Meeting in 1987.[26]

These recommendations were acted on at the December 2-3, 1985, meeting of the Rockefeller Board that appropriated funds for training in Clinical Economics at Levels One and Two. Development of a curriculum for Level Three was to take place later. John Eisenberg, professor of medicine at the University of Pennsylvania and chairman of the Subcommittee summarized the importance of this component in an editorial that also would have gladdened the heart of William Petty:

> In the same way that clinical epidemiology has bridged the care of individuals with the health of populations, there is emerging a parallel approach to placing clinical decisions in a larger context—using economic analysis to assess clinical strategies. This sister discipline, which can be called clinical economics, is being practiced by physicians and other analysts who are interested in how well resources are used. Clinical economics enables the evaluation of efficiency to join studies of efficacy and effectiveness in assessing medical practice.[27,28]

Much progress had been made but there were still a few lingering doubts within the Foundation's administrative hierarchy about the long-term viability of the INCLEN program. After all, these were rather unusual approaches in an arena that for seven decades had been packaged into three almost independent sectors: biomedical laboratory research, medical education, and public health. Accordingly, in the Spring of 1985 the Foundation's senior officers commissioned yet another review of the Health of Populations component. The three reviewers were Gerard N. Burrow, at that time Professor of Medicine, Faculty of Medicine, University of Toronto and now Dean of the School of Medicine, University of California, San Diego; Thomas Grayston, Professor of Epidemiology, School of Public Health, University of Washington; and Dean T. Jamison, Ph.D., an economist who at that time was Chief of Policy Analysis in the Education and Training Department of the World Bank, Washington, D.C., and who is now a professor on the faculty of the School of Public Health, University of California, Los Angeles. Their report was highly supportive and commended the innovative nature of the program. They applauded its concentration on training a critical mass of clinicians in epidemiological, economic, and statistical concepts and methods, and the intensive follow-up by the preceptors of Fellows who had returned home.[29] They were high in their praise for the dedication and commitment of the CERTCs' faculties to the individual Fellows and to the CEUs.

The reviewers commented both on the diversity of definitions of clinical epidemiology extant and the apparent variations in the emphases in the Health of Populations and its INCLEN program over the years. These variations were in large measure caused by the shifting sands within the Foundation and our attempts to explain this strange business to various constituencies; some differences undoubtedly stemmed from the diverse views and interests of the officers themselves, as well as differences among the faculties of the CERTCs. Dean Jamison placed the matter in readily understandable context with the following array that accords completely with my own thinking about these matters (see Table 8.1.).[30]

Jamison pointed out that "classical" epidemiology, big "E" in David Sackett's terminology, has focused on Cell I.A, the upper left-hand corner, and that a narrowly interpreted application of "clinical" epidemiology, little "e" according to Sackett, has tended to focus on Cell II.B, the lower right-hand corner.

Several other constructive suggestions were offered:

- Links with "classical" epidemiology programs should be forged and strengthened, as should those with Ministries of Health and other appropriate government agencies;
- Adequate time and energy as well as funding must be provided to maintain and strengthen the follow-up of returned Fellows through visits to the CEUs from their preceptors at regular intervals;
- In selecting research projects for the Fellows, more attention should be paid to making certain that they were feasible with the resources at the disposal of the Fellow's CEU; that the problem was of importance—preferably of international importance; and that the results were published in

TABLE 8.1. Elements of a Quantitative Approach to the Health of Populations.

Level of Observation/Interaction	Objective of Analysis	
	A. Descriptive	B. Prescriptive
1. Community	Incidence, prevalence,and etiology of disease; structure, capacity, and finance of health services	Evaluation of strategies for environmental, and mental and behavioral change; evaluation of strategies for provision and finance of curative and preventive services
2. Individual	Determinants of clinician-patient behavior and interaction, including demand for services and compliance	Dynamic evaluation of diagnostic, prognostic, and therapeutic alternatives in light of legal and economic environments, and objectives and constraints for individual patients

peer-reviewed journals—preferably "international" journals. Not only are prestige, status, and academic advancement dependent on first-rate research but so is funding for future research.

If it is true that: "People and populations have 'problems' and universities and governments have 'departments'," so it must follow that disciplines and professions cannot be constrained by artificial boundaries, such as those wrought by the schism. Just as "classical" epidemiologists have tended to expand their interests downward and toward the right in this matrix, so are "clinical" epidemiologists expanding their horizons upward and toward the left. In the "real" world there are no boundaries to the pursuit of understanding and "truth."

With many issues clarified, INCLEN was now poised to take on its full global scope envisaged originally. Africa and the Indian subcontinent had received only limited attention to date. Accordingly, the following steps were taken:

- On October 12-13, 1985, a Clinical Epidemiology Seminar was held in Srinigar, Kashmir, India, sponsored by The United States Agency for International Development (USAID) as part of a program to encourage the development of epidemiology in that country. The participants included administrators and key department chairmen from selected medical schools. In addition to orienting and educating Indian academics, the Seminar assisted the INCLEN faculty in selecting suitable institutions where CEUs might be developed. This initiative and the subsequent expansion of INCLEN in India with a 5-year, $2.1 million grant were accomplished through the tireless efforts of W.B. Rogers Beasley, M.D., at the time Director of the USAID Health Program in India and later a Senior Scientist attached to the Foundation's Division of Health Sciences in New York.

- The Special Programme for Tropical Disease Research (TDR) of the World Bank, the United Nations Development Program, and the World Health Organization announced that it would begin formal cosponsorship of the Annual INCLEN Meetings, in addition to supporting a number of Fellows for training in clinical epidemiology at the CERTCs. This development was the result of the direct involvement of Richard Morrow, M.D., Secretary of the Scientific Working Group on Epidemiology of the TDR Programme.

- The Foundation in collaboration with the International Development Research Centre (IDRC) of Canada, each agency paying half the cost, began support of a special CERTC at the University of Toronto to provide an annual 3-month course in clinical epidemiology for senior medical school faculty and health services administrators, including those working in the public health sector. This highly effective innovation was later to be known as the Toronto Management Training Short Course.

- The Foundation began providing INCLEN with funds for Multicenter Collaborative Research Programs. These had to be initiated by the Fellows and were designed to foster cooperative investigations among CEUs, as well as with CERTCs.

- The Foundation also appropriated funds to enable Content Resource Experts to visit CEUs to help Fellows design research projects. There is little point in designing elegant epidemiological studies for biological, social, or psychological problems which do not incorporate the best thinking about substantive issues associated with them.

- To monitor the development of biostatistics (in addition to health statistics) in the CEUs, help select candidates for training, and maintain communication among the CERTCs with respect to curriculum development, a subcommittee (originally established at the first INCLEN Meeting in Hawaii in 1983) was reaffirmed with Professors Annette Dobson (Newcastle), Michael Gent (McMaster), chair, and Charles Goldsmith (McMaster).

- The core establishment for each CEU had by now been expanded from five to six clinicians trained in epidemiology, one biostatistician also trained in clinical epidemiology who might or might not be a physician, and a Health or Clinical Economist, trained to at least Level Two and preferably Level Three, who also might or might not be a physician. To this group would be added a Social Scientist, as discussed later.[31]

By the end of 1985 leadership had changed at the University of Newcastle. Professor Richard Heller who had joined its Asian and Pacific Centre for Clinical Epidemiology the previous year succeeded to the CERTC Directorship when Stephen Leeder moved to the University of Sydney's Westmead Hospital. Altogether, 80 young clinical faculty members had been trained at the three CERTCs, 70 had been funded by the Rockefeller Foundation and 10 by other agencies. The Asian and Pacific component of INCLEN had been expanded to seven CEUs with the addition of Gadjah Mada University, Yogyakarta, Indonesia. This medical school previously had been supported by the Rockefeller Foundation to develop a program in community medicine. As a result of a longtime interest in Indonesia, the Australian International Development Assistance Board (AIDAB) undertook to support Gadjah Mada's new CEU. The Latin American component now consisted of the three CEUs mentioned earlier at Escola Paulista, São Paulo, Brazil, Javeriana University, Bogota, Colombia, and the University of Chile, Santiago, and a newly designated Unit at the General Hospital of the Autonomous University of Mexico, Mexico City. There were also the three smaller, quasi-official, CEUs at Universidad de la Frontera, Temuco, Chile, the Universidad Federal do Rio de Janeiro, Brazil, and the Institute of Nutrition, Mexico City. In all the Foundation had invested almost $5.0 million in INCLEN by the end of 1985.

Of greater importance, however, was the fact that within the Foundation, including its Board, there now was genuine enthusiasm and widespread support for the potential of INCLEN to effect important changes in medical education and health services in the developing world. A recent Trustee Task Force on Development had recommended that the Foundation place greater emphasis on helping African nations. More specifically, the officers received authority to proceed with the development of an African component of INCLEN beyond the earlier tentative efforts to develop a CEU at the University of Ibadan, Nigeria, and the then tangentially involved unit in the Faculty of Medicine, Addis Ababa University, Ethiopia. USAID had now also committed itself officially to supporting the development of clinical epidemiology in selected Indian medical schools.

For the latter expansion another Commission, composed of representatives from the CERTCs and the Foundation, visited nine medical institutions in India from March 3 to 14, 1986. Three of these medical schools were selected for development of CEUs: the College of Medicine, Trivandrum, Kerala; Government Medical College, Nagpur, Maharasta; and King George Medical College, Lucknow, Utter Pradesh. In addition, available USAID funds would permit special training efforts to be made at two other prominent Indian medical institutions: the All-India Institute of Medical Sciences, Ansari Kagar, New Delhi; and Christian Medical College and Hospital, Vellore, Tamil Nadu. The Rockefeller Foundation would also continue its support to the first CEU established in India at the Institute of Child Health, Madras Medical College; it was to become an integral part of a new Advanced Centre for Clinical Epidemiology Research and Training (ACCERT) formally inaugurated in April 1988. This Unit provided a bridge between two parallel clinical epidemiology programs, one at the Institute of Child Health and the second at the Tuberculosis Research Centre; both had been evolving since 1985. The combined CEU is also fortunate in being able to draw on the substantial resources of the renowned Institute for Research in Medical Statistics at Madras.[32]

"INCLEN IV" was held in Shanghai, April 6-11, 1986. This was the first Annual Meeting in which I participated following my retirement from the Foundation. One innovation was a 2-day premeeting workshop on Clinical Economics at which I gave the opening talk. Included were several allusions to Sir William Petty! The object of the Workshop was to provide all Fellows trained at CERTCs before the introduction of more formal teaching in health economics, with at least Level One training as described previously. From the evaluation forms completed after the workshop it was apparent that this and more were achieved.

INCLEN IV was attended by 117 persons, and some 57% of the 77 scientific papers presented were out-of-hospital or community-based studies. For the first time, invited content experts gave talks on their fields of interest and acted as discussants of papers. As reasonably impartial critics, they pronounced the research presentations overall to be of unusually high standard. As in all educational and scientific endeavors, however, there is always ample room for improvement.[33]

At the Shanghai Meeting it was announced that a fourth CERTC was to be established at the University of North Carolina, Chapel Hill, and on June 20, 1986, a grant for this purpose was approved by the Rockefeller Board. The need for additional training capacity was a consequence of the accelerated expansion of INCLEN in India and Africa. Projected needs were for 24 more Fellows for India and 32 for Africa, in addition to current commitments to the Asian and Pacific Region and Latin America.

The selection of the University of North Carolina had been made by another Commission also composed of representatives of the current CERTCs and the Foundation. Following invitations sent to key centers of clinical epidemiology in North America and Europe the Commission considered five universities: the Johns Hopkins, North Carolina, and Yale in the United States; and Oxford and Southampton in England. North Carolina, Yale, and Southampton all had been considered between 1978 and 1983. The latter two were thought to have limited resources for the demands of an international training program on their smaller but unquestionably first-rate clinical epidemiology faculties. North Carolina was now the unanimous choice of the selection Commission because of the size (15 clinical epidemiologists, second in size only to McMaster which then had about 30) and the quality of its clinical epidemiology group. In addition, the new CERTC would have an integral position within the Division of General Medicine and Clinical Epidemiology of an excellent Department of Internal Medicine.

Strong features included the long-standing close association between this group and their colleagues in the Departments of Epidemiology and Biostatistics in the School of Public Health, the presence of a well-established Health Services Research Center linking both schools, as well as first-rate groups in the social sciences and health economics. One of the best outreach regional health programs in the United States, and extensive international experience, added to the attractiveness of Chapel Hill as a site for a CERTC. Finally, Robert and Suzanne Fletcher, the new Co-Directors, were co-authors of one of the first textbooks in this field: *Clinical Epidemiology: The Essentials*,[34] then co-editors of the influential *Journal of General Internal Medicine* and now co-editors of the *Annals of Internal Medicine*. I elaborate on these matters to illustrate the kinds of interests and resources that a well-balanced health sciences center should assemble if it seeks to excel in population-based medicine, in addition to molecular and clinical medicine.

I was not involved in the 1986 decision to select Chapel Hill, but based on our preliminary assessments, and had John Knowles lived and our original plans for developing a larger number of clinical epidemiology centers in North America taken effect, the University of North Carolina would undoubtedly have been chosen. I derived a special pleasure in seeing this preeminent group selected for two reasons. First, the Fletchers were graduates of my former department at the Johns Hopkins University, and second, this selection recalled my own 10 happy years in the Department of Internal Medicine at Chapel Hill. During that tenure, I had undertaken early investigations in what are now labeled clinical epidemiology and health services research together with colleagues such as the late John Cassel, founding chairman of the Department of Epidemiology, the late Bernard Greenberg, professor of biostatistics and subsequently Dean of the School of Public Health, T. Franklin Williams, currently director of the U.S. National Institute on Aging, and Michel Ibrahim, now professor of epidemiology and Dean of the School of Public Health at Chapel Hill.

INCLEN's governance had been modified over the last year or two and now took on a more formal structure. At a meeting of the International Epidemiological Association in Vancouver in 1984, the Executive Committee had been transformed into the CERTCs' Advisory Committee. Consisting of the directors of the CERTCs and representatives of the Rockefeller Foundation, it meets twice a year. In addition, a broader based Council was created that included all the sponsors or directors of the CEUs, the directors of the CERTCs, and representatives of all the funding agencies; it meets during each Annual Meeting. The CERTCs' Advisory Committee defines overall operating policy for the Network. Among the latter's actions during 1986 was a tightening of requirements for attendance by Fellows at the Annual Meetings. Henceforth invitations would be issued to First Year Fellows who had been home for at least 4 months. Fellows who wish to attend a second Annual Meeting must present data from a study completed after their return home from training and also a "second-generation" abstract, that is, one based on the design for a second research project being planned. Fellows wishing to attend a third or successive INCLEN Meeting must submit an abstract describing a research project started and completed after their return home and also an abstract describing a new (third) research protocol. All research abstracts were to be judged competitively and accepted subject to availability of travel funds. Fellows from non-Rockefeller Foundation-sponsored CEUs would be eligible to attend provided they paid their own expenses.

At the June 20, 1986, meeting of the Rockefeller Board, McMaster was awarded its third major grant for the continued support of its CERTC. In October of that year another important event was the extended tour made by yet another Commission (again composed of representatives of the CERTCs and the Foundation) to medical schools in eight African countries: Cameroon, Egypt, Ethiopia, Kenya, Nigeria, Tanzania, Zambia, and Zimbabwe. Its mission was to assess the potential for developing CEUs and to interview prospective Fellows. Initially three new CEUs were selected: the Faculty of Medicine, University of Nairobi, Kenya; the Center for Health Sciences, University of Yaounde, Cameroon; and the Godfrey Higgins School of Medicine, University of Zimbabwe. The University of Addis Ababa, Ethiopia, also was now formally recognized as part of the African Network and of INCLEN. Two other institutions were added later: the Faculty of Medicine,

Makerere University, Kampala, Uganda, and the relatively new Faculty of Medicine of the Suez Canal University, Ismailia, Egypt. All told there were to be 6 CEUs in Africa.[35]

By 1986 the criteria for site visits were tightened, and a standardized visit report form introduced. All Fellows were to receive a site visit from their own preceptor about 6 months after their return home. Subsequent visits to returned Fellows would continue to be made annually but not necessarily by each student's original preceptor. Although each CERTC would have Fellows trained at all four CERTCs, it was agreed that long-term follow-up for each CEU would be the responsibility of only two CERTCs. This pattern of assignments would ensure diversity of exposure to different preceptors, minimize the potential for providing conflicting "advice," and enable more efficient scheduling of travel to several Units within a region. Nurturance and support of the CEUs through these site visits are among the most important features of the INCLEN program. Not only do they provide backing for the Fellows but they enrich the preceptors' experiences in the developing world.[36] For urging and promoting this arrangement, McMaster should receive much of the credit.

During 1986 four Multicenter Collaborative Research Grants were awarded competitively. These linked participating CEUs to one another and to major research groups in other settings. Two types of studies were recognized: the first uses a multidisciplinary approach in which members of different disciplines in separate institutions collaborate to study the same problem, and the second involves investigators in several institutions who agree to follow a common protocol and to work within a defined decision-making and management structure. The initial studies selected were antibiotic usage in six countries; behavioral antecedents of diarrheal disease; incidence of cryptosporidial diarrhea; and study of sociocultural perspectives in clinical epidemiological research.[37,38]

INCLEN now consisted of 5 CEUs in Southeast Asia, 2 in China, 6 in India, 7 in Latin America, and 7 in Africa for a total of 27 plus the four CERTCs. The administrative load on the two officers at the Foundation's offices in New York was enormous. Accordingly, with Trustee approval, an INCLEN Executive Office was opened early in 1987 at the University of Pennsylvania. The purpose was to receive and manage Fellowship applications, coordinate site visits, centralize CEU records, and facilitate communication within the Network.[39]

The year 1987 saw further consolidation following the rapid expansion of the previous 2 years. The Annual Meeting, "INCLEN V," held at Oaxaca, Mexico, January 25-30, 1987, was attended by 144 persons, including many of the CEUs' deans and sponsors, representatives of international funding agencies, and content experts. The newcomers and non-INCLEN participants provided "rave reviews" for the scientific program (personal communication, Scott B. Halstead, February 1987). The latter was enhanced by a special research report section devoted to Clinical Economics. A successful Biostatistics Methods Workshop was also conducted. Altogether 72 scientific papers, selected competitively by a committee of the CERTCs' faculty, were presented; of these papers about half could be considered community based. Recalling that the INCLEN Fellows who undertook these investigations are hospital-based clinicians in, for the most part, conventional medical schools with little research tradition in their clinical departments, this must surely represent a substantial expansion of their perspectives. Here are representative topics:

- A study of risk factors for persistent and recurrent respiratory factors in children;
- Long-term protective efficacy of Hepatitis B vaccine in children;
- Mental health in malnourished children's families;
- Health and sociocultural aspects of opium among Hilltribe children;
- A multivariate study of factors affecting Diphtheria, Pertussis and Tetanus (DPT) immunization status of children;
- Tobacco, alcohol, and coffee consumption in patients with cancer of the digestive tract;
- A sample survey of health services in rural Anhui.[40]

The *INCLEN Newsletter*, now published twice a year, included periodic reports from all CEUs. Accounts of the space, facilities, and material support were provided; virtually all CEUs now had adequate, sometimes quite generous, quarters. Three organizational patterns were apparent. First was the CEU's location within a clinical department, more often than not, the department of medicine. A second arrangement involved a multi-department affiliation to a common central office with the director usually reporting to the dean of the medical school. Only one Unit had been set up as an independent department of clinical epidemiology and that was at the West China University of Medical Sciences (Sichuan) where its status as a National Training Center, as well as certain local competitive aspirations, seem to have favored this arrangement. All the CEUs had active sponsors; often there were two. Eighteen sponsors attended the Oaxaca Meeting; several had also taken advantage of the 3-month INCLEN Management Training Short Course at the University of Toronto. The latter, which by this time had evolved into a major exercise, was another element in the strategy for healing the schism. The goal was to provide midcareer senior medical executives from ministries of health, hospitals, medical schools, and other health agencies with an understanding of epidemiological concepts and skills. The expectation is that these skills will enhance their capacities for decision making, management, and evaluation and enable them more effectively to support clinical and population-based research, as well as improve policy making in all sectors of the health enterprise. INCLEN was building an understanding of the population perspective at all levels of the academic hierarchy and to a more limited extent in ministries of health.

At every INCLEN Annual Meeting a representative of each CEU, and a faculty member of each CERTC, reported to the participants on problems and progress. By 1987 virtually all the CEUs had given one or more courses or workshops in design, measurement, and evaluation—among the central concepts and skills of clinical epidemiology—for their own school's faculty. Most had given several of these, and a majority had given national or regional courses or workshops; some, as at West China University of Medical Sciences (Sichuan), lasted as long as 4 months. These were in addition to journal clubs, clinical rounds, and other educational venues. Some of the larger exercises took place when one or more preceptors from the CERTCs made a site visit.

Major textbooks on clinical epidemiology and biostatistics were translated into Chinese, Indonesian, Portuguese, and Spanish by CEU members. Other teaching material has been similarly translated. A specially written Chinese textbook, *The Guide to Clinical Research Design,* prepared by Wang Jialang, an INCLEN Fellow and now a member of the Sichuan faculty, was published in March 1986. The first printing rapidly sold out; reprinted within several months, some 5000 copies have now been sold. Work is under way on another text to be called *Clinical Epidemiology.*

The fruits of all this, and perhaps the best evidence of progress, were the growing demands on CEU faculty for consultations about research design within their own institutions and externally. In addition to the M.Sc. training in clinical epidemiology being offered by two universities in Thailand mentioned earlier, Escola Paulista de Medicina in Brazil had plans to do the same. Educational strategies and methods varied, but in most settings formal undergraduate curriculum time was provided and elective courses offered. Not a few CEUs were using small-group, problem-solving, learning methods of the types espoused initially by the McMaster and Newcastle CERTCs.

The Rockefeller Board of Trustees now backed INCLEN enthusiastically. At the April 1, 1987, meeting they awarded two grants totaling $1.45 million to continue and expand all of the *Network's* activities. To foster more direct involvement with other organizations whose interests and missions are similar to INCLEN's, several cooperative ventures were undertaken. Based on the quality of their papers presented at INCLEN V, six Fellows were funded to attend the triennial Scientific Conference of the International Epidemiological Association in Helsinki, Finland, August 8-13, 1987. Four more Fellows were similarly selected and financed to attend a meeting of the International Society of Technology Assessment in Health Care in the Netherlands, May 20-27, 1987. Finally, Professor Michael Gent of McMaster addressed the Vth International Congress of the World Federation of Public Health Associations in Mexico City. He described the goals, structure, and accomplishments to date of INCLEN. At the same meeting, Elizabeth Merino Conde, M.D., a returned INCLEN Fellow, presented a paper on "The Development of a Clinical Epidemiology Unit at the General Hospital in Mexico City." Both presentations provided further evidence of INCLEN's continuing efforts at healing the schism, "spreading the gospel," and promoting better understanding of the epidemiological concepts and methods essential for improving the public's health.[41]

INCLEN's research standards were constantly rising but there was still much room for improvement. At its meeting in Nairobi, September 7-8, 1987, the CERTCs' Advisory Committee Meeting tightened further the requirements for acceptance of papers to be presented at the Annual Meetings. For those Fellows who had attended two or more INCLEN Annual Meetings, it was decided to evaluate their papers separately from those of more recently returned Fellows; the more senior Fellows could be held to higher standards. The abstracts submitted would be evaluated by the faculty at each of the four basic CERTCs; the scores would be averaged and the top 25 or 30 papers accepted for presentation. This approach had the advantage of involving a larger and more diverse body of critics, as well as acquainting them with the range of topics being investigated and the appropriateness of the methods employed. Where deficiencies in the abstracts were found to contribute to a poor score, these were to be discussed between the Fellow and his or her preceptor with a view to improvement.[42]

Requirements for site visits were also tightened. CEU Directors and sponsors were asked to contribute information beforehand. For each Fellow all research projects were to be listed according to their stage of development. The categories included those being planned, those developed but unfunded, those funded and in progress, those completed, and those in various stages of publication (i.e., in preparation, submitted for publication, in press, or published). This information was subsequently placed on a new computer database that had been established at the University of North Carolina CERTC.[43]

One component of each CEU discussed at Hawaii was still missing. To complete the links with the community and foster understanding by physicians, and eventually by politicians and policy makers, of the impact of social and cultural factors on health and disease, each CEU required a social scientist. The schism between medicine and public health is typified by the virtual exclusion of social scientists from leadership positions in most medical schools, especially in developing countries. Participation by token social and behavioral scientists in teaching first-year medical students and in departments of community, preventive, or social medicine and in departments of family medicine or general practice has increased gradually in North American and British medical schools. Their integration into the academic fabric, let alone its power structure, is still to come. Social scientists have fared much better in schools of public health where their views have contributed materially to teaching and research. As in the case of epidemiology, medicine owes a debt of gratitude to these schools for nurturing and developing the social sciences' potential for helping to understand and ameliorate health and disease.

Bridges between the CERTCs' major clinical departments and the parent universities' social science departments needed to be built. Professor Michael Heller of the University of Newcastle took the initiative to advance this essential function of INCLEN. He employed H. Nichlos Higginbotham, a social scientist, to prepare an initial training plan suitable for incorporation into each of the CERTCs. At the Oaxaca Annual Meeting this basic plan resulted in the CERTCs' Advisory Committee appointing a Health Social Science Subcommittee. This was chaired by Higginbotham, who subsequently was appointed a Senior Lecturer at the University of Newcastle. The Subcommittee's membership varied but eventually included representatives from all four CERTCs, each of which either appointed or identified a colleague in its university to undertake development of the social science component. The Rockefeller and other foundations were represented on the Subcommittee, and there were two advisors: Professors Mark Nichter and Steven West from the University of Arizona and Arizona State University, respectively. Extensive review of contemporary training programs in what the Subcommittee proposed calling Health Social Science, as well as extensive considerations of Third World needs, resulted in the strong recommendation that such a program be established.[44] The Health Social Science Subcommittee issued its final proposal in February 1987.[45] Earlier versions of their deliberations had discussed three levels of competence, including the preparation of social scientists at the Ph.D. level for work in CEUs, but initially they recommended that, as in the case of Clinical Economics, a start should be made with two levels of instruction:

> Level One. The focus of training clinical epidemiology Fellows is to provide a basic understanding of social factors in health and disease, and of the methods appropriate for studying these in various cultures. Curricula will emphasize preparation of data collection materials with Fellows learning how to conduct 'pilot' interviews to gather information necessary for designing formal survey instruments.
>
> Also included are topics such as the application of the social sciences to health education and behavior change, patient-provider relationships and communication, and quasi-experimental and qualitative research approaches. As such, this material is not a radical departure from the current clinical epidemiology course work. Rather, it reflects an extension of additional options to research design (e.g., greater emphasis on observational studies) and ways of conceptualizing health problems (e.g., belief systems, cultural values, and social factors in health behaviors). Further, it is recognized that these areas overlap to some degree with topics already taught by other specialists; e.g., health economists and policy analysts. This not only emphasizes the evolutionary nature of this aspect of training, but also that other faculty can readily assist in this portion.
>
> Level Two. The aim is to equip Social Science Fellows with the expertise necessary for them to collaborate effectively with their CEU colleagues. Upon completion, they will have knowledge of epidemiology, biostatistics, computing, and health economics. In addition, they will have special expertise in qualitative and other nonexperimental research techniques; cultural factors in designing and validating questionnaires; social, cultural, and psychological determinants of health, disease, and risk behavior; how cultural beliefs influence the planning of community interventions; and the principles of behavior change, at the level of the individual, community, and government.[46]

At its June 19, 1987, meeting the Rockefeller Board allocated funds to initiate the formal training of one Health Social Scientist for each CEU. This was an important expansion of the Foundation's interests for it presaged a new commitment to examining the social and cultural determinants of health and disease, originally excluded by the Foundation, as observed in Chapter 4. Virchow's oft-repeated aphorism was now being taken seriously; it was a far cry from the seemingly restrictive views of disease causation held by Welch, Rose, and Gates 75 years earlier. As stated in the docket document presented to the Board, Clinical Fellows and Social Scientists trained to Level One are expected to:

- Broaden their search for causal factors by taking the sociocultural and behavioral dimensions of illness into account;
- Learn how to use intensive community study methods, including participant observation and questionnaires, and how to cross-check the validity of field survey protocols;
- Design techniques to construct valid measures of social, cultural, and psychological variables;
- Understand the principles of behavior change applicable to individuals at high risk of certain diseases;
- Draw upon social scientists' ethnographic knowledge of community dynamics to plan, execute, and evaluate health interventions; and
- Understand factors influencing the dissemination and adoption of research results among policymakers, organizations, and populations.[47]

Edwin Chadwick and Lemuel Shattuck, the two laymen whose social sensitivity and activism did so much for "redefining the unacceptable" in their day, would have been happy, as would Frank, Osler, Paul, and Ryle. My own satisfaction with this initiative was augmented by the prospect that there now would be more aggressive investigation of Factor "X" and that, in due course, not only physicians, but administrators, politicians, and the public would come to appreciate the ubiquitous nature and fundamental importance to the entire health endeavor of the Placebo and Hawthorne effects.

In addition to introducing Level One training for all current INCLEN Fellows, the program called for accepting three Level Two Health Social Science Fellows (also to be known as INCLEN Fellows) starting in 1988, and eight per year for the following 3 years. Before selection, the latter were to have completed training to the master's or doctorate level in one of the major social sciences (anthropology, psychology, or sociology). The purpose of the new INCLEN Fellowships was to provide intensive training in clinical epidemiology and related Health Services Research for social scientists; it was not to make social scientists out of epidemiologists. Ideally the social scientists would be members of a separate social science department, faculty, or group outside the medical school; they would have disciplinary identity and a clear career structure. The objective is to build bridges between social scientists and clinicians. Where possible a senior social scientist is encouraged to act as a sponsor for the Health Social Science activities of the CEU. A good example is to be found at Mahidol University, Bangkok, where the Dean of the Faculty of Social Sciences and Humanities is the sponsor. He has already developed several joint projects with the CEU at the Mahidol University's Siriraj Hospital Medical School (personal communication, Nichlos Higginbotham, October 28, 1989).

Great attention is being paid to the integration of Biostatisticians, Clinical Economists and Health Social Scientists into the CEUs, to their career structures, peer relationships, and future advancement. Links of all three groups to other colleagues in these disciplines in other schools and departments of each CEU's university are seen as essential; it is not always easy to accomplish. INCLEN's overriding objective is to foster the rational direction of society's resources to improve the health of populations; it has no interest in building barriers, fomenting jurisdictional disputes, or promoting turf battles. The University of Newcastle received a third 3-year grant to support its CERTC at the September 6-7, 1987, meeting of the Foundation's Board. The Newcastle CERTC, now renamed Centre for Clinical Epidemiology and Biostatistics, was enlarged to include additional economists, social scientists, and later a chair in environmental and occupational epidemiology.

Still another expansion of the Network was started in 1987. It became evident to the INCLEN Commission visiting Africa that more than 15 Francophone countries would be excluded from participation because English is the language of instruction in all current CERTCs. Caroline Dupuy, M.D., and Charles Mérieux, M.D. of the Fondation Mérieux learned of the problem. They arranged for an INCLEN Workshop to be held at Annecy, France, October 30-November 1, 1988. A faculty drawn from all the CERTCs worked with more than 60 participants from medical schools in France, including a large contingent from the academic medical community in Lyons. In addition there were participants from the Université de Montréal, Canada.

Early expressions of skepticism (the usual experience when epidemiological concepts are introduced to traditional clinicians) were followed by unbounded enthusiasm as an outcome of skillful indoctrination of the novitiates by means of critical appraisal of the learning material. With the help of the Fondation Mérieux, collaborating with the Rockefeller Foundation, a Francophone CERTC will be established at Université Claude Bernard and its Hospital Eduoard-Herriot in Lyons. Subsequently five young clinical faculty have been accepted for training at the four original CERTCs. There would now be a total of six CERTCs in the developed world—the original four, plus Toronto, and now Lyons. Thought is also being given in Canada to establishing yet another Francophone CERTC at l'Université de Montréal to serve other universities in Québec, elsewhere in the Western Hemisphere, and perhaps in other countries.[48]

There was further tangible evidence of INCLEN's numerical, in addition to its intellectual, progress: a course in Clinical Research and Design offered by the CEU at Shanghai Medical University was attended by 100 physicians. This faculty also gave eight Consultant Seminars at other medical institutions in China. Suez Canal University introduced an M.Sc. degree course in research design, and the CEU at the Madras Medical College was allocated the entire first floor of a new 10-story building for its work.[49]

A number of the Fellows had now been back in their CEUs for several years. In addition to the regular site visits of preceptors, it became increasingly evident that Continuing Education and Distance Learning components were needed. An initial survey of CEUs found that 16 of them were interested in the former method of learning, and 13 in the latter. Accordingly a Subcommittee of the CERTCs' Advisory Committee was established to develop specific plans for making these two activities more widely available.

Nor was technological support for the Network neglected. Among the problems facing many of the CEUs was the need for access to adequate computing equipment. The returning biostatisticians trained at the CERTCs generated added pressure to provide these essential tools. For the most part, this boiled down to making available microcomputers with adequate memory and storage. There was a need to standardize hardware and software. The Biostatistics Subcommittee subsequently recommended that all components of INCLEN adopt IBM or 100% compatible microcomputers as the hardware of choice; encouragement was given to standardizing around several software packages, including statistical programs for analyses.

In addition to frequent personal interactions through the annual meetings, workshops, seminars, and site visits, more frequent exchanges of information were recognized as desirable. Accordingly electronic communication through E-Mail was pioneered using the COSY Network at the University of Guelph, Ontario, a system with broad capacity for networking among universities in developing countries. Although slow at first, the use of this modality is being adopted by more and more of the CEUs. In addition, McMaster University introduced CD-ROM technology for MEDLINE searches and a service that provided hard copies of articles requested by the CEUs. Of much greater potential has been the emergence of FAX (facsimile) transmission, a technology available to a growing number of the CEUs. All these technologies are demonstrated at INCLEN Annual Meetings.

In 1987 Thailand was in many ways developing as a prototype that demonstrated in practical form INCLEN's original aspirations and objectives. Their national Clinical Epidemiology Club, the M.Sc. courses, the regular National Clinical Epidemiology Workshops, and the creation of THAICLEN were mentioned earlier. Three other medical schools in Thailand decided to establish CEUs: Chiang Mai University; Ramathibodhi Hospital Medical School, Mahidol University; and Prince of Songkla University. More recently, they have formed a consortium to reform medical education in the entire country which, among other matters, committed each school to include clinical epidemiology in its curriculum. With some help from the Rockefeller Foundation, but financed largely by other agencies including AIDAB, IDRC, WHO, and the universities themselves, eight Fellows from the three new universities were accepted for training in clinical epidemiology in 1987. Of equal interest was the funding of an additional three Fellows from two Thai Army Hospitals and one clinician working in the Outbreak Investigation Unit, Division of Epidemiology of Thailand's Ministry of Public Health.

This last appointment was the result of another Rockefeller Foundation initiative. Scott Halstead, based on his long experience in Thailand before joining the Foundation, was able to arrange sponsorship of a novel experiment that would have gladdened the hearts of the likes of William Farr and members of the London Epidemiological Society. The objective was to link directly the decision-making process for health matters with epidemiological research. A new National Epidemiology Board of Thailand was inaugurated in January, 1988. The development of the Board followed 2 years of preparatory work. This was a major exercise requiring extensive analyses, much of it carried out by the INCLEN CEUs, to create a list that placed the country's health problems in priority.

Professor Prawase Wasi (mentioned earlier), chairman of the Department of Medicine at the Siriraj Hospital Medical School of Mahidol University and sponsor of its CEU, was President of the Board. Composed of 7 members from the Ministry of Health and 10 members from outside the Ministry, the Board appointed a five-person Executive Committee, a Fact Finding Commission, a Policy Development Commission, and three other working commissions on Communicable Diseases, Environmental Health, and Community Health. The latter three groups were charged with responsibility for framing research questions, conducting competitions for research funding, and for awarding and monitoring contract research. Professor Charas Suwanwela, by this time Dean of Medicine, and subsequently President of Chulalongkorn University and sponsor of its CEU, was a member of the Executive Committee of the Board and Director of its Environmental Health Commission.[50] The first major report from the Board, sponsored by the Rockefeller Foundation, was a *Review of the Health Situation in Thailand: Priority Ranking of Diseases.*[51] Integration of ideas and action at last seemed feasible.

Other CEUs are being encouraged to examine this model and adapt it to the needs of their own countries. The Rockefeller Foundation prepared a brochure setting forth the history of such enterprises and invited applications from Ministries of Health in countries with an INCLEN CEU.[52] Several of these, in addition to Thailand, are taking steps to establish such boards. Perhaps, for the first time in 75 years, there is now the prospect that strong and meaningful ties can be established between Ministries of Health and at least some of their countries' medical schools. This must surely be a step toward the goal of making the latters' priorities and advice about resource allocation accord more closely to the distribution of the public's health problems.

To strengthen this initiative and provide yet another opportunity to learn from Thailand's remarkable progress in the application of epidemiological thinking throughout its health establishment, "INCLEN VI" was held, again in Pattaya, Thailand, on January 24-30, 1988. Early negotiations proceeded smoothly so that the meeting could be held in conjunction with another of the *International Epidemiological Association*'s (IEA) Regional Meetings, again in Southeast Asia. And once more, the UNDP/WB/WHO Special Programme for Tropical Disease Research agreed to cosponsor and finance the joint meeting.

A third negotiation was conducted with the International Field Epidemiology Training Program (FETP) of the U.S. Centers for Disease Control (CDC), which had units in India, the Philippines, Taiwan, and Thailand. Planning for the collaborative meeting involved primarily the well-developed unit in Thailand attached to the Ministry of Health; the initial reaction of the Thais was enthusiastic. The field or "shoe-leather" epidemiologists from CDC at first were reluctant to participate in a meeting with "clinical" epidemiologists. Alexander Langmuir, whom we met in Chapter 5, founder of CDC's Epidemic Intelligence Service, would have jumped at this opportunity. He placed major emphasis on attracting bright young clinicians to careers in epidemiology and public health. Like his colleague from

Scotland, the late Robert Cruickshank, professor of bacteriology at the University of Edinburgh and first president of the IEA, Langmuir would have seized the prospect of contributing to this major international meeting for "spreading the gospel." In due course, participation of the FETP was agreed, and in the event, they and their colleagues from CDC were actively involved in that and subsequent INCLEN annual meetings. This highly successful pioneering exercise in tripartite cooperation was another attempt at healing the schism.

Attended by almost 500 persons, "INCLEN VI" was reported to have been, once more, a highly successful. There were three parallel meetings, each open to those primarily involved in one of the other two. The INCLEN registration alone included 176 persons from 24 countries. All 26 CEUs were represented with 17 of the older established Units giving progress reports, and the 10 newer CEUs meeting with the CERTCs' faculties. The excellent arrangements for the meeting were carried out by the Division of Epidemiology of the Ministry of Health, and it was opened formally by the Minister of Health, the Honorable Terdpong Jayanandana. IN-CLEN was spreading its wings; in 5 years it had moved from a small gathering of 22 persons in Hawaii to this large international conference.[53]

In commenting on this second Pattaya meeting, Scott Halstead emphasized the ubiquitous power of epidemiology to guide scientific responses to the people's health needs when he wrote:

> From the Rockefeller Foundation's perspective, I hope the point was made persuasively that epidemiology can be applied from a number of perspectives. Good health requires the composite efforts of field epidemiology, outbreak epidemiology, epidemiological studies of treatment modalities, and studies of cost effectiveness of medical care. There is much to be gained [by cooperation among] these various members of the greater health team.[54]

The scientific meeting included addresses by international leaders in many applications of epidemiology; special attention was given to field epidemiology and the training program in Thailand. More than 100 scientific papers covering completed research or planned research were presented, and as has been the tradition at the Annual INCLEN Meetings, discussion of each was introduced by a member of a CERTC faculty or a senior consultant, usually a content expert. By all accounts the papers continued to improve in quality and expand in breadth of coverage; again about half could be classified as community based. Of the 46 papers involving completed research, some 70% recommended a useful change in the practice of a curative or preventive intervention. Here are the titles of illustrative papers to indicate the range of topics covered:

- Cost-effectiveness of methods of screening for diabetes mellitus;
- A drugstore survey of patterns of antibiotic use in Makati, Metro Manila;
- Diarrhea concepts and management in a rural area in Mexico;
- Incidence and risk factors for diarrhea in children under 5 in a Bangkok low socioeconomic community;
- Injuries from motorcycle use in Khon Kaen, Thailand;

- Patterns of vocabulary attainment among urban and rural children of the 9th region, Chile;
- Risk factors for obstructive airway passage disease among women in Bogota, Colombia;
- Well-controlled and less well controlled hypertension in stroke patients in Yogakarta, Indonesia;
- Effectiveness of religious health workers in improving compliance with tuberculosis chemotherapy in the Philippines;
- The effectiveness of rice-electrolyte solution in the management of acute diarrhea in Egypt;
- The multicenter study of mental disorders in Brazil: the São Paulo survey.[55]

There were other activities at the Pattaya Meeting. In addition to the Health Social Science Subcommittee Workshop, and progress reported by the E-Mail Group (subsequently known as the Telecommunications and Informatics Subcommittee), the biostatisticians met. They reexamined their role in the CEUs and saw the need for strengthening integration into each Unit's activities. The ratio of one biostatistician to six epidemiologists may need rethinking; one to three may be a more reasonable ratio—certainly that is the case if the experience at McMaster is a guide. As the group reiterated the dependence of epidemiology on statistics, one could not help recalling the seminal contributions of the early French and British statisticians discussed in Chapter 2. There were also suggestions for increasing the number of methodological papers presented at the meetings, including those by CERTC faculty and consultants. The need was reemphasized for further improvement in the design of research projects and preparation of the papers presented. Several participants expressed reservations about the relevance and quality of some of the Network's projects.

More specific statistical issues were also raised. One consultant statistician argued for much larger sample sizes than those customarily used or indicated by the usual sample size calculations. Often the most important medical questions are not being identified, a matter that may involve both statistical and medical considerations. The impact of a study in a developing country may differ substantially from that of a comparable study in a developed country; a large medical effect demonstrated by a study may offset the demand for studies that might otherwise require large numbers in the samples. Finally there needed to be greater attention paid to the career structures for biostatisticians in the CEUs. The following points were made:

- Preference should usually be placed on selecting statisticians with mathematical rather than medical backgrounds for INCLEN Fellowships;
- Important criteria for selection of statistician Fellows should be a demonstrated interest in medical problems, and an ability to communicate with consultees;
- Basic training in certain clinical areas may be desirable for some INCLEN statisticians, but this should not be a part of the INCLEN training program itself;

- Newly formed CEUs should be encouraged to select a statistician for training quite early in their development, perhaps around the time the third Fellow is chosen;
- Selection of a statistician for the CEU should be seen as a long term investment. An evolutionary period of several years may be needed for him or her to develop good working relationships and skills in the various areas of clinical research;
- Collaborative statistical work on applied rather than theoretical problems should be rewarded. Career incentives and structure should be built on this premise;
- Wherever possible, the statistician should be given a faculty position, preferably in the medical schools associated with the CEU.
- The work of statisticians which leads to publications should be recognized by authorships.[56]

Another important group at INCLEN VI was that devoted to Continuing Education and Distance Learning. They agreed on the following recommendations:

- Each CEU should be encouraged to hold weekly self-directed, problem-oriented, continuing education (CE) sessions. One CEU member should take prime responsibility for organizing these. CERTC faculty should be asked for their help from afar, and the mini-library would be an important resource;
- A demand for a series of modules on advanced epidemiology and biostatistics topics for use by CEU members has emerged, and detailed proposals should be sought for the development and utilization of such a series;
- Short courses on particular topics in various regions should be tried out. There is considerable expressed demand from CEUs for these;
- Each INCLEN Annual Meeting should include one or more formal Continuing Education sessions, These may be in the form of a 1- to 2-day workshop before the meeting or in sessions during the meeting. The issue of CE should also appear for discussion on the meeting agenda;
- Site visit forms should be amended to include information on the CE activities of the CEU. The site visits should include time for discussion and the items for this identified in advance;
- CEUs should consider whether or when they wish to begin their own training programs in clinical epidemiology. Continuing discussion should identify whether there is a need for Distance Learning modules or formal courses to which CERTC faculty and materials might contribute.[57]

On March 29, 1988, the Foundation's Board appropriated another $1.4 million to further the development of INCLEN, bringing the total appropriations from the Foundation to almost $10.0 million since inception of the Health of Populations component in 1979. At the end of 1988 it was anticipated that 96 clinical epidemiologists, 9 biostatisticians, and 6 clinical economists from 15 countries would have completed training. Besides the Rockefeller Foundation, 10 other international agencies had supported the training of 41 additional Fellows at the INCLEN CERTCs; 29 were from the *INCLEN CEUs*, and 12 from affiliated or nearby institutions. By this time the new CERTC at Université Claude Bernard had been officially designated. In 1988 the highly successful 3-month Toronto Management Training Short Course had 28 applicants for the course of whom 12 were accepted. The six modules about which the course is built are Research Design, Information Sciences, Management Skills, Biostatistics and Data Management, Health Policy, and Medical Education.[58,59]

Antibiotics consume the largest portion of the budgets for drugs in the developing world and are a major factor in costs everywhere. More importantly, their indiscriminant use poses major health hazards to individuals and populations. Both patients and physicians are influenced in their use by behavioral factors (including Factor "X"). These, in turn, are strongly conditioned by social and cultural belief systems and traditions and, therefore, understanding them is of fundamental importance for improving matters. Under the leadership of Calvin M. Kunin, M.D., Professor of Medicine, Ohio State University, representatives of the Multicenter Study Group on Antibiotic Use and the Health Social Sciences Subcommittee had a preliminary meeting on June 30, 1988, to map future strategies. As a consequence, the CERTCs' Advisory Committee, meeting on September 8-9, 1988, decided that the original Multicenter Study Group on Antibiotic Use would be broadened in scope and elevated in importance within *INCLEN* by the establishment of a Pharmacoepidemiology Task Force under the direction of Kunin.[60]

Progress on other fronts was reported from a number of the CEUs in the course of the year. At Universidad de la Frontera, Temuco, Chile, the CEU acquired new and larger space and developed links with the Chilean National Health Service. At Christian Medical College, Vellore, India, new space was also provided in the main hospital. Plans were even discussed for creating INDIACLEN. The CEU at West China University of Medical Sciences provided extensive teaching for undergraduates, postgraduates, and students from other provincial institutions. This group also took the lead in 1988 for organizing a highly successful National Conference on Clinical Epidemiology, held at Chengdu in April 1989. At this meeting CHINACLEN was established—another manifestation of the spread of epidemiological thinking within countries. In Indonesia, Tonny Sadjimin, M.D., one of the earliest graduates of the McMaster program as well as recipient of a Ph.D. in epidemiology from the University of Western Ontario, headed up the CEU at Gadjah Mada University, Yogyakarta, and soon organized INDOCLEN among the medical schools of Indonesia. Further evidence of constructive collaboration with ministries of health occurred in Indonesia when Sadjimin was asked by his government to supervise two FETP trainees.

Although INCLEN's development has been phenomenal, it was not without its risks. Claims cannot yet be made for its ultimate success, only for its aspirations, progress toward stated objectives, and favorable subjective judgments by those not directly involved. The sponsors and participants are, of course, delighted, but they are not entirely disinterested. "Tincture of enthusiasm," and the Hawthorne effect, all play important roles in attempts to effect change, even among those who regard themselves as critics of all they read, most of what they hear, and even some of what they see. The March 29, 1989, docket item for the Rockefeller Foundation Board had this to say about the risks inherent in the INCLEN experiment:

> The principal risk [is] that in some CEU institutions clinical epidemiology may not become firmly established because the Fellows are hampered by inadequate research funding, because they are not permitted sufficient time for research and teaching, or even because they are transferred elsewhere. Ultimately, INCLEN must be judged by the improvements it effects through the practice of clinical epidemiology on health research, health care, and incidence rates for preventable or curable diseases....

> Interim evaluation will continue to be based on the degree to which CEUs succeed in attaining an administrative identity, making an impact on undergraduate and post-graduate medical training, and establishing defined research goals on priority health problems, or resource-consuming health services.[61]

The 1989 Annual Meeting took place in Goa, India, January 22-27; it was "INCLEN VII." Again cosponsored by the Rockefeller Foundation, the UNDP/WB/WHO/Special Programme for Tropical Disease Research and the USAID, the meeting was attended by almost 300 persons, including 85 Fellows from the CEUs, the content experts, several deans of schools of public health, and faculty from the department of international health of the Johns Hopkins School of Hygiene and Public Health that now has an advisory status with INCLEN. Workshops before and during the meeting were held by the groups concerned with Biostatistics, Clinical Economics, Health Social Sciences, Pharmacoepidemiology, Cardiovascular Disease, Pediatric Respiratory Diseases, Thromboembolic Stroke, and Telecommunications and Informatics. The first Scientific Writing Workshop was also held, and critiques of individual manuscripts were offered to interested Fellows. Another topic that attracted a number of participants was Occupational and Environmental Epidemiology; this group was encouraged by the CERTCs' Advisory Committee to conduct a survey of CEUs to determine the extent of interest in further developing a field of growing global importance.

Because INCLEN is an educational as well as a research modality, a special session was devoted to methods for refining the educational objectives of CEUs and assessing progress toward their attainment. Two new ideas were advanced: first, that each CEU should have an "education correspondent," and second, that a handbook should be prepared on the "Role of the CEU in Education." These ideas were given greater specificity by their proponents Professors Chitr Sitthi-Amorn, M.D., of Chulalongkorn University, Bangkok, and Victor R. Neufeld, M.D., of McMaster. One criterion proposed for assessing a CEU's educational accomplishments would be periodic surveillance of the burden of illness in the population served. Trends in the health status of the community would be followed over time as a guide to helping the medical faculty place health problems in some rational priority as a guide to curriculum development and revision. Both the ideas and the methods had been developed by a Task Force of the Network of Community-Oriented Educational Institutions for Health Sciences.[62] These ideas were well received and would be acted upon. INCLEN was now well on the way to becoming institutionalized.[63]

A new departure was the requirement that, following a Fellow's initial participation in an annual meeting when a study protocol can be presented, only completed research could be accepted for presentation at the annual scientific meetings. In spite of this limitation more papers than ever were presented, 87 all told, of which about 45% were community based. Stimulating hospital-based academic clinicians to devote consistently almost half of their collective research efforts to studies of patients and populations beyond hospital walls must surely represent a change in medical priorities, especially in the developing world. In addition another 62 new research proposals were systematically discussed with preceptors and content experts; formerly these activities had been part of the scheduled presentations.[64]

In her 1982 Program Review, Professor Carol Buck had made specific proposals with criteria for evaluating progress by each of the CEUs and by INCLEN as an entity. The issue of evaluation was again raised at the Hawaii meeting when the principal objectives for INCLEN were enunciated by the Faculties involved. An outline based on Carol Buck's strategy was developed at that time but had yet to be implemented. At INCLEN II an outline of "Criteria for Success of a *CEU*" was presented by Peter Tugwell of McMaster and endorsed. The substantial expansion of the Network in India with its numerous (well over 100) medical schools provided an excellent opportunity for a structured evaluation. Accordingly an India INCLEN Assessment Team was established in January 1988 with Mark C. Steinhoff, Associate Professor of International Health and Pediatrics of the Johns Hopkins University, as Coordinator. An extensive baseline protocol was prepared with interviews and document analyses conducted at the original three medical schools selected to join INCLEN, and at three relatively similar schools that might be used for comparison purposes. The intent is to repeat the survey in 1992 and again after 10 years.[65]

Robert and Suzanne Fletcher, professors of medicine and clinical epidemiology and co-directors of the CERTC at the University of North Carolina, spent 5 weeks in 1989 preparing a thorough plan for the overall evaluation of INCLEN. Their approach was similar to those proposed by Buck and Tugwell but now included much greater detail and heirarchical specificity.[66] They related INCLEN'S agreed-upon objectives to criteria for evaluation. That the Fletchers have grasped the true potential of the program and the essence of the arguments advanced in earlier chapters of this volume, is illustrated by the following statement:

> In most Third World countries, as in developed countries, power and influence to change medical care resides primarily with physicians. An important period in the development of professional attitudes is the time during medical education. Within medical education institutions, clinical departments of schools of medicine are more influential than departments of social and administrative medicine, and there are few schools of public health. The clinical departments set the agenda for the curriculum,

medical students' perceptions of what is important in medicine, and the allocation of resources. Therefore any program aimed at developing more effective management of health services around the world should include medical educators and the clinical departments of medical schools. Only with such an approach would practicing physicians become convinced of the importance of the population perspective of health, and of health services at the organizational level.[67]

My conclusion from the analyses presented in Chapters 4 and 5 was that, other accomplishments aside, departments of community, preventive, or social medicine, and schools of public health have, for the most part, failed in their efforts to provide all physicians with the population perspective. In fostering INCLEN's approach it behooves us, therefore, to be specific about the way in which its impact is to be assessed; the Fletchers have done this. Without unduly burdening the reader by describing the major measures and indicators proposed, an outline of the criteria to be used should interest medical educators:

Fellows

1. Fellows should have active, successful research careers including:
   - Completion of the research project begun during INCLEN training;
   - Publication of original research;
   - Funding for research;
   - Time for research.
2. Fellows should teach what they have learned in INCLEN.
3. Fellows should continue to work as clinicians and as clinical role models.
4. Fellows should participate in the activities of their CEU.
5. Fellows should be promoted in academic rank.

Clinical Epidemiology Units (CEUs)

1. CEU faculty should have the best personnel and physical arrangements:
   - At least the prescribed complement of Fellows;
   - Adequate space;
   - Support staff;
   - Easy access to computer facilities;
   - Easy access to rapid international communication systems;
   - Rapid access to basic references for clinical epidemiology;
   - Capacity to perform literature searches.
2. The CEU should have an effective management system.
3. The CEU faculty, as a group, should have successful and balanced research programs:
   - Proportion of publications that include clinical epidemiology contents and methods;

- The balance with respect to:
  - Hospital versus community sample;
  - Communicable versus noncommunicable disease;
  - Various kinds of research questions;
  - Various kinds of research designs;
  - International versus local journals;
  - Order of authorship;
  - Local versus multicenter studies;
  - Original research versus other publications;
  - Priority health problems versus less important ones;
  - Funding for research.
4. CEU members, taken together, should teach clinical epidemiology, biostatistics, clinical economics, and the health social sciences.

Institutions

1. The medical school should include "clinical epidemiology" (broadly defined) in its curriculum.
2. The medical school's patient care programs should reflect insights gained through clinical epidemiology.
3. The CEU faculty should be involved in institutional health care and educational policy decisions.
4. The CEU faculty should be involved in the research of faculty and students outside the CEU.
5. The institution should conduct an ongoing analysis of the priority health problems in its region.

Regions

1. The CEU faculty should be involved in:
   - Health policymaking with local and regional policymakers;
   - Regional research policy;
   - Regional education.

International

1. INCLEN graduates should participate in international bodies that are concerned with:
   - Health policy;
   - Clinical and health services research policy;
   - Medical educational policy.

The data for accomplishing this evaluation are now being accumulated. In the meantime, we do have one useful measure of achievement. Since the first trainee returned home to a CEU, as of October 5, 1989, 302 journal articles have been published by INCLEN Fellows; these are apart from books, book chapters, translations, and conference presentations. The majority of the papers were published in local or, more frequently, national or regional medical publications. More than 60, however, were published in major English language journals, most frequently in specialty journals. Eleven papers and one "letter-to-the-editor" were published in international medical journals such as the *British Medical Journal*, the *Lancet*, and *New England Journal of Medicine*, and in the *American Journal of Epidemiology* and the *International Journal of Epidemiology*.[69] All these journals are known to have high editorial standards based on peer review by biostatisticians and senior epidemiologists. INCLEN Fellows are on the Editorial Boards of 18 national medical journals and are planning 2 new journals in clinical epidemiology and research design. In addition to the texts written by Professor Wang Jialang of Chengdu, Professor Chitr Sitthi-Amorn of Chulalongkorn (one of the participants in the 1980 Cambridge Workshop) has written a volume entitled *Clinical Epidemiology: A Population Targeted Approach to Health Reform*.[70]

On the educational front, three INCLEN medical schools are involved in curriculum redesign exercises. Clinical Economics Fellows are now returning to their home CEUs, but such has been the interest generated by one Fellow that, in the course of 5 months, he gave 100 lectures on the principles of cost-effectiveness analysis and related matters. Strategies for savings in health care costs that do not imperil the quality of care may well turn out to be INCLEN's most powerful agent for effecting behavior changes and priorities by physicians, policymakers, politicians, and eventually the public.

There is, of course, no way of knowing whether all these articles, positions on editorial boards, curriculum exercises, and lectures might not have evolved without INCLEN. The output does appear to be substantial and although, as in all aspects of INCLEN's activities, there is much room for growth and improvement, the fact that clinicians are engaged in these extended activities must attest to a reasonably high level of commitment and competence at this time.

Another significant contribution to foster our mutual objectives was taken with the inauguration of *Bridge*, an international newsletter linking the producers and users of Health Systems (another code term for Health Services) Research, and Clinical Epidemiology. Supported by the Rockefeller Foundation, it is a joint undertaking of the World Health Organization, including its Regional Office for the Americas, the Pan American Health Organization, the Foundation for Health Services Research, and INCLEN.[71] The first issue was distributed to 1400 readers in the United States and to 1600 in other countries, including translations into Spanish and Arabic; subsequent issues were almost twice that size. The distinguishing feature of this newsletter is the focus on research as a means of empowering those in the Third World to ask and investigate questions bearing on their own health problems and health services. Rather than copy the policies and practices of the developed world, many of questionable benefit even in their original settings, investigators in the Third World acquire the capacity to develop their own solutions and order their own priorities.

By the end of 1989, 148 Fellows from the 26 CEUs had been trained: 33 internists, 24 pediatricians, 15 obstetrician/gynecologists, 5 family physicians, 2 psychiatrists, 1 anesthesiologist, 11 biostatisticians, and 4 health social scientists.[72] Another 35 Fellows have been accepted for 1989-1990, and an additional 12 for the 3-month Management Training Short Course at the University of Toronto CERTC. Three of the trainees are faculty members for the newly established Francophone CERTC at Université Claude Bernard at Lyons. The full Faculty complement for each of the 27 CEUs of about 10 core staff all told will amount to some 270 faculty who must be trained; that means training should proceed until 1992 or 14 years after the Health of Populations component started. Additional time will be required to train faculty for the Francophone CEUs that have yet to be selected. In 1989 the sponsors of the CEUs, each of which receives annual support from the Rockefeller Foundation, included: 14 deans, 3 associate deans, 5 department chairmen, 2 hospital directors, and 3 research directors. Their responsibilities have been refined further so that they now undertake to:

- Assist is the selection of Fellows who have research aptitude, leadership capacity, are in tenure track positions, and who, on return, will have positions with clinical teaching and research responsibilities;
- See that Fellows have 20% or more of their time protected for research;
- Create an administrative structure for management of the CEU;
- Set aside convenient space for the members of the *CEU* to work and hold discussions;
- Ensure that returning Fellows not be transferred for a period of at least 5 years.

The educational programs at the four basic CERTCs (excluding Toronto and Lyons) are not standardized but they have agreed that they will all cover common elements. The duration of training is 9 to 16 months and leads to an M.Sc. or M.S. degree. Five to seven Fellows are accepted by each CERTC annually. Tutorials and small-group seminars are used extensively, but there are also more formal exercises in epidemiology, biostatistics, and research design. Using their own clinical experiences and data from their own countries, which they bring with them, each Fellow undertakes an exercise that places the health problems of his or her own municipality, region, or nation in priority order—explaining the rationale behind the order. Finally, written designs are prepared for a research project to be carried out by the Fellow on return home and supported by the initial $5,000 start-up grant.

The close of 1989 marked the start of another phase for INCLEN. It was time to consider the establishment of CERTCs within the developing countries themselves so that they can continue training indigenous colleagues for other medical schools within their countries and even their regions. China, Thailand, and India have already taken steps in this direction. Yet another Bellagio Meeting was held (October 8-13, 1989) to discuss the criteria for selecting additional CERTCs in developing countries. Other decisions were made with respect to the future role of the present CERTCs in supporting the entire Network.[73]

One important development concerns the institutional future of INCLEN: At some point, it must become independent of the Rockefeller Foundation. Much progress had been made in this direction, and, as noted, 10 national and international agencies were already supporting parts of the Network by 1989; the Executive Office, established at the University of Pennsylvania, was managing the day-to-day activities of INCLEN. Toward the end of 1988, INCLEN, Inc. was created; this new corporation, which is tax exempt in the United States, is undoubtedly eligible for similar status in other countries. It has its own Board of Trustees, and in due course will have its own Executive Director and full-time headquarters staff with responsibility for all recordkeeping, selection procedures, fund-raising, disbursements, and general institutional support.

One model that could serve as a prototype was used to build on the original "green revolution" initiatives. Like several other major twentieth-century innovations, it too had its origins at Bellagio. The Foundation supported the establishment of agricultural research and training centers located in Mexico, Colombia, Chile, India, and the Philippines. The first of these, the International Rice Research Institute in the Philippines, was established in 1960 with support from the Government of the Philippines and the Ford and Rockefeller foundations. By 1980 there were 13 such institutes in the developing world. They cover, in addition to rice, wheat, maize, potatoes, livestock, and animal diseases, the problems of agriculture in tropical and semiarid countries, and plant genetics. Starting in 1971 this network, supported by an informal consortium of governments, international assistance agencies, and the Rockefeller, Ford, and Kellogg foundations, was known as the Consultative Group on International Agricultural Research (CGIAR). In 1981, the Consortium, with more than 30 governmental and institutional members, spent $139 million for the capital and operating costs of these Institutes.

Still in being, a related but separate and autonomous, nonprofit technical assistance agency, the International Agricultural Development Agency, was established by the Rockefeller Foundation in 1975. It was later transformed into the International Services for National Agricultural Research with headquarters in the Hague. The purpose of this entity was to provide long-range advice (but not financial support) for developing countries adopting and adapting research findings of the CGIAR System's Institutes to the needs of those countries in which the latter were located and in other countries.[74]

There is much to be learned from the long history and experiences of these highly productive agricultural institutions that can be applied to INCLEN. For the concepts and methods embodied in INCLEN to endure, broader involvement of governments, international assistance agencies, and foundations is required. Of greater importance, however, is the need to create a self-perpetuating global institution to carry on the work now barely begun. Possible solutions may emerge from the report of the Commission on Health Research for Development.[75,76] One of the principal objectives of the Commission is to stimulate governments and international assistance agencies to support and foster the use of epidemiological and related research in developing countries—research with a label that stresses its importance: Essential National Health Research. The Commission emphasizes the urgent need to develop and promote strategies that will encourage policymakers and politicians to demand more research of this kind, especially as it relates to economic evaluation of medical interventions and priorities for health services.

INCLEN remains a hypothesis until final evaluations are completed. Enough time should elapse to be certain that the enthusiasm of the pioneers (the Hawthorne and Placebo effects, Factor "X") has faded or been factored in to the final assessments and that any changes for the better are enduring. Sometime after 1999, 20 years after INCLEN's inception, a judgment can be advanced. Under INCLEN's auspices, there are only 27 schools in the developing world and 6 (including Toronto and Lyons) in developed countries which, to varying degrees, embrace the population perspective through epidemiological approaches, especially in their clinical departments. Other medical schools in North America (e.g., Harvard University, University of Texas, San Antonio; University of Washington, Seattle; Yale University), Europe, and Australasia have established active programs in clinical epidemiology—some, as noted earlier, several years before the advent of INCLEN. What INCLEN is attempting to demonstrate is that the horizons of medical faculties in the Third World can be expanded and that training in population-based research empowers young faculty to understand, and it is hoped eventually to cope with, the health problems of entire communities. INCLEN has trained many more Fellows than other programs with related objectives, but much more is urgently needed in both the developed and developing worlds.

Further encouraging evidence of change is to be found in the progress made by the North American Health of the Public program launched in 1986 by the Pew Charitable Trusts and the Rockefeller Foundation. The goals are similar to those of INCLEN. From 89 applicants, six universities were selected initially: Columbia, the Johns Hopkins, North Carolina, New Mexico, Tufts, and Washington at Seattle; four of these have both medical schools and schools of public health. As an embryonic network these six programs aim to redirect priorities for medical education and health research in their respective institutions to accord more directly with the needs of the public each serves. There is also the longer term prospect that some or all of them may be able to provide training in clinical epidemiology and related population-based disciplines to candidates from the Third World in addition to domestic trainees.[77,78]

Forty-four medical schools worldwide are members of the Network of Community-Oriented Educational Institutions for Health Sciences—yet another innovative approach to redirecting medical education so that eventually populations will be served by more balanced health care systems (see Chapter 7). An additional 72 institutions are associate members. The sixth biennial meeting of the Network held at Maastricht, the Netherlands, (September 17-19, 1989), was attended by more than 300 participants, including 40 medical students and several Ministers of Health. As active Network members, the faculties of these schools are committed to reordering institutional priorities so that educational, research, and patient care objectives are related directly to the health problems of their populations.[79] With the possible exceptions of McMaster in Canada and Newcastle in Australia, nowhere is the transition reasonably complete from strategies that rely solely on the biomedical and clinical approaches to those that include the population perspective. Even in these two exemplary institutions there is much that remains to be accomplished.

Other entities are trying to *heal the schism* in the Third World. Examples include the World Health Organization's Special Programme for Research and Training in Tropical Disease Research; WHO's Programme of Health Systems Research and Development that provides fellowships, workshops, short courses, and research grants; the Community Epidemiology and Health Management Network with its short courses and grants, and the fellowships and institutional support of the International Health Policy Program. There is now the prospect that these and other organizations will join together in a coordinated fashion under the umbrella of the Commission on Health Services Research for Development.

"INCLEN VIII" held at Puebla, Mexico (January 18-26, 1990), included joint activities with the Field Epidemiology Training Program, the World Bank, the Commission on Health Research and Development, and representatives of other organizations interested in healing the schism. To this end some 10 international networks and consortia dedicated to improving the public's health in Third World countries signed *A Declaration of Agreement* (*The Puebla Declaration*) in which they committed themselves to furthering the goals set out by the Commission in support of Essential National Research for Development.[80] This development has the power to promote cooperation instead of competition among those with similar, if not identical, objectives in the Third World.

The plethora of terms used to describe this fairly straightforward arena might startle the likes of William Petty. We now have Clinical Epidemiology, Clinical Economics, Health Economics, Health Services Research, Health Systems Research, Public Health Research, Health Care Evaluation and Assessment, Outcomes Research, Medical Audit, Functional Assessment, Health Policy Research, Technology Assessment, Decision Analysis, Cost-Benefit and Cost-Effectiveness Analyses, and probably others. Are all these labels really necessary?[81] Is not the essential element in each of these activities the study of groups or populations, in addition to the study of cells and individuals? Why cannot they all be encompassed by the term population-based studies? This is the perspective that has to be restored to its original place alongside the biomedical and clinical perspectives.

In the meantime, given the urgent needs for help, especially in the developing world, the seeming inability of the present arrangements to cope adequately with determining health priorities, allocating resources, restraining costs, improving access, and raising quality, there is little to lose in retrying an old approach in a new configuration. At the very least INCLEN should serve to introduce more young physicians to the population perspective and help them to understand better the work of other epidemiologists and public health workers in general. Above all it empowers them with the concepts and skills required to ask and answer questions scientifically and to make their own choices. Demands may even increase for further graduate education in these fields, not only within medical schools but from schools of public health. Scott Halstead summarized the current status of INCLEN when he wrote:

> The excitement being created by INCLEN may reflect merely the relative weakness of the biomedical research communities in developing countries and the attractions of a remedial program. To this observer, the task-orientation, strong methodologic basis, and population orientation of clinical epidemiology has created in many Fellows, for the first time in their careers, a sense of being in control of frighteningly complex health care systems. This may be the dynamic by which disciplined research can serve as a vector for social change.[82]

References

1. Bishop FM. Prevention: wave of the future. J Community Health 1980;5:221-227 (222).
2. White KL. Contemporary epidemiology: perspectives and uses. Epidemiol Bull (Pan American Health Organization) 1984;5:13-16, (13).
3. Ibid, p. 16.
4. Buck C, Llopis A, Nájera E, Terris M. *The Challenge of Epidemiology: Issues and Selected Readings*. Scientific Publication No. 505. Washington, D.C.: Pan American Health Organization, 1988:984.
5. Ibid, p. 815.
6. Ibid, p. 981.
7. Ibid, p. 984.
8. *INCLEN Newsletter*, # 2, August, 1984. New York: Rockefeller Foundation, 1984:5.
9. Ibid, pp. 2-3.
10. Ibid, p. 4.
11. Second Annual Meeting. *Minutes of the CERTC/RF Meetings*, January 29-February 3, 1984. New York: Rockefeller Foundation, April 1984:24 (unpublished).
12. Ibid, p. 2.
13. *INCLEN Newsletter, Volume 10, # 2*, December 1989, pp. 8-9.
14. *INCLEN Newsletter, #2*, August 1984, p.16.
15. Second Annual Meeting. *Minutes of the CERTC/RF Meetings*, January 29-February 3, 1984. New York: Rockefeller Foundation, April 1984:3.
16. *Report of the Second Annual Meeting of the International Clinical Epidemiology Network*. Pattaya, Thailand, January 29-February 3, 1984. New York: Rockefeller Foundation, 1984:18 (unpublished).
17. Memorandum from Scott B. Halstead to Richard W. Lyman, March 1, 1984. New York: Rockefeller Foundation, 1984:1.
18. Ibid, p. 22.
19. Second Annual Meeting. Minutes of the CERTC/RF Meetings, January 29-February 3, 1984. New York: Rockefeller Foundation, April 1984:16.
20. *Report of Second Annual Meeting of the International Clinical Epidemiology Network*, Pattaya, Thailand, January 29-February 3, 1984. New York: Rockefeller Foundation, 1984:21.
21. Memorandum from Scott B. Halstead to Richard W. Lyman, March 1, 1984. New York: Rockefeller Foundstion, 1984:3.

22. *Third Annual INCLEN Meeting: Program*, Cavite, The Philippines, January 27-February 1, 1985. New York: Rockefeller Foundation, 1985 (unpublished).
23. Sackett DL, Haynes RB, Tugwell, P. *Clinical Epidemiolgy: A Basic Science for Clinical Medicine*. Boston: Little, Brown, 1985.
24. Report of the Health Economics Subcommittee as Agreed at *INCLEN III*, January 27-1 February, 1985, Cavite, The Philippines. *The Role of Economic Analysis in the International Clinical Epidemiology Network*. New York: Rockefeller Foundation, 1985, pp.4-5. These findings were reaffirmed in the minutes of the same Committee at Holderness, New Hampshire, September 2-4, 1986 (unpublished).
25. Ibid, p. 13.
26. Ibid, p. 2.
27. Eisenberg JM. From clinical epidemiology to clinical economics. J Gen Intern Med 1988;3:299-300.
28. Eisenberg J. Clinical economics. JAMA 1989;262:2879-2886.
29. Burrows GN, Grayston T, Jamison DT. *Mid-term Evaluation of the International Clinical Epidemiology Network*. 29 May, 1985. New York: Rockefeller Foundation, 1985 (unpublished).
30. Ibid, p. 4.
31. *INCLEN Newsletters* # 4, November 1985; # 5, July 1986; # 6, July 1987; and Dockets for the Rockefeller Foundation Board of Trustees' Meetings on December 2-3, 1985, April 2, 1986, and June 20, 1986.
32. *INCLEN Newsletter* # 5, July 1986.
33. *Fourth Annual INCLEN Meeting: Program and Abstracts*, Shanghai, China, April 6-11, 1986. New York: Rockefeller Foundation, 1986 (unpublished).
34. Fletcher RH, Fletcher SW, Wagner EH. *Clinical Epidemiology: The Essentials*, 2d Ed. Baltimore: Williams & Wilkins, 1988.
35. *INCLEN Newsletter* # 6, July 1987, p. 1.
36. Ibid, pp. 8-12.
37. Ibid, p. 2.
38. University of Toronto *CERTC* Faculty: Multicenter collaborative research: A summary document of the collaborative research workshop held January 1989 in Goa, India. Toronto, University of Toronto, October 12, 1989 (unpublished).
39. Ibid.
40. *Fifth Annual INCLEN Meeting: Program and Abstracts*, Oaxaca, Mexico, January 25-30, 1987. New York: Rockefeller Foundation, 1987 (unpublished).
41. *INCLEN Newsletter* # 6, July 1987, p. 9.
42. *INCLEN Newsletter* # 7, December 1987, p. 2.
43. Ibid, p. 2.
44. Proposal for the *INCLEN* Health Social Science Training Component attached to letter to Scott B. Halstead, M.D., New York: Rockefeller Foundation, February 18, 1987.
45. Health Social Science Subcommittee. *Proposal for the INCLEN Social Science Training Component*. New York: Rockefeller Foundation, 1987 (unpublished).
46. Proposal for the *INCLEN* Health Social Science Training Component attached to letter to Scott B. Halstead, M.D., New York: Rockefeller Foundation, February 18, 1987.
47. Social Science Training in *INCLEN*. Docket for the Rockefeller Foundation Board of Trustees' Meeting on June 19, 1987.
48. *INCLEN Newsletter* # 7, December 1987, pp. 4-5.
49. Ibid, pp. 15-18.

50. Ibid, p. 3.
51. National Epidemiology Board of Thailand—Fact Finding Commission: *Review of the Health Situation in Thailand—Priority Ranking of Diseases.* Bangkok: The Board, 1987.
52. Rockefeller Foundation. National research and policy boards: Information booklet, (Mimeographed). New York: Rockefeller Foundation, January 1988.
53. *Sixth Annual INCLEN Meeting: Program and Abstracts*, Pattaya, Thailand, January 24-30, 1988. New York: Rockefeller Foundation, 1988 (unpublished).
54. Ibid, p. 2.
55. Ibid.
56. *INCLEN Newsletter* # 8, June 1988, pp. 9-10.
57. Ibid, p. 11.
58. Ibid, p. 24.
59. University of Toronto *CERTC*: Toronto executive short course: Proposed management module. Toronto: University of Toronto *CERTC*, October 9, 1989 (unpublished).
60. *INCLEN Newsletter* # 9, November 1988, pp. 11-12.
61. Clinical Epidemiology Docket Item for the Rockefeller Foundation Board of Trustees Meeting, March 29, 1988, p.5.
62. Network of Community-Oriented Educational Institutions for Health Sciences, Task Force II: Priority health problems in medical education—Final summary report, (Mimeographed). McMaster University, September 1989.
63. *INCLEN Newsletter Vol. 10, # 1,* June 1989, p. 2.
64. *Seventh Annual INCLEN Meeting: Program and Abstracts*, Goa, India, January 22-27, 1989. New York: Rockefeller Foundation, 1989 (unpublished).
65. Steinhoff M, Murthy N, Nichter M, Pereira S. *Baseline Assessment: The India INCLEN Program.* Fort Aguada, Goa, India, January, 1989 (unpublished).
66. Fletcher RH, Fletcher SW. *A Plan for Evaluation of the International Clinical Epidemiology Network (INCLEN).* Bellagio, Italy: Rockefeller Foundation Study and Conference Center, March 1989 (unpublished).
67. Ibid, p. 8.
68. Ibid, pp. 34-39.
69. Computer printout of all publications by *INCLEN* Fellows, October 5, 1989, New York: Rockefeller Foundation, 1989.
70. Chitr S-A. *Clinical Epidemiology: A Population Targeted Approach to Health Reform.* Bangkok: Chulalongkorn University, 1989.
71. Foundation for Health Services Research. Washington, D.C.: *Bridge*, Number 1, Spring 1989 and Number 2, Summer/Fall 1989.
72. Halstead SB, Tugwell P, Bennett K. The International Clinical Epidemiology Network (*INCLEN*): A progress report. J Clin Epidemiol (in press).
73. Rockefeller Foundation. The International Clinical Epidemiology Network (*INCLEN*): Design for the Future. Papers prepared for the Meeting at the Bellagio Study and Conference Center, October 9-11, 1989;44:579-589.
74. *Annual Reports, 1974-82.* New York: Rockefeller Foundation.
75. Anon. Independent International Commission in Health Research Development. Lancet 1987;ii:1076-1077.
76. Commission on Health Research for Development. *Health Research: Essential Link to Equity in Development.* New York: Oxford University Press, 1990.
77. Schroeder SA, Zones JS, Showback JA. Academic medicine as a public trust. JAMA 1989;262:803-812.

78. Duban S, Hickey M, Kaufman A. Grantwatch-Health of the public: an academic challenge. Health Affairs 1990;9:159-160.
79. The Network of Community-Oriented Educational Institutions for Health Sciences. *A Short Description of its Aims and Activities.* Maastricht, The Netherlands, University of Limburg: The Network, 1987, and personal communication from Professor Victor Neufeld, Chairman of the Network, September 30, 1989.
80. The Puebla Declaration. Washington, D.C.: Foundation for Health Services Research, 1990; Bridge, No. 4, Spring, p. 5.
81. White KL. On confusing the name with the thing! Washington, D.C.: Foundation for Health Services Research, 1989; Bridge, No.3, Winter, pp. 2-3.
82. Halstead SB. Epidemiological research: a vector for social change. Address presented at *INCLEN VI*, Pattaya Beach, Thailand, January 23, 1988 (unpublished). I am indebted to this address for numerous other facts and figures scattered throughout this chapter.

9
Back to the Future

Change is the order of the day! Industries, banks, governments, the military, even churches and sometimes universities, restructure ever more frequently. Mergers, acquisitions, takeovers, divestments, closures, bankruptcies, changed policies, and fresh managements are the instruments of change. Rapid dissemination of new knowledge and old wisdom keep shifting the opportunities, expectations, and values to which the social institutions of our global village must respond. The health and medical enterprises are no exceptions; change has occurred in the past and it will in the future. The the medical establishment's problems are among the most daunting—even threatening—because of the profession's traditional top-down, elitist, "doctors know best" stance. But that too will change, or be changed.

To the public health component of our collective endeavor, society owes a great debt of gratitude for its persistent efforts at "redefining the unacceptable." Often in the face of enormous obstacles, those laboring in this vineyard persisted in drawing attention, for example, to the influence of social factors on health and disease, to mounting health hazards, and to large pockets of contemporary neglect and deprivation. Contributing both knowledge and energy, many in schools of public health and health departments have pointed out the destructive imbalances and resource misallocations that plague efforts to provide rational health services in both the developed and developing worlds. They have even stressed the distortions in contemporary medical education and the mindless adherence to a constricted biomedical paradigm for both explaining disease causation and assessing the benefits of interventions.

Above all, we are especially indebted to the schools of public health for stabilizing and nurturing epidemiology (and the other population-based disciplines) as fundamental sciences for the entire health enterprise. True, epidemiology had its conception and childhood in clinical medicine, and different decisions along the way might have produced different results, but the fact remains that for more than seven decades epidemiology has flourished and evolved primarily in schools of public health. Useful as they have been, however, these arrangements may need to be reexamined. Redefining the unacceptable is an exercise that can be applied internally within the health system as well as externally.

252

Nor is the old top-down approach to the provision of health services acceptable in either developed or developing countries. No other service sector in society operates without a clear assessment of its "market" (to use commercial parlance), its "catchment area" (to use health services jargon), or its denominator (to use epidemiological and demographic terminology). The World Health Organization (WHO) and UNICEF deserve credit for making explicit this sea change in expectations and values. In 1978 the declaration of Alma Ata proclaimed the goal of "Health for All by the Year 2000." Largely ignored by most medical academicians in developed countries, this slogan articulated in simple terms the hopes of desperate millions in the Third World to which the health establishment must respond.[1]

Exactly what population should a medical school and its related institutions serve, with services, education, and research? Is it the municipality, the county, region, province, the country, or the world? Who decides and on what basis? Some health problems must be more important than others. Some must cause more days lost from work or school, more days in pain, in bed, or in hospital. Some must "cost" individuals and society more than others, by whatever measure we choose to use. Not for long is it likely the public or its politicians will accept pleas for more money unsupported by population-based analyses. Soon it should be unacceptable for a hospital or health facility to set priorities without a firmly grounded population-based information system. Similarly, medical schools will ignore at their peril the public's expectations when they determine the numbers and types of physicians they graduate. Nor will it be acceptable for clinical research agendas, in contrast to truly fundamental research, to disregard the health problems of those who do the suffering and foot the bills. The health establishment will soon be surrounded by the twenty first-century paradigm shift, based largely on the information revolution.[2,3] Exactly what are the goals of "public health" and of "medicine"? It was Albert Einstein who observed that the greatest difficulty confronting the twentieth century revolved around the persistent ambiguity of our "goals" as we perfect the "means."

From every corner of the health field the need for change crowds in. "Popsie" Welch's landmark point has been made! Large segments of the world's population and the world's health problems had been too long neglected by the medical school over which he presided in Baltimore. In many ways, the early twentieth century public health pioneers have triumphed. The task now is to translate that message back into the language and activities of the entire health establishment. No longer can ephemeral academic *schisms* be allowed to disrupt the worldwide goal of dedicating all our efforts to improving the public's health. Franklin Paine Mall (1862-1917), a preeminent scientist and first professor of anatomy at the Johns Hopkins, had this to say:

> Medical research must pass from the study of disease to that of health. The lesson of the Nineteenth Century, the greatest lesson of that century, is that the object of medical study is for the maintenance of health rather than the cure of disease.[4]

Abraham Flexner saw the need to bring the biological sciences into medical education. Flexner seems to have overlooked, however, crucial aspects of medical history. Among those whose contributions were sketched in Chapter 2, he seems to have ignored the teachings of Petty and Frank and, although he mentions Rudolf Virchow in his autobiography, there is no reference to the latter's central message.[5] Flexner seems to have been unaware of Pierre-Charles-Alexandre Louis, of John Snow, of the London Epidemiological Society, and of the efforts of many prominent clinicians to incorporate the study of groups or populations, as well as the study of individuals, cells, and organs, into their research and teaching. As I observed in Chapter 1, however, he was fully aware in 1910 that more than schooling in the natural sciences would be required if medicine were to fulfill its mission.

Nevertheless, the schism did occur. Schools of public health exist throughout the world; their ratio to the population in the United States is greatest. Perhaps this is the best of all possible arrangements, and yet the problems reviewed in Chapter 1 suggest that there is much room—and urgent need—for improvement. The primary concern is not with the key roles of anthropologists, biologists, chemists, economists, engineers, social scientists, statisticians, and many others in improving the public's health. The concern in this volume and the International Clinical Epidemiology Network (*INCLEN*) initiative are with recruiting a larger proportion of the best young *medical* minds into this essential endeavor, and with ensuring that all physicians fully understand and appreciate the importance of the population perspective. Is it really feasible to make substantial progress in resolving the gargantuan problems facing governments and their ministries of health throughout the world without the full cooperation of the collective medical profession? Can there be effective "public health education" without fundamental changes in "medical education"?

Within the Rockefeller Foundation, John B. Grant, M.D., a renowned officer for 42 years who is mentioned in the Preface, seems to have had substantial doubts about the direction of medical education at midcentury. In the memorandum he prepared in 1956 he proposed an imaginative scheme for realigning medical education within an expanded medical center, analogous to what are now referred to as Health Sciences Schools or Centers. Under his plan both undergraduate and postgraduate education for public health work (macro level) and for individual patient care (micro level) would be provided by an enlarged faculty. The "...professorships in the applied fields of public health [would] become chairs in a medical center instead of in a school of public health or in a medical school as such."[6] What might have happened if his views had prevailed within the Foundation at that time?

A third of a century later the population perspective can no longer be ignored. Epidemiology is a fundamental science for both medicine and public health.[7] The fact that there is an ever-widening array of potential applications for epidemiological concepts and methods should not be an excuse for balkanizing its collective efforts. Disciplinary hubris seems especially unbecoming for a scientific endeavor. Like its analogues in several other branches of scientific inquiry, epidemiology owes its origins and the continuing renewal of its intellectual capital to a long line of statisticians who provided the fundamental methods for identifying and measuring bias and error and, I would add, the capacity to study Factor "X" (see Chapter 6).

The task of epidemiology is largely that of transmitting fundamental scientific precepts to all those who work throughout the health establishment. There is great diversity in the possible applications of epidemiology to contemporary health problems. There are censuses; there are population-based, household, and community sample surveys, including interview, questionnaire, serological, nutritional, and anthropometric surveys; there are surveillance and monitoring functions; there is outbreak, action, or field epidemiology; there are analyses of secondary data for clues to causation, or to emerging problems; there are case-control and cohort studies and randomized clinical trials; there is evaluation of the risks, benefits, and outcomes of individual and collective maneuvers; and with the help of the epidemiologists' intellectual cousins, the economists, there is estimation of the costs, relative effectiveness, and benefits of health interventions and services of all types. There are ivory tower and armchair epidemiologists, there are shoe-leather epidemiologists, environmental and occupational epidemiologists, and hospital epidemiologists—and then there are clinical epidemiologists. The distinctions are not helpful and are probably transient. The first array describes some of the current applications of epidemiology; the second where they are working.

In establishing the Health of Populations component and INCLEN we chose to focus on clinical epidemiology for three reasons. The first was to emphasize its historical origins with the work of clinicians, most recently through the initiatives of the late John Paul, professor of medicine at Yale University. The second reason was to start with the Fellows' point of departure, that is, hospital-based clinical practice, and gradually to extend their horizons to encompass ambulatory and primary care, "nonpatients," and the population in the community. The third reason was to emphasize the opportunities for clinicians to use epidemiological concepts and methods to improve their own research, teaching, and patient care. It was not our intention to establish clinical epidemiology as a discrete specialty of medicine or of epidemiology. The papers presented at the first eight annual INCLEN meetings attest to the breadth of interest and the growing interactions between research based in institutional settings and that based in the community. After all, the health problems we are attempting to address, and the people who experience them, know nothing of these artificial boundaries. More epidemiologists of all types are needed as well as much more epidemiological and population-based thinking throughout medicine and public health.

Five fundamental shifts—revolutions, if you prefer—in approaches to understanding health and disease favor spread of the population perspective throughout the health enterprise. First, there is the *Information Revolution*. As major contributors to that revolution in medicine, epidemiologists are supported by those dedicated to generating useful information of all types: interpersonal, observational, experimental, bibliographic, and statistical.[8] The first two categories are a consequence of renewed interest in patient-physician relationships, and growing recognition of the need to understand that all therapeutic transactions require effective bilateral communication. If it is important to understand the distribution of perceived health problems at the population or macro level, it is of equal—even greater—importance to understand them at the individual or micro level. Listening, understanding, counselling, and explaining, including awareness of Factor "X", are essential dimensions for fulfilling the tasks of the great majority of health professionals.[9]

Aggregated data or health statistics—"people with the tears wiped off"—are only as valid and reliable as the initial observations and records on which they are based. Clinicians need to become familiar with the means by which health statistics are generated. They are the lifeblood of many epidemiological exercises that impact on resource allocation and the management of health services. Then there is the widening view that the skills of critical appraisal, based as they are on statistical and epidemiological methods, must be applied more vigorously and rigorously to the avalanche of publications that threaten to obscure the occasional nuggets of credible knowledge, and even rarer glimpses of wisdom.[10] The *Information Revolution* is bound to extend the scientific base of the health enterprise to embrace the population perspective.

The epidemiologists' second ally is that vast (and controversial) activity involved in mapping the human genome. For medicine and public health, it is the contemporary equivalent of the Manhattan Project. I am in no position to assess the medical and social impacts of this quantum leap in our knowledge of where we start and how me must live to achieve the potential of our "talents," circumscribed by the limits of our inheritance. The implications are truly revolutionary, not only for medical interventions but also for behavioral, educational, nutritional, occupational, social, and especially environmental modifications. Physicians, health departments, employers, educators, the public, and its politicians will all need to cope with this breathtaking new penetration into the origins of living matter and its boundaries. Epidemiologists are bound to become partners in defining the intricate distributions of our genetic heritage that may determine individual and collective health risks. Molecular biology, especially once the human genome is mapped, must surely turn increasingly to the study of populations, as Professor Janice Egeland Ph.D. of the University of Florida and her colleagues attempted to demonstrate (unsuccessfully, as it turned out later) in the case of bipolar affective disorders.[11] The *Genetic Revolution* is a not-so-secret exercise that should foster better appreciation of the population perspective's utility.

The third ally is the unifying revolution that our knowledge of the immune system is bringing to the health endeavor. True, we have long talked about host, environment, and agent, but in spite of Jenner's and Pasteur's pioneering efforts most of the talk in medical circles during the past half century has been about the agent, as discussed in Chapter 3. Now the talk is turning much more to the other two components of the triad. Not only is the individual's genetic inheritance conditioned by past exposures to a wide variety of animate and inanimate stimuli, but the way he or she perceives these and feels about them is acknowledged to be of vital importance in determining later responses. The powerful new field of psychoneuroimmunology (an unfortunate bit of jargon), aided and abetted by the neurosciences and the behavioral sciences, is now codifying both the characteristics of diverse stimuli and the pathways through which these experiences are mediated. The messages and signals as well as the messengers' biochemical and electrophysical properties are now being examined.[12-14]

As with individuals so with populations. Stimuli affecting groups of individuals (populations) such as poverty, unemployment (or the threat of it), famines, natural disasters, catastrophes, occupational "stress," domestic strife, and even the utterances of charismatic leaders need to be measured and factored into the establishment of health priorities as we continue "redefining the unacceptable." The rapidly unfolding insights provided by the *Immunological Revolution* are bound to favor acceptance of the population perspective.

The fourth ally is the growing body of popular and political concern with the local and global environments. Their importance stems from the fact that the environment is the most malleable of all possible points for intervention. The potential for changes in the human genome must be limited, at least during the foreseeable future. Human behavior, although the most important factor to change, is also the most difficult. Educating, training, and learning to control our immune systems is likely to increase in importance as knowledge grows, but now we are only at the threshold of untold possibilities. Bugs and worms will be with us for centuries to come, but their importance as the sole locus for intervention is likely to decrease as other factors are found to gain in prominence.

That leaves the environment, a concern fostered by the sanitary idea, as one of the most fruitful areas for intervention. Whether we start with the peace, tranquility, and the possible flow of Factor "X" associated with recreational parks, forests, green swards, art galleries, music, and poetry, or whether we start with our collective efforts to stop destruction of tropical rain forests and the release of fluorocarbons that threaten us with global warming, modification of our environments is achieving an ever higher priority throughout the world. Between the extremes are auditory and visual pollution, despoiling of beaches, careless oil spills, reckless disposal of hazardous and toxic wastes, and destructive working conditions. No one committed to improving the public's health can overlook the importance of our biological, chemical, and social environments on the health status of individuals and populations. The *Environmental Revolution* requires wider understanding of the population perspective by the entire health establishment.

Finally there is the *Managerial Revolution.* Health services, systems, and institutions of all kinds are now being "managed," some more effectively and efficiently than others. Individual and group practices, clinics, hospitals, hospices, nursing homes, health maintenance organizations, insurance entities of all types, as well as regional and national health services, now find it essential to size their operations to the populations served and organize their personnel to satisfy the public's expectations. Without the population perspective and a full appreciation of epidemiological concepts and skills, attempts at rational management are futile.

Binding together the dramatic changes being wrought by these five revolutions is the growing prospect for widespread acceptance of a twenty-first-century paradigm to guide our understanding of health and disease.[15,16] The term bio-psychosocial is certainly awkward, but there do not seem to be other labels readily available, except for a chronological eponym (i.e., twenty-first century paradigm), or the one Jan Smuts introduced 60 years ago—holistic.[17] The inexorable advances of science and the integrative capacity of scholars to synthesize ideas from diverse fields foreshadow the urgent need for medical schools to broaden their perspectives beyond the molecular and clinical, important as these are.

The starting place for reform, therefore, is the medical school. To effect change these institutions will need to be led by deans and department heads who, without necessarily being experts in all three, understand and embrace the population perspective in addition to the molecular and clinical perspectives. Schools partic-ipating in INCLEN have succeeded in attracting a number of such individuals to positions of leadership. Some critics of this approach assert that an expanded concern for the public's health on the part of medical school faculties will result in medical dominance and clinical elitism. That view assumes that the priorities and resource allocations of this new breed of academic leaders will be limited to the biomedical perspective and the hubris that too often accompanies it. It also assumes that academic medicine cannot change its paradigms, perspectives, priorities, and practices to accommodate the new knowledge that daily crowds in. A public health, population-based, or bottom-up perspective and a twenty-first-century, biopsycho-social, or holistic paradigm are now needed. INCLEN is showing the way, for not only what the late Sir Theodore Fox, editor of the *Lancet*, called "The Greater Medical Profession" but for what now can be called "The Greater Health Professions."[18,19]

Like it or not, for better or for worse physicians are the lead figures in implementing (or resisting) society's efforts to control, cure, and ameliorate disease. The task is to change physicians' perceptions, attitudes, and knowledge. Those whom their fellow citizens call physicians are endowed with substantial rights, privileges, obligations, status, and perquisites. The name is unlikely to change; their ideas, attitudes, methods, and practices will inevitably change. By starting with the medical school, however, the school's faculty is not restricted to physicians. Flexner introduced natural scientists into medical schools; that was all to the good. In addition, as he implied, we now need anthropologists, biostatis-ticians, economists, engineers, psychologists, and sociologists, to name the more obvious. The twenty-first-century paradigm requires no less.

There are at least five specific innovations that medical schools might consider introducing. These are directed at helping to broaden the faculty's and students' perspectives and at recruiting an adequate proportion of the best minds in medicine and related professions to careers devoted to improving the public's health:

- First, through faculty discussions and consensus building, each medical school could develop a detailed Mission Statement for undergraduate, postgraduate, and continuing education, for research, and for service. The statement should be based on an analysis of the health problems of the populations targeted, what might be done about them, and what new insights may be emerging that will permit useful interventions at the micro (i.e., individual), or macro (i.e., community) levels.[20]

- Second, each medical school could establish a Clinical Epidemiology Unit in one or more of the major clinical departments, using the *INCLEN* model as described in Chapters 7 and 8.

  Depending on the scope of the *CEU* and the availability of other resources in the school, a Department of Epidemiology, Biostatistics, and Health Statistics might be established. Such a department would not substitute for the *CEU* but rather support it by teaching research methods, supporting research in other departments, and by collaborating with investigators throughout the school. This department could also conduct substantive and methodological research of its own. There is the opportunity and responsibility for the faculty to provide training for their colleagues in other departments, and for young physicians undergoing postgraduate specialty training.

- Third, each medical school could establish a Health Analysis and Intelligence Unit attached to the Dean's Office (or in the case of a Health Sciences Center to the Vice President's or Vice Chancellor's Office). As the ombudsman for the school, the faculty, and affiliated hospitals and health care institutions it would provide timely health statistics and related information required for updating the school's Mission Statement. Much of this might be accomplished by stimulating public and private agencies to collect ever more meaningful data from which useful information or "intelligence" could be developed to guide institutional policies. After describing the underlying assumptions, the Unit should array the available information in some order of priorities for education (undergraduate, postgraduate, and continuing), for research, and for service.

  Another responsibility for the Health Analysis and Intelligence Unit would be to inform the faculty, medical students, practitioners, health agencies, institutional and other managers, politicians, and the public about the population's health problems and what is being done about them. Through Newsletters, Bulletins, "one-pagers," E-mail, and the media, perhaps couched in different languages for the several audiences, information should be widely and regularly disseminated. This should not be a public relations exercise but a serious educational effort to generate understanding at all levels about what can be done individually and collectively to improve health and control disease.[21]

- Fourth, each medical school could establish a Department of Occupational and Environmental Health. Initially this might be a component of a Clinical Epidemiology Unit. The dimensions of contemporary environmental problems probably will require at least some schools to create a new department. This department would be analogous to the original, nineteenth-century, Departments of Hygiene in many European medical schools. The importance of the biological, physical, chemical, psychological, and social environments is widely accepted; it is imperative that medical schools imbue both faculty and students with an understanding of their critical impacts on health and disease. In addition to the educational function, there is the urgent need to help industry and society generally with the pressing problems of maintaining or regaining a healthful environment. Schools of Engineering will continue to have major responsibilities for training professionals such as sanitary, civil, and industrial engineers who will work in the health field. Medical schools, however, will need to provide much of the biological, epidemiological, and clinical education for those who choose these important careers. The example of the original combined Y-shaped course developed at the Harvard Medical School and the Massachusetts Institute of Technology discussed in Chapter 4 comes to mind.

- Fifth, managers of hospitals, health care institutions, and "systems," and of health ministries and health departments at all levels require deeper understanding than many exhibit of the biological, psychological, and social vagaries of health and disease, as well as of the traditions and cultures of the health professions. A cursory glance at most hospitals and health departments in both the developed and developing worlds shows that they are "administered," not "managed." They should be led, run, or operated so that a defined set of goals and objectives is achieved.

University departments of administrative medicine have not been conspicuously successful. Most programs in hospital administration and, more recently, of health services administration, focus on *how* to run institutions, rather than on *why* they exist and whether they make an important and appropriate difference to the health of the populations served. A feasible alternative is to encourage Schools of Business and Industrial Management and Schools of Public Administration to provide specialized graduate courses for physicians and others who wish to embark on careers in "managerial medicine"—a field of growing importance. To suggest that "business" schools be involved, is not necessarily to endorse the profit motive as the guiding principle for organizing and managing what is both a private, and, increasingly, a publicly-financed, enterprise. It is, however, to endorse the need for a thorough understanding of management concepts and skills, in addition to the population perspective, epidemiological concepts and methods, and the need for better use of information. Medical schools should provide the clinical, epidemiological, and biological components in the education of this critical category of health professionals.

Schools of Business or Industrial Management or Public Administration could also provide instruction for medical students in such subjects as the organization of health care systems—including hospitals and health economics (where this is not covered by health or clinical economists in a CEU).

These five suggestions take it for granted that the medical school has a strong Department of Psychiatry (including Social Psychiatry) and Behavioral Sciences. This department should provide the scientific underpinning for understanding the many psychological, social, and cultural dimensions of health and disease. Pursuit of greater understanding and awareness of the ubiquitous character and therapeutic potential of Factor "X" should be among its major responsibilities. It is also assumed that Schools of Nursing and of Social Work will be expanding their epidemiological capacities and their programs in community and home nursing, and that they will become part of enlarged Health Sciences Faculties. The inevitable result of these innnovations will be much greater emphasis on primary care in medical education and research. There will be recogniton of the fundamental necessity for medical schools to provide adequate numbers of appropriately trained general physicians to take care of the great majority of the population's health problems.

If all this were to come to pass, what is to be the fate of Departments of Miscellaneous Medicine? Most, if not all, of their faculty members could find new and happier homes in one or more of the new units or departments described. Their status will be different—indeed, much stronger—because their mandates will have been defined clearly in the institution's Mission Statement. No longer will they be marginal faculty striving for their place in the scheme of things by redefining the unacceptable with results that fall on deaf ears. The faculty and their works will be institutionalized within the fabric of the medical (or health sciences) enterprise; they will participate in gradually constructing their own institution's essential guidance system.

Biostatisticians, epidemiologists, economists, anthropologists, psychologists, and sociologists, together with traditional fundamental scientists and the clinical faculty, will have a common institutional allegiance, defined by a common Mission Statement and supported by timely population-based information. Under these arrangements, extensions of the concepts underlying INCLEN, graduate degrees in epidemiology, biostatistics, and health statistics, health services research, and environmental and occupational health will be provided by these expanded Schools of Health Sciences, depending on their priorities and resources. Other health-related graduate degrees would be provided by Schools of Engineering, Business, and Industrial Management, Public Administration, Nursing, and Social Work.

Two more essential functions could readily be undertaken by medical schools. First is the vital field of tropical medicine. Diseases of the tropics, in addition to their genesis in poverty and deprivation of many types, are associated with a wide range of microorganisms, parasites, and assorted vectors. In the tropics, these are "local" diseases. The issue is more the site of the population suffering from the disease than the methods of investigation. Departments of microbiology, parasitology, and pharmacology, as well as their newer analogues, of cell biology, molecular biology, and immunology, are appropriate sites for investigation of these all-too-prevalent scourges. INCLEN's CEUs are studying many of these problems. Travelers' diseases can be managed in designated specialty clinics.

Nutrition is another vitally important factor influencing the health of populations in both the developed and developing worlds for better and for worse. Medical schools have been negligent in the conduct of research and teaching in this essential field. A few departments of biochemistry, and even clinical departments, have programs in nutrition; many more should. Again, INCLEN's CEUs are tackling many of these problems.

Constructive decisions were taken by the University of Toronto and the Government of Australia when several years ago they merged the faculties of their schools of public health with those of their medical schools and redeployed financial support.[22,23] Neither of these two countries now has a school of public health, but they do have numerous well-supported and well-attended undergraduate and postgraduate programs in what might be called "the new public health."

Although not without considerable controversy and much personal anguish at the time, the changes now seem to be regarded by the great majority of those directly concerned as having substantially improved matters (personal communications from persons at the universities of Toronto and Sydney and elsewhere in the two countries). For example, the Associate Dean for Community Health at the University of Toronto originally opposed the merger of the School of Hygiene with the Faculty of Medicine; he is now a staunch supporter and writes:

> ...[T]here has been a tremendous resurgence of creativity within Community Health—
> a series of major thrusts [are] being developed in collaboration with other Health
> Sciences [Faculties], as well as with the Faculty of Medicine, the Institute of
> Environmental Studies, Engineering, Law, Management Studies, with the wider area
> health units, the Canadian Public Health Association, etc.. I am personally convinced
> that Public Health can never be self-contained in the universities, professional groups,
> and the community at large (personal communication, Professor John E. Hastings,
> March 27, 1989).

From Australia comes word that since a 1986 Review for the Federal Minister of Health there have been dramatic changes in the number of institutions and individuals involved in training for public health. Final answers are by no means available yet, and there are still questions to be asked about selection procedures and the quality of instruction. Nevertheless, the Public Health Association of Australia, in a recent Review of Postgraduate Public Health Training in Australia had this to say:

> Until 1986 only two universities offered formal postgraduate courses in public health.
> By January 1988 eleven institutions of higher education offered fourteen Master
> programs in public health. Additional courses are being developed so that by January
> 1989 there will be at least seventeen Master of Public Health courses in Australia. In
> 1987 approximately 120 new students were accepted into postgraduate public health
> courses. In 1988 at least 275 new students entered these courses....Thus there has been
> a massive expansion of public health training and Australia can now be considered
> well-served in the number and geographic spread of courses.[24]

Of the 14 courses offered in 1988, 8 are in medical schools. This certainly contrasts favorably with the two medical schools offering such courses before 1986. No data are provided on the composition of the student bodies, nor do we know how many are physicians, especially young physicians.[25]

The population perspective for which schools of public health have acted as faithful custodians for the past 75 years now should prevail throughout the health enterprise. The faculties of these schools have enriched a vital legacy left them by clinicians. The issue is not the perspective itself but how best to apply it more widely. That achievement must surely involve effective leadership, credible information and, above all, political will—both within academia and at all levels of government. For three-quarters of a century, faculty from schools of public health have been at the forefront in "redefining the unacceptable." Clinicians used to be at the forefront of that major social endeavor; now they have an opportunity to resume their social responsibilities. At the very least, the matter deserves debate. The public needs to know the outcome of that debate in unequivocal language.

In 1978 John Knowles called attention to the separation of medicine and public health and to the need for reasserting the importance of the population perspective throughout the health establishment. Since then, the Rockefeller Foundation, together with many other foundations and organizations, has made its contribution to defining the origins and dimensions of the *schism* and has initiated one specific approach to *healing the schism*. I have described its genesis and early development in some detail to illustrate the enormity of the problems being tackled. The task is far from over. Johann Peter Frank might now paraphrase Victor Hugo's aphorism by reaffirming that "there is nothing so irresistible as an idea whose time has come—again!"

References

1. Director-General of the World Health Organization and Executive Director of the United Nations Children's Fund. *Primary Health Care*. Geneva and New York: WHO and UNICEF, 1978.
2. Foss L, Rothenberg K. *The Second Medical Revolution: From Biomedicine to Infomedicine*. Boston and London: New Science Library, Shambhala, 1987.
3. Kuhn T. *The Structure of Scientific Revolutions*. Chicago: University of Chicago Press, 1970.
4. Sabin FR. *Franklin Paine Mall: The Story of a Mind*. Baltimore: Johns Hopkins, 1934:279. Quoted by Eisenberg L. From circumstance to mechanism in pediatrics during the Hopkins century. Pediatrics 1990;85:42-49.
5. Flexner A. *I Remember*. New York: Simon and Schuster, 1940.
6. Seipp C, ed. *Health for the Community: Selected Papers of Dr. John B. Grant*. Baltimore: Johns Hopkins, 1963:129-131.
7. White KL, Henderson MM, eds. *Epidemiology as a Fundamental Science: Its Uses in Health Services Planning, Administration and Evaluation*. New York: Oxford University Press, 1977.
8. White KL. Information for health care: an epidemiological perspective. Inquiry 1980;17:296-312.
9. White KL. *The Task of Medicine*. Menlo Park, California: Henry J. Kaiser, Jr., Family Foundation, 1988.
10. Warren KS, ed. *Selectivity in Information Systems: Survival of the Fittest*. New York: Praeger Scientific, 1985.
11. Egeland JA, Gerhard DS, Pauls DL, et al. Bipolar affective disorders linked to DNA markers on chromosome II. Nature (London) 1987;325:783-787.

12. Ader R, Cohen N, eds. *Psychoneuroimmunology*. New York: Academic Press, 1981.
13. Krieger DT. Brain peptides: what, where, and why? Science 1983;222:975-985.
14. Pelletier KR, Herzing DL. Psychoneuroimmunology: toward a mind body model. Advances 1988;5:27-56.
15. Wulff HR, Pedersen SA, Rosenberg R. *Philosophy of Medicine: An Introduction*. Oxford: Blackwell, 1986.
16. Comfort A. A bridge to the twenty-first century. Lancet 1989;ii:1512-1513.
17. Smuts JC. *Holism and Evolution*. London: Macmillan, 1926.
18. Fox TF. The greater medical profession. Lancet 1956;ii:779-780.
19. Royal Society of Medicine and the Josiah Macy Jr. Foundation. *The Greater Medical Profession*. New York: Josiah Macy Jr. Foundation, 1973.
20. University of Saskatchewan. *Towards a New Beginning: Review of the College of Medicine*. Saskatoon: University of Saskatchewan, 1989.
21. White KL. Health care: limits and opportunities for health sciences centers. In: Squires BP, ed. *Proceedings of the Conference on Health in the '80s and '90s and Its Impact on Health Sciences Education*. Toronto: Council of Ontario Universities, 1983.
22. Community Health Task Force. *Final Report*. University of Toronto, 1988.
23. White KL. *Australia's Bicentennial Health Initiative: Independent Review of Research and Educational Requirements for Public Health and Tropical Health in Australia*. Canberra: Minister for Health, 1986.
24. Public Health Association of Australia. *Public Health Training*. Canberra: Public Health Association, 1988:1.
25. Ibid, p. 52.

Author Index

Subject Index